Janet Wilkie

Guidelines in Clinical Anaesthesia

To Meriel and Brian

Guidelines in Clinical Anaesthesia

PETER HUTTON
BSc, PhD, MB, ChB, FFARCS

GRISELDA COOPER
MB, ChB, FFARCS

FOREWORD BY
CEDRIC PRYS-ROBERTS
MA, DM, PhD, FFARCS
Professor, Sir Humphry Davy Department of Anaesthesia, University of Bristol

BLACKWELL SCIENTIFIC PUBLICATIONS

OXFORD   LONDON   EDINBURGH
BOSTON   PALO ALTO   MELBOURNE

While every effort has been made to check drug dosages in this book, it is still possible that errors have been missed. Furthermore, dosage schedules are being continually revised and new side-effects recognized. For these reasons the reader is strongly urged to consult the drug companies' printed instructions before administering any of the drugs recommended in this book.

© 1985 by
Blackwell Scientific Publications
Editorial offices:
Osney Mead, Oxford, OX2 0EL
8 John Street, London, WC1N 2ES
23 Ainslie Place, Edinburgh, EH3 6AJ
52 Beacon Street, Boston
  Massachusetts 02108, USA
667 Lytton Avenue, Palo Alto
  California 94301, USA
107 Barry Street, Carlton
  Victoria 3053, Australia

First published 1985

Set by HiTech Typesetters Ltd, Oxford and printed and bound in Great Britain by William Clowes & Sons Beccles, Suffolk

DISTRIBUTORS

USA
  Blackwell Mosby Book
    Distributors
  11830 Westline Industrial Drive
  St Louis, Missouri 63141

Canada
  Blackwell Mosby Book
    Distributors
  120 Melford Drive, Scarborough
  Ontario M1B 2X4

Australia
  Blackwell Scientific Publications
    (Australia) Pty Ltd
  107 Barry Street, Carlton
  Victoria 3053

British Library
Cataloguing in Publication Data
  Hutton, Peter
  Guidelines in clinical anaesthesia.
  1. Pathology   2. Anaesthesia
  I. Title   II. Cooper, Griselda
  615′.0024617   RD82

ISBN 0-632-01389-3

Contents

Foreword, vii

Preface, ix

1 Cardiovascular disease, 1

2 Pulmonary function, chest disease and anaesthesia, 102

3 Disorders of nerve and muscle, 137

4 The liver, 167

5 Nutritional disorders, 194

6 Endocrine and metabolic disease, 209

7 Renal disease, 248

8 Diseases of the connective tissue, bones and joints, 274

9 Haematology, 301

10 Psychiatry, 335

11 Anaesthesia and old age, 355

12 Miscellaneous conditions, 371

Appendix: General further reading, 386

Abbreviations, 387

Index, 391

Foreword

Anaesthesia, like every other branch of clinical medicine, is becoming more and more complex and specialized. During the early years of training, the anaesthetist is faced with increasing pressures to acquire a variety of technical skills, while at the same time consolidating and expanding the basic science background gained a few years previously in medical school. The Faculty of Anaesthetists has consistently emphasized the importance of the basic sciences as the cornerstone of its training programmes and its examinations. Medicine, and its application in anaesthesia, has also been an important component of training for the final FFARCS examination. Now with the introduction of the new programme of examinations, the timing of these training components has changed, so that medicine becomes an important component of both Parts 1 and 3 of the new examination.

But a knowledge of the principles and practice of medicine is not simply a passport to examination success, it is a vital part of the everyday practice of anaesthesia and its allied specialty of intensive care. Gone are the days when only the fittest patients were subjected to anaesthesia and surgery, when the decisions were made by physicians who had little knowledge of the problems of anaesthesia and the postoperative period. Nevertheless, they established good guidelines for the perioperative management of patients with conditions such as diabetes, thyrotoxicosis or pre-existing steroid therapy.

Now the anaesthetist must be his own physician, prepared to diagnose, investigate and treat the medical conditions which are coincident in so many surgical patients. Clearly the anaesthetist cannot hope to match the overall medical knowledge of the specialist physician, and must therefore aim for selective proficiency. To this end the trainee anaesthetist must first learn of the significance of pre-existing medical conditions, how to assess and minimize operative risk, to recognize possibilities for interactions between pre-existing drug therapy and the drugs used during and after anaesthesia, and how to select and time preoperative interventions to minimize postoperative complications. Next comes the choice of general or regional anaesthetic techniques available for the surgical procedure, and the influence of the patient's medical condition on this choice. Finally, postoperative care of the medical patient may require hours or days of co-operative attention between anaesthetists, physicians and surgeons.

This book provides an excellent background for all these purposes. The authors, with their respective backgrounds in bio-engineering, clinical and academic anaesthesia, have sought to emphasize the practical aspects of medical management of the surgical patient. Beyond this they have achieved a balance between the theoretical and practical basis of medical management, in a way which has not been previously achieved in books of this nature. But there is also plenty here for the seasoned veteran in anaesthesia who needs for example a reference to the current management of the Type 1 diabetic patient, the hypertensive patient treated with calcium channel blockers, or the patient with a phaeochromocytoma. For the medical student and intern, the perspective of medicine in relation to anaesthesia will be clarified.

Cedric Prys-Roberts

Preface

It is far better to cure at the beginning than at the end.

Persius AD 34–62

This book was written because we felt there was a need for it. It is intended primarily for anaesthetists in training and particularly for those preparing for the examinations of the Faculty of Anaesthetists. We would anticipate it to be of equal value to anaesthetists studying for postgraduate examinations in North America, Europe and Australasia.

The object of the book is to examine the way in which coincidental diseases or other problems affect the process of anaesthesia. Considerations of this nature are becoming more important both as people live longer and as fewer patients are rejected as 'unfit' for surgery. Failure to appreciate the impact of intercurrent illness was one of the factors singled out by the Lunn & Mushin report (1982)* as being contributory to anaesthetic mortality. Our book does not, and is not intended to, describe how to give anaesthesia for specialized surgical procedures: many excellent texts which do so already exist.

The book chapters are arranged according to organ systems with an additional section headed 'Miscellaneous conditions' for a small number of topics which do not classify easily. The pattern each chapter takes is that which we felt was the most appropriate for the subject matter. The background pathology and physiology of diseases are explored sufficiently to explain their relevance to anaesthesia and then the pre, intra, and post-operative care is discussed. This is done both in general terms and in relation to specific conditions. It is assumed, to prevent repetition in the text, that all patients will routinely have at least their pulse, blood pressure and ECG observed regularly but, where appropriate the principles and objectives of monitoring techniques are considered in depth. An attempt has therefore been made to integrate and provide a logical basis for all the ways in which co-existing illness requires modifications to be made in anaesthetic technique.

* Lunn J.N. & Mushin W.W. (1982) *Mortality Associated with Anaesthesia.* The Nuffield Provincial Hospitals Trust.

The extent to which any particular aspect of a topic should be pursued was frequently difficult to decide upon. It was never our intention to compete with specialist monographs and ultimately we were guided by what we thought represented an 'above average' blend of theoretical and practical knowledge. Because of this, a number of readers and critics will doubtless, in their view, find us too detailed in some areas and deficient in others.

For several reasons no references are quoted in the text. Firstly, the book is intended to be useful in everyday anaesthesia and including references makes it difficult to achieve a concise format. Secondly, the majority of the information is available, although presented in a different manner in diverse standard textbooks. Thirdly, it was never our objective to produce a reference source book. Finally, much of what is written reflects our own day to day practice. Selected references of papers and monographs specific to the text are, however, given at the end of each chapter and it is hoped that these will, for the interested reader, be articles which have a useful content and will allow a relatively rapid access to other more specialized sources. In addition, there is an appendix containing a list of standard reference texts which we ourselves have used in the past, and in the preparation of this book, to check certain facts and to obtain the details of some original references.

In researching various aspects of anaesthesia we have been surprised to find how frequently standard textbook recommendations depend upon relatively few anecdotal case reports. In these instances we have described what we feel is a logical approach and said what we would do in the given circumstances. Naturally, we are not assuming that this is the only approach or solution possible.

Because there is little point in repeating what is already covered adequately in other textbooks, certain topics have been omitted. The most obvious of these are the care of the pregnant woman close to term and the special problems of neonates and children.

We would be pleased if readers found the book of use as a concise, up-to-date guide. Used daily, junior anaesthetists will, we hope, be able to find advice on what to look for in the preoperative visit and to anticipate the likely anaesthetic problems. On occasions it may help them to know when to ask for help or when to discuss the case with a senior colleague.

In the preparation of this book many people have given freely of their knowledge during casual conversation but a special word of appreciation must go to Professor C. Prys-Roberts, Dr B.T. Cooper, Dr P.R. Harrison and Dr S.E. Goodman for giving constructive advice on Chapters 1, 4, 7 and 12 respectively. There were also useful discussions with Dr P.J. Simpson, Dr S.A. Masey and Dr C.R.

Monk. Finally, our very grateful thanks go to Lynne Breeze for converting the manuscript into typescript, and to Mr Per Saugman and Mr J. Robson of Blackwell Scientific Publications Ltd for piloting it through the press.

Sir Humphry Davy Department of Anaesthesia, University of Bristol

Peter Hutton
Griselda Cooper

1/Cardiovascular disease

Part I: General principles
Preoperative assessment
  History
  Examination
  Investigations
Common drugs and their problems
Perioperative management
  The risks and timing of surgery
  The principles of cardiovascular
    monitoring
  Anaesthetic considerations
Postoperative phase

Part II: Individual conditions
Ischaemic heart disease
Cor pulmonale
Cardiomyopathies
Hypertension
Dysrhythmias, conduction defects
  and pacemakers
Valvular heart disease
Congenital heart disease

Cardiovascular disease is so prevalent that no anaesthetist can hope to avoid dealing with those so afflicted. The incidence in the general population increases with advancing age; 6% have cardiovascular disease in the fifth decade, 23% in the sixth decade and 45% in the seventh decade. Cardiac disease causes more than twice as many deaths annually as all types of cancer. Moreover, of great importance to anaesthetists, there is an increased mortality and morbidity during and following surgery.

Patients with cardiovascular disease have frequently been investigated and treated prior to presenting for surgery so the extent of their disability is well documented. Not uncommonly, however, the occult condition first becomes apparent when the patient is examined preoperatively. It is important to be aware of any underlying anatomical or physiological malfunction because what is quiescent in daily life can become life-threatening in the perioperative period. This chapter first describes briefly the essentials of the history taking, examination and investigation of the cardiovascular system. The principles of the anaesthetic management of patients with cardiovascular disease are then discussed in general terms without reference to any named disorder. Finally, the features relevant to individual conditions are considered in more detail.

The material has been arranged in this manner in an attempt both to prevent repetition and to allow a general philosophy of anaesthesia to be developed which, with suitable modification, can easily be adapted to suit any particular patient. Inevitably, on occasions it has been difficult to decide whether to place certain details under

1

'General principles' or 'Individual conditions'; where necessary the text has been cross referenced.

PART I. GENERAL PRINCIPLES

Preoperative assessment

History

Severe cardiovascular disease may be totally asymptomatic. The cardinal symptoms are dyspnoea, chest pain and oedema. The objects of the history are to gauge the level of functional incapacity, to evaluate whether the symptoms are improving, static or worsening, and to give a clue to the underlying pathophysiology.

Dyspnoea is an uncomfortable awareness of breathing which, when secondary to cardiovascular disease, is a symptom not of any specific cardiac lesion but of some forms of heart failure. The commonest cause is an abnormally high pulmonary venous pressure which, because of the resultant increased pulmonary blood volume, leads both to a decrease in compliance and to a deterioration in alveolar gas transfer. In longstanding cases this can end with irreversible interstitial changes.

The most frequent and significant presentation of the dyspnoea of cardiac origin is shortness of breath on exertion. Less commonly, dyspnoea can be caused by the tissue anoxia of low cardiac output states. The mechanism of this response is uncertain but is thought to be similar to the 'air hunger' of the shocked patient.

To assess the severity of the disease determine the degree of exertion which brings on the dyspnoea, bearing in mind the patient's general physical condition, work history, and recreational habits. Dyspnoea on effort is generally the first symptom of left ventricular failure (LVF). Try to distinguish this from an intrinsic pulmonary cause where the onset of dyspnoea is usually (but not invariably) more gradual. Acute LVF is characterized by orthopnoea (dyspnoea on lying flat) or paroxysmal nocturnal dyspnoea (PND) (acute onset of dyspnoea which wakes the patient and forces him to sit up). The history, the presence of cyanosis and of crepitations on auscultation, help to differentiate it from bronchial asthma.

Pain in the chest has many causes other than myocardial ischaemia (e.g. pericarditis, pleurisy, pneumothorax, pulmonary embolism, oesophageal pain, peptic ulcer, biliary colic, aortic aneurysm, bone fractures or secondaries, collapsed vertebrae), but, when present, suspect and identify or eliminate a cardiac origin. Ischaemic pain is typically felt over the lower sternum, is gripping, aching or pressing in character with radiation to either the arm, the neck, the jaw, the abdomen or the back of the chest. The severity can be from mild to agonizing and it may slowly wax and wane. Pain secondary to cardiac ischaemia is considered in more detail in 'Functional disease of the myocardium'.

The pain which occurs when ischaemia is sufficiently severe and prolonged to cause infarction differs from angina in being more intense, persisting at rest and lasting for over an hour. In the elderly, myocardial tissue may infarct without any of the accompanying symptoms of ischaemia ('silent infarct').

Oedema in cardiac failure has multiple causes which are not fully understood. Contributory factors are an increased venous pressure secondary to a failing right ventricle and an impaired renal blood flow. The latter promotes secondary aldosteronism and excessive reabsorption of salt and water by the renal tubules. This tissue fluid gravitates to the dependent parts of the body and is detected in the feet and legs in the ambulant and over the sacrum in those confined to bed. The differential diagnosis of peripheral oedema includes renal disease, cirrhosis, deep vein thrombosis (DVT) and poor lymphatic drainage.

Ankle swelling occurs in many normal middle-aged people who have been standing for most of the day. It is also seen in pre-menstrual women when sodium and water retention are maximal.

Cardiac syncope and palpitations are predominantly symptoms of cardiac dysrhythmias. They can be difficult to differentiate from anxiety neurosis on history alone and are best confirmed by an elec-trocardiogram (ECG) taken during symptoms. Syncope and dizzi-ness associated with neck rotation and extension are indicative of vertebrobasilar insufficiency. This is important to discover because it has obvious implications in the positioning of the anaesthetized patient's head.

Other conditions may either reveal or produce cardiovascular pathology. The most important of these to elicit are diabetes mellitus (see Chapter 6), strokes and transient ischaemic attacks (see Chapter 3) and rheumatic fever (see 'Valvular heart disease').

Examination

Specific findings are described later under the appropriate section heading in 'Individual conditions': only the principles of examina-tion are outlined here. Examine the patient with his legs horizontal and the upper body at 45°.

Begin with general observations. Look for cachexia (chronic severe heart failure), stunted growth in children (shunts), obesity (makes symptoms worse), the stigmata of genetic defects associated with congenital heart disease (e.g. Down's syndrome), the presence of peripheral and central cyanosis, and breathlessness. Following this, systematically examine the hands and arms, move to the neck and face, then to the precordium and back, and finally check the lower limbs. At some stage the retinae should be examined and the blood pressure (BP) taken, the counsel of perfection requiring the latter to be done in both arms and with the patient both supine and standing. Many texts suggest that the BP be taken at the end when the patient is at his ease, but taking it early can make other physical signs easier to interpret. Comments on the methods and accuracy of indirect blood pressure measurement can be found in 'The principles of cardiovascular monitoring' (p. 23).

In the hands, look for anaemia, clubbing, splinter haemorrhages, peripheral cyanosis and vasodilation. Make a preliminary assessment of the rate and rhythm of the pulse in both radial arteries and compare the arrival of the pulse wave with that in the femoral artery (delay implies aortic coarctation). Hold the arm up and feel for a collapsing pulse (Table 1.1). This has a fast upstroke but the peak is not sustained and there is an early and rapid pressure drop. If the examiner's fingers are placed lightly over the radial artery he feels a 'tapping' sensation. With his fingers curled around the volar surface of the forearm the peak of the pulse may often be felt within the forearm muscles. To produce a collapsing pulse there are two requirements, an elevated stroke volume and a very low resistance peripheral vascular bed. In 'shock states', although there is often a very rapid peripheral run off, the stroke volume is insufficient to produce a powerful rapid upstroke and the pulse is then described as 'thready' (see Table 1.1).

Examine the internal and external jugular veins with the patient reclining at 45° and his head supported on a pillow. It is essential that the skin and sternomastoid muscles (which lie on top of the internal jugular veins) are relaxed or the venous pulses will be obscured. The internal jugular veins are immediately lateral to the carotid arteries and can usually only be seen on expiration in thin people or in those with abnormal venous pulsation. The external jugular vein traverses the roof of the posterior triangle of the neck. Although useful on occasions for recording the mean jugular venous pressure (JVP), because of its valve-like entry into the subclavian vein it is a poor demonstrator of jugular venous waves. With the patient reclining at 45° the top of the right atrium is in the same horizontal plane as the sternal angle. The vertical height of the venous column above this level is the JVP or central venous pressure (CVP) and it is normally less than 3 cm H_2O.

Table 1.1. Abnormal pulses.

Name	Pulse waveform	Characteristics	Significance
Plateau		Low systolic Low or low normal diastolic Slow rise, 'plateau'	Aortic stenosis
Collapsing		High systolic Low diastolic Rapid rise Rapid fall	Aortic incompetence Persistent ductus arteriosus A–V fistula Pregnancy Fever Severe, acute anaemia Hyperthyroidism
Thready		Low systolic Low diastolic Normal rise time	All the causes of shock Deliberate hypotension Low cardiac output from severe mitral, pulmonary or tricuspid stenosis
Bisferiens		Two impulses felt with each beat.	Combined aortic stenosis and incompetence (very rare)
Alternans		Alternate large and small amplitude beats. Not felt but noted when taking BP	Left ventricular failure (mechanism unknown)
Paradoxus		Excessive decrease in pulse volume with inspiration	Powerful inspiratory effort needed to overcome airways obstruction (asthma) Reduced diastolic volume (tamponade, constrictive pericarditis)
Absent radial		Usually unilateral	Previous cardiac surgery. Arterial embolism. Trauma. Congenital defect (check ulnar)

It may be impossible to measure the JVP clinically in a patient who is very breathless, if the accessory muscles of respiration are in use or if there is a large difference between the pressure in inspiration and expiration (as in asthma or chronic obstructive airways disease). Superior mediastinal obstruction causes a non-pulsatile overfilling and is accompanied by congested facies. Do not make the

5

mistake of missing a grossly elevated JVP because the upper fluid level is concealed behind the angle of the jaw.

The CVP wave is shown in Fig. 1.1. Its mean value changes with the phase of breathing or intermittent positive pressure ventilation (IPPV). The interpretations of its abnormalities (which are often difficult to identify clinically) are listed in Table 1.2.

Feel the carotid pulse noting the rate, rhythm and the pulse volume and character and its change with ventilation.

The rate and rhythm are easy to assess. Atrial fibrillation (AF) can be distinguished from ventricular ectopic beats (VEs) because the dysrhythmia intensifies with exercise, whereas VEs tend to disappear with exercise. The character of the pulse wave, despite apparently crystal-clear textbook descriptions is often very difficult to interpret clinically. A summary of named pulses and their significance is given in Table 1.1.

Percuss and auscultate the lung bases and feel for sacral oedema. Inspect the chest for asymmetry and the presence of abnormal pulsations. Palpate for the apex beat, heaves and thrills. Percussion of the heart is of little value except the absence of cardiac dullness implies

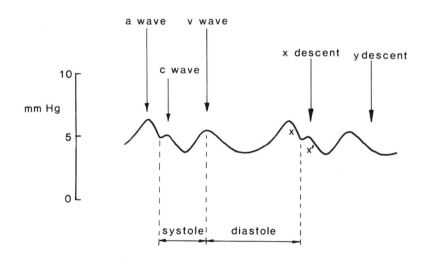

THE CENTRAL VENOUS PRESSURE WAVE

Fig. 1.1. Two peaks (a and v) and two troughs (x and y) are seen during every cardiac cycle. The a wave is the result of atrial contraction and precedes the carotid pulse. The v wave follows the carotid pulse and represents the rise in atrial pressure due to continued venous filling whilst the tricuspid valve is closed. The c wave is an inconstant and variable feature which is associated with transmitted arterial pulsation and/or deformation of the atrium with bulging of the tricuspid valve during early systole.

Table 1.2. Abnormalities of the CVP wave.

Abnormality	Character	Significance
Absent 'a' wave	Absent pulsation before carotid pulse	No co-ordinated atrial contraction, atrial fibrillation
Large 'a' wave	Occurs prior to systole with every cardiac cycle	Powerful atrial contraction to force blood through narrow orifice (tricuspid valve stenosis or atresia) or into stiff hypertrophied ventricle (pulmonary valve stenosis or pulmonary hypertension)
Large 'v' wave	Occurs prematurely, immediately after carotid pulse.	Represents reflux of blood into the right atrium during right ventricular systole because of tricuspid incompetence, usually secondary to cardiac failure.
'Cannon' waves	Large, abrupt waves synchronous with the carotid pulse (i.e. at the timing of the 'c' wave)	Implies atrial contraction against a closed tricuspid valve. If regular it is due to a nodal rhythm and retrograde atrial conduction: if intermittent, complete heart block.

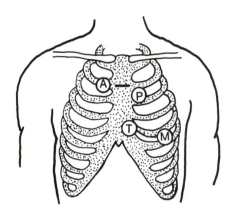

Fig. 1.2. The classical areas described for auscultation of the *A*ortic, *P*ulmonary, *T*ricuspid and *M*itral valves. The sternal angle is marked (—).

hyperinflated lung tissue between the heart and chest wall. Then auscultate the neck (for carotid bruits or the radiation of aortic systolic murmurs) and the whole of the precordium, not just the classical areas for valve murmurs (see Fig. 1.2). Listen in expiration and inspiration. Murmurs can be accentuated by exercise and mitral stenosis is best heard with the patient rolled on to the left side.

Note any liver tenderness or enlargement in the abdomen and listen for bruits over the renal arteries. Lastly, look at the lower limbs for evidence of arterial insufficiency. Feel for oedema and for the popliteal, posterior tibial and dorsalis pedis arteries.

The two commonest abnormalities seen through the ophthalmoscope are hypertensive and diabetic retinopathy.

Investigations

Full blood count (FBC). This should be normal. If the haemoglobin concentration (Hb) is low, tachydysrhythmias may cause angina; if the Hb is high it could be a response to arterial desaturation from a right to left shunt or polycythaemia with the hyperviscosity syndrome.

Urea and electrolytes (U & E's). These should be normal. Depending upon the drug, diuretics can cause hypokalaemia (common) or hyperkalaemia (rare).

Liver function tests (LFT's). These can be abnormal in chronic right ventricular failure (RVF) which is sometimes called cardiac cirrhosis (see 'cirrhosis', Chapter 4).

Cardiac enzymes. These are considered in 'Ischaemic heart disease' (p. 44).

Chest X-ray (CXR). This investigation is mandatory in any patient with a history of cardiovascular disease, whatever the age. It can be used to obtain an assessment of heart size, to provide evidence of the effects of heart disease on the lungs and to detect calcium on the heart-valves, pericardium and aorta. The standard film is a posterior-anterior (P-A) exposure with the tube 6 feet from the patient and the plate against the anterior chest wall taken at full inspiration. This minimizes distortion. Under these conditions, the transverse diameter of the normal heart shadow is less than half the transverse diameter of the thorax. Penetrated P-A and lateral films make calcium easier to see and oblique films (often with barium swallow) outline the left atrium. Cardiac features of the adult CXR are shown in Fig. 1.3.

Portable X-rays are antero-posterior (A-P) films taken with a divergent beam. They do not show the normal proportions of the thorax and its contents, are frequently rotated and not in inspiration, and need care in interpretation.

A system for reading CXR's is detailed in Chapter 2. CXR findings particular to individual cardiac conditions are described when appropriate later.

Electrocardiogram

The ECG is probably the most useful single routine clinical investigation, even in the absence of symptoms. The principles of interpre-

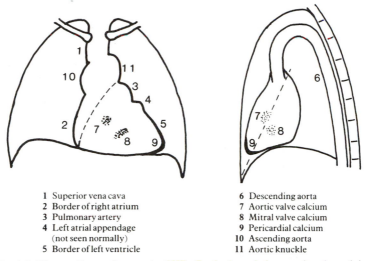

1 Superior vena cava	6 Descending aorta
2 Border of right atrium	7 Aortic valve calcium
3 Pulmonary artery	8 Mitral valve calcium
4 Left atrial appendage	9 Pericardial calcium
(not seen normally)	10 Ascending aorta
5 Border of left ventricle	11 Aortic knuckle

Fig. 1.3. The cardiac outline on the CXR. On the lateral view aortic valve calcium is mainly above a line (shown dotted) joining the carina to the anterior sterno-diaphragmatic angle and mitral valve calcium is mainly below it. On the P–A view, the aortic valve lies in the centre of the heart and is obscured by the spine. Mitral valve calcium is visible to the left of the spine. The dotted line on the P-A view shows the limits of the right ventricle.

tation are described here. Abnormalities of specific conditions are detailed as they arise in the text.

Check all recordings for paper speed (25 mm/sec) and sensitivity (1 mv/cm). A 12 lead ECG has three bipolar limb leads (I, II and III), three unipolar limb leads (aVR, aVL and aVF) and six unipolar chest leads (V_{1-6}). The definitions of the various named components of the ECG are shown in Fig. 1.4.

The P wave represents atrial depolarization. It is most easily seen in leads V_1 and V_2, but when abnormal, the most significant changes in shape may be best seen in leads II and V_{4-6}. The normal P wave is less than 0.1 second in duration and less than 2.5 mm in height. There is no atrial repolarization wave seen because it is small and obscured by the QRS complex. Abnormalities of the P wave are:
- absent—no co-ordinated atrial contraction (see later, Fig. 1.23).
- too tall — right atrial hypertrophy (see later, Fig. 1.38(a)).
- too wide and/or bifid — left atrial hypertrophy delaying conduction and causing atrial asynchrony (see later, Fig. 1.38(b)).
- inverted, too close to, or following the QRS — abnormal focus initiating atrial contraction (see later, Fig. 1.24).

The P-R interval (see Fig. 1.4) is the time taken for excitation to spread from the sino-atrial (S-A) node, through the atrial muscle and atrioventricular (A-V) node, down the bundle of His and into the ventricular conducting system. Most of the time is taken up with

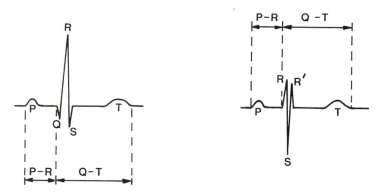

Fig. 1.4. QRS terminology. The first positive deflection is labelled R. The second positive deflection is labelled R'. A negative deflection preceding an R is labelled Q. A negative deflection following an R is labelled S. The identifying letter is unrelated to the underlying event, R in a left sided lead being equivalent to S in a right sided lead. The Q–T interval varies with heart rate, the normal upper limits being 0.5 seconds (12.5 mm on the trace) at 40 beats per minute and 0.28 seconds (7 mm on the trace) at 150 beats per minute.

A-V node delay. The normal P-R interval is 0.12–0.2 seconds (3 to 5 small squares). Abnormalities are:
- too short — nodal rhythm, delta wave in the QRS, (see later, Figs 1.24, 1.35).
- too long but fixed — first degree heart block.
- variable — second or third degree heart block (see later, Figs 1.27, 1.28, 1.29, 1.30).

The QRS complex represents ventricular depolarization. The ventricular conducting system is shown in Fig. 1.5. Depolarization should be complete within 0.12 seconds (3 small squares) and no one lead should have a total amplitude of over 35 mm.

During normal conduction, the interventricular septum is depolarized first and activity spreads across the septum from left to right (Fig. 1.6(a)). This simultaneously produces an upward deflection (R wave) in the right ventricular leads and a small downward deflection in the left ventricular leads (Q wave). The two ventricles then depolarize together (Fig. 1.6(b)) and because of the greater mass of the left ventricle, its electrical effect swamps that of the right. A downward deflection occurs in the right ventricular leads (S wave) and an upward deflection in the left ventricular leads (R wave). When the whole of the myocardium has depolarized (Fig. 1.6(c)), the ECG returns to the baseline. Abnormalities of the QRS complex are:
- too tall—hypertrophied muscle beneath the electrode.
- too short—a reduction in active muscle (infarction) or an excess of fat or lung beneath the electrode.

10

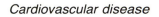

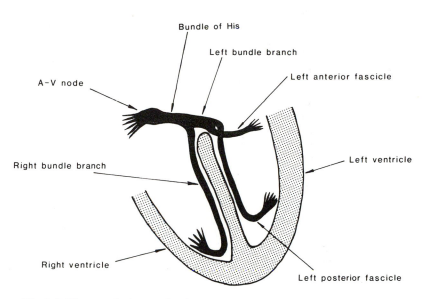

Fig. 1.5. The ventricular conducting system.

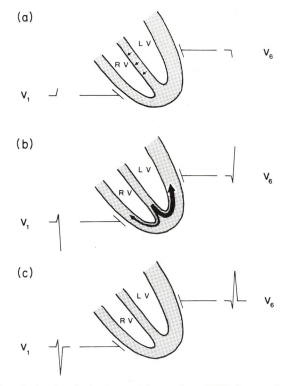

Fig. 1.6. Ventricular depolarization and the resultant ECG. See text for details.

- deep Q wave (over 2 mm)—an absence of living myocardium beneath the electrode fails to obscure septal depolarization.
- too wide—
- wrong shape— } atypical ventricular depolarization (see later Figs, 1.8, 1.9, 1.31, 1.32, 1.36).
- wrong R:S ratio—

Ventricular muscle which depolarizes in an aberrant manner also repolarizes abnormally and there may be accompanying changes in the S-T segment and T wave.

The S-T segment represents a period of electrical inactivity after the completion of depolarization and before the start of repolarization. It is not normally more than 0.5 mm above or below the isoelectric line in any lead. Changes in the S-T segment occur when events in the myocardium and pericardium produce an electrical current secondary to injured (but not dead) or abnormal cells. By far the commonest cause of marked S-T changes is myocardial ischaemia (see later, Fig. 1.18). Other causes are pericarditis, cardiomyopathy, ventricular aneurysm, and acid-base and electrolyte disturbances (especially severe hypokalaemia, see Fig. 7.1).

The 'injury current' displaces the whole ECG up or down except during the electrically quiescent S-T segment, but the visual effect is a change in the S-T segment.

The T wave represents ventricular repolarization which is dependent upon transmembrane ionic movement and the sodium/potassium pump. Not all myocardial cells repolarize after the same time interval or in the same electrical direction, and the wave as seen represents the resultant summation of all the individual cellular repolarizations. Factors which alter the mechanism of repolarization can therefore change both the shape and the position of the T wave. These include ischaemia, infarction, ventricular hypertrophy, conduction defects, electrolyte disturbances (NB potassium, see Fig. 7.1), drugs (NB digoxin, Fig. 1.10), myocarditis, cardiomyopathy, pericarditis, septicaemia, hypothyroidism, and pulmonary embolism.

Repolarization in the healthy heart occurs in the same electrical sequence and along the same pathways as depolarization. The T wave is thus usually upright in those leads in which the QRS complex is upright and vice versa. The normal T wave is always upright in leads I and II. Inversion in V_1 and V_2 is a normal variant.

The Q-T interval represents the time period from the beginning of ventricular depolarization to the end of repolarization. It normally varies with heart rate (see Fig. 1.4) and when abnormalities occur they are usually secondary to electrolyte changes (NB prolonged Q-T in hypocalcaemia).

Individual leads and cardiac axis. Each of the leads reflects the activity in a particular part of the heart:

• Leads I, aVL, V_5, V_6 give information about the left side of the heart.

• Leads V_5 and V_6 are specific to the left ventricle.

• Leads V_1, V_2 give information about the right ventricle.

• Leads V_3, V_4 give information about the interventricular septum and the anterior wall of the left ventricle.

• Leads II, III, aVF give information about the inferior surface of the heart.

Together aVR, aVL, aVF, I, II and III provide a 'clock face' view of cardiac electrical activity in the frontal plane of the body (Fig. 1.7) and can be used to assess the direction of the mean frontal cardiac axis. (They say nothing about electrical vector activity at right angles to the coronal plane.) The cardiac axis is the direction of the mean electrical vector which results from all the individual cellular depolarizations during the production of the QRS. It is therefore in the approximate direction of the lead with the tallest R wave or at right angles to the lead in which the R and S waves are equal. There are only 6 leads available for assessment and the axis can therefore only be obtained to the nearest 30° on visual inspection. This means that firm statements can only be made when the axis deviation is considerable. Current cardiological opinion suggests that the importance of the electrical axis has been overemphasized in the past.

In practice, axis deviation which might indicate pathology is determined by applying 'rules of thumb' to the heights of the R and S waves in leads I, II and III.

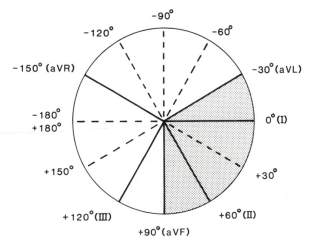

Fig. 1.7. The frontal plane cardiac axis. The range of the normal axis is shown shaded.

13

Left axis deviation is significant when there is a deep S wave in III and the S wave is of greater amplitude than the R wave in II (Fig. 1.8). It is usually caused by a conduction defect (especially left anterior hemiblock, Fig. 1.33) rather than by left ventricular hypertrophy. Minor degrees of left axis deviation are found in any condition in which the heart is more horizontal than normal (e.g. short fat subjects, pregnancy, all the causes of a raised diaphragm), and rarely are associated with tricuspid atresia and ostium primum atrial septal defects.

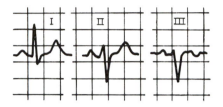

Fig. 1.8. Left axis deviation.

Right axis deviation is significant when there is a deep S wave in I and the largest R wave is in III (Fig. 1.9). This is associated mainly with right ventricular hypertrophy secondary to pulmonary hypertension or congenital heart disease. Minor degrees of right axis deviation occur in tall thin subjects (vertical heart), in those with left posterior hemiblock, and in ostium secundum atrial septal defects.

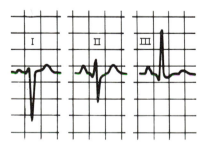

Fig. 1.9. Right axis deviation.

When examining an ECG, develop the habit of looking in turn for disturbances of rhythm, estimating the rate (divide the number of large squares between two QRS complexes into 300), and sequentially assessing abnormalities in the P wave, the P-R interval and the T wave.

Abnormalities of individual conditions are detailed as they arise in the text.

Special investigations

These are undertaken by cardiologists to increase the accuracy of diagnosis. They include exercise ECG testing, 24 hour ECG recordings, phonocardiography, echocardiography, cardiac catheterization and nuclear imaging. All require expert interpretation to assess the significance of the findings.

Common drugs and their problems

Drugs used in the treatment of cardiovascular disease have important anaesthetic implications. The response to treatment and the dosage required to abate symptoms give an idea of the severity of the disease. Do not forget that many patients fail to take their tablets correctly. Only important points about the commoner groups of drugs are discussed below.

Diuretics are prescribed to control either heart failure or hypertension. Examine the patient to see if this has been achieved. Ascertain the type of diuretic, and in particular whether it is potassium-losing or potassium-sparing.

The thiazides act on the distal convoluted tubule to induce a sodium chloride diuresis, whereas the loop diuretics (e.g. frusemide, bumetanide, ethacrynic acid) inhibit active chloride reabsorption in the ascending loop of Henle. Both thiazides and loop diuretics promote potassium loss. The resultant hypokalaemia impairs cardiac conduction (prolonged P-R and Q-T intervals, depressed ST segment and flattened T waves when severe, see Fig. 7.1) and increases the rate of spontaneous depolarization of the atria and the ventricles encouraging ectopic beats. In addition to cardiovascular complications during anaesthesia, patients may also be sensitive to non-depolarizing muscle relaxants.

Potassium-sparing diuretics (e.g. spironolactone, amiloride and triamterene) act on the lower part of the distal tubule and on the collecting duct. It is possible for patients to become hyperkalaemic on these drugs. There may then be dangers with suxamethonium administration.

Always check the serum potassium in patients who are on diuretics since abnormalities are asymptomatic until severe. The desired potassium level is 3.5–5.0 mmol/litre and corrective measures should be undertaken if it is outside this range. With chronic hypokalaemia, the total body deficit can be over 500 mmol potassium. Hypokalaemia can be treated with oral potassium if time permits. The maximum recommended replacement rate in emergencies is up to 240 mmol/day intravenously. Do this in a high dependency area with continuous ECG monitoring. If surgery is urgent, even a few hours treatment is beneficial.

In emergencies, correct hyperkalaemia with intravenous dextrose and insulin. The adverse effects of hyperkalaemia on cardiac conduction are antagonized by calcium.

Digoxin (and other cardiac glycosides) are used in the treatment of congestive heart failure and supraventricular dysrhythmias (especially AF and atrial flutter). The indications for its use have decreased since the introduction of better diuretics, vasodilators and anti-dysrhythmic agents such as verapamil, amiodarone and beta-adrenoceptor blockers.

In the failing heart, digoxin produces a positive inotropic action. It inhibits the potassium/sodium ATPase of the sarcolemma and this allows the intracellular accumulation of sodium ions. These displace bound calcium ions and make more available to take part in the contractile process.

When used to control an excess of atrial stimuli presenting to the A-V node, digoxin slows A-V conduction and prolongs the A-V refractory period thus reducing the ventricular rate. In addition, it is a very weak vagal stimulant.

Digoxin toxicity is not rare (up to 20% of patients). The commonest side effects experienced by the patient (anorexia, nausea, vomiting, diarrhoea, psychiatric disturbances) are unrelated to its cardiac actions. In the heart, almost any dysrhythmia can be produced, the most frequent being VEs, coupled beats and ventricular tachycardia (VT).

IV administration causes an increase in systemic vascular resistance from the constriction of peripheral blood vessels. This occurs before the beneficial cardiac effect (onset of action 30 minutes, peak at several hours) and may cause a worsening of left ventricular failure.

The maintenance dose is usually 250 μg daily. Toxicity is more likely in the presence of hypokalaemia, hypercalcaemia, hypoxaemia, hypothyroidism and reduced renal clearance. Where doubt exists, the serum digoxin level should be measured.

Because of its action on the sarcolemma, digoxin produces ECG changes. These are shown in Fig. 1.10. If the patient is under-digitalized, walking up the ward will increase the heart rate by more than 20 beats/minute and this may require correction before surgery.

Continue digoxin perioperatively. There is reputed to be an increased risk of bradycardia with suxamethonium. Always maintain normocapnia. Hyperventilation decreases the serum potassium which may precipitate digitalis toxicity.

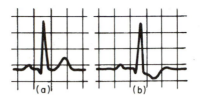

Fig. 1.10. The effect of digoxin on the lateral chest leads. (a) before digitalization; (b) after digitalization. Note S–T segment and T wave changes.

Beta-adrenoceptor blockers differ in their specificity, pharmacokinetics and side effects, but all have the property of competitively antagonizing beta-adrenoceptor stimulation, whether it be neural or hormonal, exogenous or endogenous. The drugs occupy stereospecific beta-adrenoceptors on the cell membrane and may inhibit the intracellular action of adenyl cyclase. All beta-adrenoceptor blockers reduce myocardial contractility and by blocking the catecholamine augmentation of the rate of pre-potential drift (phase 4, Fig. 1.11) in pacemaker cells, they prevent the development of a tachycardia and limit the cardiac output.

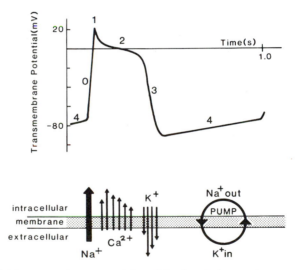

Fig. 1.11. Diagrammatic representation of the electrical events in an automatic cardiac cell. O = depolarization, 1 = overshoot, 2 = plateau, 3 = repolarization, 4 = diastolic prepotential drift. The major determinant of heart rate is the gradient of the prepotential drift towards the threshold potential. It is increased by adrenaline and sympathetic stimulation and reduced by beta-adrenoceptor blockade, vagal stimulation and hypothermia.

The major therapeutic differences between beta-adrenoceptor blockers is whether they are cardioselective or not. Intrinsic sympathomimetic activity and membrane stabilization are now thought to be of little practical importance at normal dose levels. Depressed conduction, antidysrhythmic actions and negative inotropy are primarily due to a removal of beta-adrenoceptor stimulation.

Beta-adrenoceptor blockers are widely used in the treatment of hypertension (mechanism of action unclear), angina (reduce myocardial oxygen requirements by reducing heart rate and blood pressure response to exercise), myocardial infarction (still a controversial area), dysrhythmias which depend primarily upon sympathetic activity (e.g. sinus tachycardia, paroxysmal atrial tachycardia, AF, ventricular dysrhythmias) and thyrotoxicosis (symptomatic relief).

Beta-adrenoceptor blockers are contra-indicated in heart failure (unless due to a tachydysrhythmia), heart block, bronchospasm, severe claudication and anaemia, and must be used with care in the presence of other agents which depress cardiac conduction. They mask the reaction to hypoglycaemia and may stimulate the pregnant uterus.

Always continue beta-adrenoceptor blockers perioperatively because a sudden cessation can lead to rebound sympathetic activity with hypertension, myocardial ischaemia, tachycardia and crescendo angina.

If necessary, maintain beta-adrenoceptor blockade postoperatively by intravenous infusion. The dose of propranolol required is one fifth of the usual oral dose. Alternatively, the combined alpha and beta-adrenoceptor blocker, labetalol, can be given at a rate titrated to produce the required pharmacodynamic response.

There is no contraindication to using regional blockade. There appears to be little interaction between beta-adrenoceptor blockers and halothane, enflurane or isoflurane except a predictable dose-dependent hypotensive effect.

The beta-adrenoceptor blocked patient is unable to increase his heart rate in response to haemorrhage. Prompt detection of blood loss and correction by fluid replacement are therefore essential.

Other hypotensive agents. In order to avoid blood pressure instability, continue all hypotensive agents up to the time of surgery. This is particularly important with relatively short acting drugs (e.g. guanethidine, bethanidine, debrisoquine, hydralazine, prazosin). With drugs of longer duration of action (e.g. methyldopa and reserpine) it is not as crucial. Clonidine has a particularly bad reputation for severe rebound hypertension on abrupt cessation.

Reserpine, which is not often used now, depletes adrenergic nerves of catecholamines, so indirect acting vasopressors have a limited effect.

Guanethidine, bethanidine and debrisoquine are taken into the adrenergic neurone by the noradrenaline uptake pump where they displace noradrenaline. The hypotensive effect of these agents is lost if drugs are given which inhibit the uptake pump (e.g. chlor-promazine, tricyclic antidepressants, ephedrine). Guanethidine, bethanidine and debrisoquine may produce postural hypotension with obvious implications for the positioning of the patient.

Calcium channel blockers are increasing in popularity. The two commonest drugs are verapamil and nifedipine. Their mechanism of action is interference with the calcium ion flux which occurs during phase 2 of the myocardial action potential (Fig. 1.11). In ventricular muscle, the calcium ions are obtained largely from an intracellular pool (see digoxin), but the cells of the A-V node and arterial and venous smooth muscle cells rely predominantly on the entry of extra-cellular calcium ions. Verapamil acts mainly on the A-V node (pro-longs the P-R interval) and nifedipine acts mainly on vascular smooth muscle. The major side effects of both drugs are a reduction in cardiac contractility when given in a high oral or bolus IV dosage and an exaggeration of the expected response when administered concurrently with other drugs of similar pharmacodynamic action.

Verapamil is now regarded by many as the drug of choice for supraventricular tachydysrhythmias (except the sick-sinus syn-drome). Adverse interactions with beta-adrenoceptor blockers and digoxin induce further conduction difficulties, leading to varying degrees of heart block. Potential problems for the anaesthetist exist with halothane and local anaesthetics.

Nifedipine is used mainly for angina and hypertension. In those patients who develop spontaneous episodes of chest pain associated with reversible S-T segment elevation which is caused by coronary artery spasm (Prinzmetal's variant angina, Fig. 1.18) nifedipine usually produces dramatic relief. It is also synergistic in combination with beta-adrenoceptor blockade in many patients with exercise in-duced angina, when presumably some degree of coronary spasm accompanies structural coronary artery stenosis. In the hypertensive patient, calcium antagonists, unlike beta-adrenoceptor blockers, do not appear to prevent a tachycardia and hypertension in response to noxious stimuli.

Nitrates are now thought to act primarily by relaxing vascular, and particularly, venous smooth muscle. In relieving angina, they probably achieve their effect by causing a redistribution of the coronary blood supply and increasing the collateral flow to ischaemic regions. In ventricular failure associated with a high diastolic filling pressure, their action on the peripheral vascular bed reduces both the preload and, to a lesser extent, the afterload.

19

When used for the treatment of angina, the frequency of use gives a guide to the severity of the ischaemic heart disease. The most common preparation is a short acting sublingual form but other long acting oral, IV and transcutaneous nitrate preparations are now available. The adverse effects common to all nitrates (throbbing headache, flushing, postural hypotension and reflex tachycardia) are related to vasodilatation.

Patients should take sublingual glyceryl trinitrate normally in the perioperative period and have them available at all times, including in the anaesthetic room. If myocardial ischaemia occurs under anaesthesia, they can be given crushed in sterile water and put in the nasal cavity. Remember that they will not be very effective sublingually after antisialogogue premedication. Alternatively, IV preparations are available.

Perioperative management

The risks and timing of surgery

For patients over 40 years of age undergoing orthopaedic, urological or general surgical operations, Goldman and colleagues computed a cardiac risk index which measured the chance of developing life-threatening or fatal cardiac complications. Important predictive factors are summarized in Table 1.3. The higher the score, the higher are the chances of developing cardiac complications. The highest risk group is those whose score is 26 points or more.

Hyperlipidaemia, smoking, mild hypertension, diabetes mellitus, stable angina and old myocardial infarction were notable factors found not to be significant predictors.

Table 1.3. Important predictive risk factors associated with the outcome of surgery and anaesthesia, according to Goldman *et al.*

Criteria	Points
Age over 70 years	5
Myocardial infarction within 6 months	10
Gallop rhythm or raised JVP	11
Aortic stenosis	3
ECG rhythm other than sinus	7
More than 5 ventricular ectopics/minute	7
General status (e.g. $PO_2 < 60$ mmHg, $PCO_2 > 50$ mmHg, urea > 50 mmol/litre, abnormal LFT's)	3
Intraperitoneal or intrathoracic operation	3
Emergency operation	4
Total possible	53

The problems and risks of operating on a patient who has had a recent infarct are considered in detail in 'perioperative infarction' (p. 43). Briefly, the outcome is best when the time from the infarct is over 6 months and aggressive, invasive monitoring is used to detect and hence prevent hypertension, tachycardia and hypotension during and after surgery.

Whether or not to accept a hypertensive patient for surgery has long been a contentious issue, and the problem is discussed more fully under 'Hypertension' (p. 53). If there are no complicating factors, patients with diastolic blood pressures of up to 110 mmHg can, with adequate monitoring, be anaesthetized safely. An exception to these recommendations is in patients presenting for carotid endarterectomy in whom poor preoperative blood pressure control $(\overline{BP > 170/95})$ is associated with a much higher incidence of postoperative hypertension and neurological deficit.

The object of preoperative preparation is to optimize the patient for surgery, and once this has been achieved, further delay is pointless. In emergency situations, a suboptimal cardiovascular status may have to be accepted. Based on the risks outlined above, reasonable guide lines are that elective surgery should not be performed on people who have unstable cardiac symptoms, within 6 months of a myocardial infarction or if cardiac failure or severe hypertension is untreated. A sympathetic explanation of any risks involved may be called for.

Whatever technique is chosen, the aim is to provide an adequate supply of well-oxygenated blood to the myocardium and to maintain a blood pressure and heart rate that are neither too high (increased O_2 consumption) nor too low (reduced O_2 supply). It is very useful to have a tray in theatre containing all the drugs likely to be required, so that pharmacological adjustments can be made with little delay.

The principles of cardiovascular monitoring

The appropriate monitoring depends upon the predictability of the patient's responses to all the various drugs and physiological insults he will receive during and after surgery. It is characteristic of people with cardiovascular disease that they are much less predictable than normals and therefore greater diligence is required to allow prompt correction of unwanted events. The extent of invasive monitoring used for any particular patient will always be dependent upon the viewpoint of the anaesthetist. Under the individual disorders we have, where there are likely to be differences of opinion, made what we think are sensible suggestions. This section describes the possible variables to be monitored and outlines the information one can gain from each of them.

21

STETHOSCOPY

The precordial, or oesophageal stethoscope (so common in North America but under-used in Britain) is inexpensive, reliable and re-usable. It gives information about the adequacy of ventilation, the presence or absence of bronchospasm and provides a beat by beat reaffirmation of cardiac activity. It is very easy to detect dropped beats and dysrhythmias. Unfortunately the 'mill-wheel' murmur in those at risk is a late sign of air embolism.

ECG

The 12 lead ECG (p. 8) gives a standard, comprehensive picture of the heart's electrical activity at a given point in time. It is obviously impractical to extend this detailed monitoring into the operative period and instead, a single monitoring lead is used to record ECG changes as they occur. To appreciate the value of the information gained from this requires a basic knowledge of the myocardial blood supply. The right coronary artery arises from the anterior aortic sinus and the left coronary artery arises from the left posterior aortic sinus. The distribution into their main smaller branches over the epicardium is shown in Fig. 1.12. Anastamoses between the branches are never adequate to maintain an efficient permanent collateral circulation, so all coronary arteries must be regarded as end arteries. Because of this, the area of ischaemia seen on the ECG can be related approximately to a particular coronary artery. The highest incidence of ischaemia occurs in the lateral wall of the left ventricle. This is followed by ischaemia of the septum and conducting system.

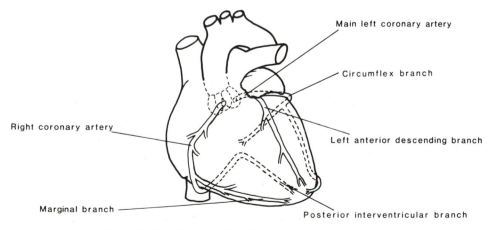

Fig. 1.12. The blood supply of the heart.

Many early studies regarded standard lead II as the best single lead for monitoring. This was because its axis parallels that of the P wave, thus making identification of the P wave easier and supposedly simplifying the differentiation of supraventricular from ventricular dysrhythmias. However, although standard lead II looks at the ventricles, it is neither sensitive nor specific, and indicates left ventricular ischaemia in only 30% of patients with known disease. More recently, the V_5 unipolar chest lead or CM5 bipolar lead (*c*hest lead from *m*anubrium to V5 position) has been recommended because it detects 87% of S-T segment changes due to left ventricular ischaemia and does not confuse the diagnosis of a dysrhythmia.

THE MEASUREMENT OF BLOOD PRESSURE

Indirect methods

All indirect methods of measurement have one feature in common. Each applies a compression cuff to a limb or digit and inflates it to a pressure sufficient to occlude flow to the distal part. They then use the pattern of return of flow as the cuff pressure is reduced to determine the systolic, diastolic and mean blood pressures. The signal used for interpretation can be palpation of the radial or brachial artery, the pressure pulsations from a single (oscillometric) or double (oscillotonometric) cuff, or the presence of flow detected by ultrasound, the Korotkoff sounds or by light reflection. Several of these techniques have now been automated.

The innate random errors of the system, the necessity for external compression, the circumference of the limb, the width of the cuff, and the type of structures compressed (quantity of fat and muscle) contribute to differences between direct and indirect measurement of blood pressure. These are minimized in the upper arm if the cuff width/arm circumference ratio is 0.4 to 0.6. Surprisingly, there are relatively few publications which compare direct and indirect readings under well controlled conditions. However, a limited number of conclusions can be drawn.

The muscles in the patient's arm must be relaxed when the measurement is taken. Otherwise, isometric exercise contracts the muscles, makes compression of the brachial artery more difficult to achieve and elevates both the systolic and diastolic readings.

If a cuff is allowed to deflate continuously, then the faster the fall in pressure and the slower the heart rate the more likely it is that the first signal detected will be at a cuff pressure below the correct one.

Using the mercury column sphygmomanometer, several studies have now shown that there is a surprising degree of variation in blood pressure interpretation among observers. This is due to differences in technique (e.g. time of cuff inflation, rate of deflation), a lack of attention to detail in signal interpretation and a tendency to show a preference for the terminal digits 0 and 5. With practice much of this error can be eliminated. Nevertheless, there still remains the observer's unconscious bias which tends to raise or lower grossly abnormal readings towards normal values.

With palpation of the radial or brachial artery as the end point, only the systolic blood pressure can be measured, and depending on the observer is below the directly measured arterial pressure by 5 to 25 mmHg.

For many years the standard method of monitoring the blood pressure was the detection of Korotkoff sounds. The phases are:

Phase 1— The first appearance of faint, clear, tapping sounds which gradually increase in intensity—'the systolic point'.

Phase 2—The softening of sounds which may become 'swishing'.

Phase 3—The return of sharper sounds.

Phase 4—The distinct, abrupt muffling of sounds which become 'soft' and 'blowing'.

Phase 5—The point at which all sounds disappear completely.

The choice of phase 4 or phase 5 as the true 'diastolic point' (for the purposes of treating hypertension) has been a major controversy. In 1975, the Medical Research Council chose phase 5 for use in their multi-centre trial. Phase 5 also reduces observer bias and gives a better agreement with direct intra-arterial pressure measurements.

It has been recommended that to optimize results, the cuff should be inflated as fast as possible to 30 mmHg above the palpated systolic pressure and deflated at a rate of 2 to 3 mmHg per heart beat. Using this technique, both the systolic and diastolic determinations tend to be below the intra-arterial reading at high levels and above it at low readings. The systolic regression line crosses the equality line at 90 mmHg and falls 20 mmHg below it at an intra-arterial pressure of 175 mmHg. The diastolic regression line crosses the equality line at 80 mmHg and falls 12 mmHg below it at an intra-arterial pressure of 120 mmHg.

The majority of automated systems use single cuff oscillometry. By definition, they have no observer bias. Each has a built-in microprocessor which both controls the cuff deflation in steps and interprets the cuff pulsations in terms of systolic, diastolic and mean pressures. It has now been demonstrated, both theoretically and experimentally, that in systems using cuff pressure oscillations, the mean blood pressure correlates well with the maximum oscillatory amplitude. In general, these machines produce similar results to the Korotkoff sounds for the detection of systolic pressure, and tend to over read the diastolic pressure across a wide range by 5 to 10 mmHg.

Studies on the Dinamap 845 have shown that it can give reliable trend information during anaesthesia provided the internal logic system is not upset by pressure fluctuations due to a dysrhythmia or external artefacts. When this occurs the systolic and diastolic readings are sensibly, deliberately suppressed and only the mean blood pressure is displayed. To avoid unnecessary trauma none of these machines should be set to read more frequently than is necessary.

The double cuff oscillotonometer has long been the favourite blood pressure monitoring instrument of many anaesthetists. When the cuff pressure is lowered slowly and the first 'change in character' of the needle movement is taken to indicate the systolic pressure, and the maximum oscillatory amplitude of the needle used as the determinant of mean pressure, a relatively high degree of accuracy can be achieved over a wide range of pressure measurements. The accuracy does, however, deteriorate with rapid cuff deflation and is subject to observer bias. It is very inaccurate when used to measure diastolic pressure.

The accuracy of all indirect measurements of blood pressure about their regression line can be increased by repeating the reading because the inherent random error by definition sums to zero. This is often done unconsciously by the observer when using the Korotkoff sounds or oscillotonometer by making recurrent small inflations during a determination cycle, in order to identify the signal more accurately.

Indirect measurement of the blood pressure is adequate for the vast majority of patients undergoing routine surgery. It becomes inadequate when the patient has cardiovascular disease, when major sudden changes in blood volume may occur, when the blood pressure is being deliberately lowered, and when very rapidly acting drugs are to be used. The exact point of transition from indirect to direct monitoring obviously differs enormously from anaesthetist to anaesthetist.

Direct measurement

The advantage of an arterial pressure line is that it provides information rapidly, on a beat to beat basis. Therefore, it is most use in those situations where there is a high degree of unpredictability or known disability of the cardiovascular system. The incidence of long term sequelae from modern cannulae in experienced hands is virtually zero, whatever artery they are inserted into. The cannula should be connected to the transducer by a short (up to 1 metre), inelastic tube. For the line to be of use, it is *essential* that the anaesthetist has confidence in its results. It should not resonate or be over damped (Fig.

25

1.13) and because of these possibilities we would recommend that the trace is *always* displayed visually, in addition to the electronic derivations of systolic and diastolic pressure. Most modern monitors have an amplifier which cuts off at approximately 20 cycles/second. This produces a 'clean' trace without loss of vital information.

In addition to the systolic and diastolic pressures and heart rate, the arterial pulse wave yields a great deal more information. The rate of rise of pressure during early systole (dP/dt) (Fig. 1.13) reflects the ability of the myocardium to develop propulsive power and is a measure of left ventricular contractility. Specialist studies use an electronically derived dP/dt to describe this upstroke, but with practice comparisons of contractility can be estimated visually from the pressure trace. This can thus be used, for example, to judge that an inotrope is necessary for the treatment of unacceptable hypotension provided the ventricular filling pressure is adequate.

In contrast to the upstroke, the characteristics of the downstroke give information about the resistance and compliance of the peripheral vascular bed. Decreased arterial pressure associated with peripheral vasodilatation can be identified by an abrupt fall of the pressure wave from its systolic peak and the absence of a sloping diastolic decay (Fig. 1.13). This occurs with sodium nitroprusside or hydralazine therapy, epidural blockade, toxic vasodilatation (hepatic failure, tetanus, septicaemia), arterio-venous fistulae and severe anaemia. An increased arterial pressure with early limitation of ejection (high dicrotic notch) and a steep diastolic run off is characteristic of high peripheral resistance occurring either pathologically

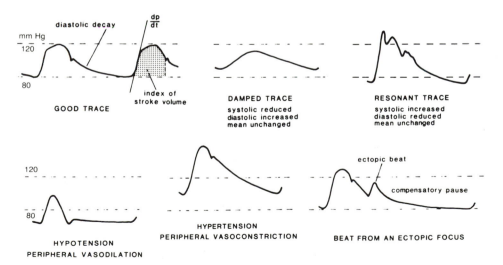

Fig. 1.13. Arterial pressure waves.

(essential hypertension) or secondary to drugs (methoxamine or phenylephrine) (Fig. 1.13).

The effect of dysrhythmias is also instantly obvious (Fig. 1.13). The myocardial oxygen consumption may be indexed by the product of heart rate and systolic pressure (see 'Functional disease of the myocardium'). Estimation of the stroke volume can be made from the hatched area under the pressure trace (Fig. 1.13).

THE CENTRAL VENOUS PRESSURE

The clinical measurement of the CVP, and a description of its component waves and their abnormalities have been given earlier (Fig. 1.1 and Table 1.2). For diagnostic purposes, the presence or absence of individual waves become of importance in atrial fibrillation, heart block, tricuspid valve disease and right ventricular hypertrophy. For monitoring purposes, in the majority of cases the CVP is required primarily as a measure of right (and, indirectly of left) ventricular filling pressure and the mean pressure is the variable which is normally recorded. All methods of recording depend upon the pressure head being referred to a point on the patient which bears a constant vertical relationship to the right atrium. Depending upon this reference point the CVP is quoted as having various 'normal values'. The most convenient and accurate position during anaesthesia, with the patient supine and horizontal, is the mid axillary line which passes through the point of the shoulder. Normal values would be from 2 to 6 mmHg. If a patient's resting CVP is required, it must be taken before anaesthesia because almost all intravenous and volatile agents produce venodilatation. This increases the volume of the capacitance vessels and reduces the CVP.

The relationship of the CVP to the left atrial pressure (LAP) is discussed later under 'The pulmonary artery catheter'.

A single reading of the CVP is of little use unless it is combined with other clinical data because a given value can be produced by a wide combination of hypo or hypervolaemic states, varying degrees of venodilatation and differing levels of ventricular performance. Consequently, it is more useful to take an accurate measurement of the CVP, infuse a known volume of isotonic fluid and watch the response. This has two main applications.

Firstly, assuming a healthy heart, it can be used to assess the degree of hypovolaemia. If 500 mls of 0.9% saline are infused over approximately 15 minutes, the CVP will either increase rapidly, increase slowly or show no response. If the measurement in a further fifteen minutes is back to its pre-infusion level, then it is likely that the patient is fluid deficient. It is, however, difficult to judge the degree of overload from an elevated response and this test is better at detecting hypovolaemic states.

Secondly, a fluid load can be used to assess ventricular response in a patient known to be approximately normovolaemic. Under these circumstances, the importance of any venous pressure measurement lies in the assumption that the venous pressure is equal to the atrial pressure and therefore varies directly with ventricular end diastolic pressure. This is in turn related (though in a grossly non-linear manner) to ventricular end diastolic volume. The heart, like any other muscle, depends upon its resting length for the contractile power it can produce (the Frank-Starling effect) and the hallmark of the failing ventricle is that it fails to empty rather than failing to fill, thereby producing an abrupt increase in atrial pressure.

Thus, volume loading the healthy patient rapidly with say 250 mls of physiological saline increases the CVP by only 1 to 2 mmHg, whereas a patient with incipient heart failure would increase his CVP from say 8 to 18 mmHg. This procedure can be undertaken with an awake or anaesthetized patient (stable before surgical intervention), in order to evaluate fully the response to volume loading and provide an index of cardiac reserve. By loading the right atrium and measuring the response of the CVP, the effects of the right and left ventricle are not separated. To isolate the action of the left or right ventricle requires the use of a left atrial or pulmonary artery catheter. Idealized left ventricular function curves and the response to an increase in the left ventricular end diastolic pressure (LVEDP) in the healthy and failing ventricle are shown in Fig. 1.14.

THE PULMONARY ARTERY CATHETER

This is often known as the Swan–Ganz catheter (after two of the originators) but should be called a flow directed balloon-tipped catheter. It is passed through a suitable vein (antecubital, internal jugular or subclavian) to the pulmonary artery under the guidance of continuous pressure monitoring. The sequence of pressure waves seen is shown in Fig. 1.15. Inflating the balloon and allowing it to occlude a pulmonary vessel gives a pressure reading which, in expiration, correlates well with LAP. This is called the pulmonary artery occlusion or wedge pressure (PAWP). The pressure wave fluctuations in the left atrium (analogous to the a and v waves of the CVP in Fig. 1.1) are heavily damped in retrograde transmission through the pulmonary venous bed and the normal PAWP trace often has poorly defined components.

Measured at the mid axillary line with the patient supine, the PAWP is normally 5 to 12 mmHg. In many cases, the PAWP

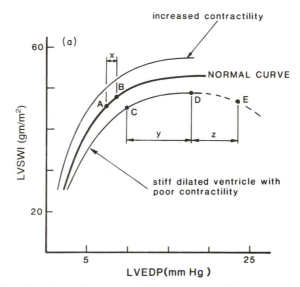

Fig. 1.14(a). Ventricular function and filling pressure. This shows the changes in left ventricular stroke work index (LVSWI) in response to changes in left ventricular end diastolic pressure (LVEDP) in both a healthy and a compromised ventricle. The data for the normal curve is taken from Prys-Roberts (1981). The effects of moving the ventricular operating point from A to B (an increase in LVEDP of x mmHg) and from C to D and D to E (increases in LVEDP of y and z mmHg) are shown in Figs 1.14(b) and 1.14(c) respectively.

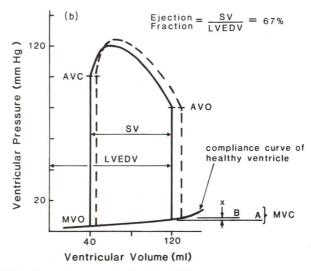

Fig. 1.14(b). Normal ventricular function. This shows the pressure-volume loop for a normal ventricle (MV = mitral valve, AV = aortic valve, O = opens, C = closes). The stroke volume (SV) and left ventricular end diastolic volume (LVEDV) used to determine the ejection fraction are marked. The effect of fluid loading which increases the LVEDP from A to B (Fig. 1.14(a)) is shown by the broken line.

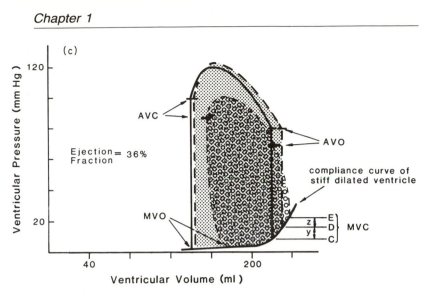

Fig. 1.14(c). Poor ventricular function. This shows the pressure-volume loop for a stiff, dilated ventricle (MV = mitral valve, AV = aortic valve, O = opens, C = closes). The change in LVEDP required to increase the LVSWI by the same amount as moving from A to B in a normal ventricle (Figs 1.14(a) and 1.14(b)) is represented by the movement from C to D. (Fig. 1.14(a)). The fall in LVSWI in moving from D to E (Fig. 1.14(a)) is shown above by the reduced area enclosed on the pressure-volume loop. A reduction in LVSWI with an increase in LVEDP (often termed decompensation) is now thought to be mainly due to mitral incompetence from a stretched valve ring, rather than overextension of the myofibrils. Because of mitral incompetence, in contracting from a LVEDP of E (above), there is no isovolumetric contraction or relaxation. Decompensation is more common in right ventricular failure where the tricuspid valve stretches easily because of the thinner ventricular wall.

approximates to (but is always slightly less than) the pulmonary artery diastolic pressure. A large difference between these two readings occurs in cor pulmonale. Working from the pulmonary artery (PA) diastolic pressure and not inflating the balloon reduces the risk of pulmonary infarction and vessel rupture. Some catheters have the facility to measure cardiac output by thermodilution.

With the catheter properly positioned as confirmed by the pressure tracing, both the PA and PAWP should show a ventilatory variation. The PAWP is lower by up to a maximum of 10 mmHg in inspiration in a spontaneously breathing subject. This ventilatory variation is increased with hypovolaemia and bronchospasm and reversed with IPPV. The digital value normally displayed by the monitor is an average PAWP derived over one or more ventilatory cycles.

Because these catheters are expensive (up to £80) and are not without serious complications (pulmonary artery rupture, dysrhythmias, pulmonary infarction, air embolism, infection and catheter knotting) they should be reserved for patients with strong indications.

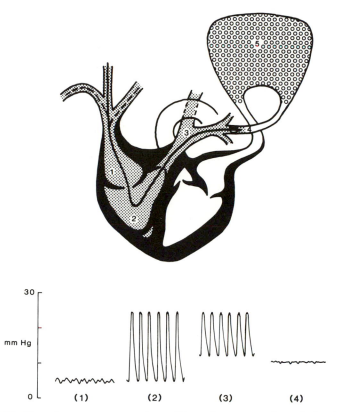

Fig. 1.15. The pulmonary artery catheter. The catheter passes through the right atrium (1) via the tricuspid valve to the right ventricle (2) and then through the pulmonary valve into the pulmonary artery (3). The wedge or occlusion pressure is that beyond the inflated balloon (4). The pressure traces are often 'noisier' than this example because of catheter tip vibration and the variation with breathing or IPPV. Note the moderator band in the right ventricle which carries conducting fibres and which, when irritated during passage of the catheter, can produce dysrhythmias.

Haemoptysis is the commonest clinical presentation of pulmonary artery rupture.

In normal man, LVEDP is approximately 4 to 5 mmHg higher than right ventricular end diastolic pressure (RVEDP), the latter being reflected in the CVP. When this relationship no longer holds, the left atrial pressure needs to be approximated by PAWP. Poor correlation between right and left atrial pressures has been noted in:

• Patients with a history of LVF or current evidence of LVF (ejection fraction below 40%).

• Patients with severe right or left bundle branch block.

• Patients with left ventricular dyssynergy (especially after myocardial infarction).

• Patients with tamponade or constrictive pericarditis.

- Patients with <u>pulmonary hypertension</u>.

The indications for a pulmonary artery catheter are increased if the operative procedure is likely to involve rapid variations in circulatory volume or peripheral resistance. The response of the left ventricle to fluid loading can be established in exactly the same way as described for the CVP.

The obvious question to ask is, under what conditions does the mean PAWP not reflect LVEDP? There is a certain amount of discussion continuing in the literature on this point but the following statements appear to be well established.

- PAWP correlates poorly with LAP at high levels of positive end expiratory pressure (PEEP) (>10 cmH$_2$O). Some workers recommend reducing it to zero temporarily prior to measurement. The relevance of this measurement taken at zero PEEP to haemodynamics with PEEP is uncertain.
- If there is an embolus distal to the balloon the reading is obviously in error.
- In LVF the LVEDP can be increased appreciably by atrial systole and the resultant 'a' waves (Fig. 1.16) are prominent both on the PA and PAWP traces. The 'a' wave peak (which reflects the LVEDP) may be up to 10 mmHg above the mean PAWP displayed on the monitor.
- In sinus rhythm with a stenosed mitral valve, there are large 'a' waves which do not reflect LVEDP because of the pressure drop across the valve.

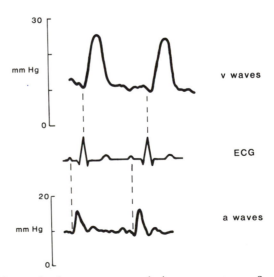

Fig. 1.16 Abnormal pulmonary artery occlusion pressure traces. See text for description.

- Giant 'v' waves occurring on the PA and PAWP traces (Fig. 1.16) are traditionally explained as being the result of mitral regurgitation. There is now, however, good evidence that they can also occur in LVF when a small, stiff, non-compliant atrium fills rapidly from a congested pulmonary circulation. Moreover, patients with severe mitral regurgitation have on occasions been found to have trivial 'v' waves on the PAWP trace.
- In severe aortic incompetence with premature mitral valve closure because of a massive regurgitant jet, the PAWP may significantly underestimate the LVEDP.

Anaesthetic considerations

There is a widespread view, held particularly by physicians and surgeons, that a regional or local block rather than a general anaesthetic is the technique of choice for patients with cardiovascular disease. There is no evidence to support this opinion and it probably represents a hangover from the time when major surgery was done on spontaneously breathing subjects and patients died 'because they could not stand the anaesthetic'.

The following arguments summarize the 'pros and cons' of each technique. In some instances, it is possible to combine them and enjoy the benefits of both.

REGIONAL ANAESTHESIA

Advantages. The main advantage is that profound anaesthesia is possible with a drug which is then slowly absorbed into the general circulation causing little systemic effect. Further advantages are that if the patient is kept awake there is no ventilatory depression in the immediate postoperative period and complete analgesia abolishes the sympathetic response to pain.

Disadvantages. As a sole anaesthetic technique, regional blocks are only suitable for operations on the extremities or below the umbilicus. Spinal and epidural techniques, because of vasodilatation, drop the blood pressure and can easily cause myocardial ischaemia. Therefore, always have a vasopressor drawn up. At the thoracic level the sympathetic nerves to the heart (T_2–T_4) may be inactivated producing a bradycardia requiring atropine or sympathomimetics. If the local anaesthetic is inadvertently administered intravenously, it can have catastrophic effects on a compromised cardiovascular system. This is particularly true of epidural, brachial plexus and Bier's blocks where the quantity of local anaesthetic is large. Bupivacaine is more dangerous than lignocaine because of its long duration of action and its affinity for the myocardium (because of high fat solubility).

The psychological stress of having the operation awake may itself induce an angina attack. This is particularly likely to occur if sensitive patients are kept in an uncomfortable and embarrassing position in the presence of thoughtless theatre personnel, or if the patient has little confidence in the block.

If the anxious patient is given a sedative premedication or increments of IV sedatives peroperatively he may become confused and the airway can become difficult to control. Both can result partly from, or contribute to, hypoxia. This must be corrected immediately and may require general anaesthesia and intubation.

Regional blocks are no excuse for inadequate monitoring. If chosen, meticulous technique and anticipation of events are all important.

GENERAL ANAESTHESIA

Advantages. There is no question that monitoring and the discussion and treatment of abnormalities is easier when the patient is asleep. The surgeon is often more relaxed and, hopefully, able to work faster. The changes in heart rate and blood pressure are more easily controlled. The use of IPPV ensures adequate oxygenation and allows control of the $PaCO_2$

Disadvantages. Induction of anaesthesia depresses the blood pressure by the direct pharmacological effect of anaesthetic agents (both intravenous and inhalational) and by the loss of baroreflex control. Spontaneous breathing techniques with high concentrations and/or prolonged administration of a volatile agent as the main anaesthetic agent can produce marked hypercapnia and hypotension.

PREMEDICATION

The primary objective is to reduce anxiety and the consequent secretion of catecholamines. The choice of drugs is a personal one. Very anxious patients may benefit from a benzodiazepine in the days before surgery. Take care to avoid excessive ventilatory depression from opioids or a tachycardia from atropine. Ensure access to glyceryl trinitrate where appropriate.

INDUCTION

Preoxygenate to minimize the chance of hypoxia. Always have good intravenous access, monitor the ECG and use a tipping trolley so that hypotension can be treated rapidly by increasing venous return. The decision whether or not to invasively monitor the BP and CVP etc. during induction depends on the individual case.

Many induction sequences are satisfactory. The key is to give the drugs slowly to minimize adverse cardiac effects. Etomidate is the induction agent which causes the least change in blood pressure and cardiac output. Thiopentone and methohexitone both cause a moderate decrease in blood pressure (20–30%) but this can be lessened by using a small dose given slowly after fentanyl 4–5 μg/kg. Ketamine may produce undesirable hypertension and tachycardia.

In emergencies suxamethonium will be necessary but may have the adverse side effect of bradycardia. Of the non-depolarizing muscle relaxants pancuronium, despite the occasional occurrence of hypertension and tachycardia, is probably the best choice. Gallamine produces a tachycardia and curare and alcuronium hypotension. Vecuronium on preliminary studies, may have advantages because of its particular cardiovascular stability. There have been several good reports of atracurium but (in doses over 0.4 mg/kg) it has, on occasions been found to cause hypotension and bradycardia.

If intending to intubate, take over the ventilation when possible. Avoid obstructing the venous return by clumsy application of the facemask or by hand ventilation with high pressures.

Laryngoscopy and intubation under light anaesthesia stimulate the sympathetic nervous system such that hypertension and tachycardia may cause myocardial ischaemia. The main stimulus is that of laryngoscopy rather than the passage of the tube into the trachea. Several techniques have been used to reduce the physiological response to this stretching of the pharynx. Local anaesthesia of the larynx and pharynx will prevent afferent neural input but must, of course, be accomplished without laryngoscopy. Laryngoscopy under deep anaesthesia, or following high dose fentanyl, reduces the response because of central nervous depression. Beta-adrenoceptor blockade and sodium nitroprusside do nothing to attenuate the neural or hormonal response but prevent its peripheral actions from being apparent. IV lignocaine has also been used but its mode of action is not well defined.

By far the most convenient method of suppressing the response to laryngoscopy, if there are no contraindications, is pre treatment with a beta-adrenoceptor blocker. Those patients who are maintained on their pre-existing treatment with beta-adrenoceptor blockers show markedly attenuated responses to laryngoscopy and intubation.

Intubate gently without forcing the tube. Watch the ECG for signs of ischaemia and, if necessary, deepen anaesthesia.

MAINTENANCE

Spontaneous breathing using volatile agents may only be suitable for short operations because the dose necessary to achieve surgical anaesthesia causes an increase in $PaCO_2$ and depression of the myocardium. Halothane primarily depresses myocardial contractility producing a dose-dependent hypotension. As the anaesthetic progresses some 'adaptation' or 'accommodation' occurs when the systemic vascular resistance decreases and cardiac output is maintained, thus supporting tissue oxygenation. Halothane depresses conduction at the S-A node and may cause junctional rhythm. It also precipitates ventricular ectopic activity, particularly in the presence of a high $PaCO_2$ or catecholamines. Enflurane has similar depressant properties but a lower propensity to produce dysrhythmias in the presence of hypercarbia and catecholamines. Isoflurane reduces arterial pressure more than halothane but it does so by dilating resistance vessels rather than by impairing myocardial contractility. Cardiac output is well maintained and the threshold for dysrhythmias in the presence of hypercarbia is higher than with halothane. Superficially, the properties of isoflurane would appear to make it the agent of choice for use with a compromised myocardium. Its ability to dilate the coronary arteries may, however, be reduced or absent in those branches whose lumens are reduced by disease. When the healthy adjacent vessels dilate, it has been suggested that there might be an inverse-steal effect shunting blood away from an area of borderline perfusion.

IPPV with a relaxant, O_2, N_2O and an opioid is the most commonly used maintenance technique. IPPV reverses the intrathoracic pressure gradients and reduces cardiac output by increasing pulmonary input impedance and causing asynchrony of the right and left ventricles. The usual acceptance of an Inspiratory:Expiratory ratio of 1:2 comes from early studies which demonstrated that, under these conditions, compensation for the inspiratory haemodynamic perturbations could be provided during expiration. The normal physiological response to IPPV is both peripheral and pulmonary venoconstriction and this reduces the cyclical changes in venous return to the right ventricle and left atrium. This compensatory mechanism is reduced by poliomyelitis, polyneuritis, spinal cord transection, autonomic neuropathy, ganglion blockers, beta-adrenoceptor blockers and high spinal or epidural anaesthesia. Under general anaesthesia, the degree of vasoconstriction possible is inversely proportional to the depth of anaesthesia.

Minimize ventilator effects by achieving low inflation pressures, a sufficient expiratory period and an adequate circulating volume.

PEEP should only be used to improve oxygenation in the presence of pulmonary pathology. Its action on the circulation depends on the degree to which its effect is transmitted to the blood vessels across the stiff, damaged lungs. The major acute cardiovascular effects of PEEP are to slow venous return to the right atrium and to raise the impedance to right ventricular ejection. The reduction in cardiac output can be catastrophic in the presence of hypovolaemia. Despite the improvement in oxygenation, because PEEP has such a deleterious effect on cardiac output, the concept of 'best PEEP' has arisen, which is the amount of PEEP at which the oxygen flux is maximal.

CARBON DIOXIDE

The response to hypocapnia produced by hyperventilation is largely independent of the agent used. Typically, it results in a 0.5–1% reduction of cardiac output per mmHg reduction in $PaCO_2$, the heart rate and mean arterial pressure being unchanged. There is also evidence that hypocapnia reduces coronary blood flow. The hyperdynamic cardiovascular response to hypercapnia under anaesthesia is strongly affected by sympathetic activity and is markedly reduced by effective beta-adrenoceptor blockade. Without beta-adrenoceptor blockade, cardiac output increases approximately 1% per mmHg increase in $PaCO_2$ under halothane anaesthesia and up to 3.5% with nitrous oxide and enflurane.

Consequently, it is sensible to ventilate to normocapnia or to only very mildly hyperventilate patients who have any form of cardiovascular disease because of the unpredictability and intensity of the response to changes in $PaCO_2$.

CHANGES IN BLOOD PRESSURE

Treatment of intraoperative deviations of blood pressure and heart rate should be directed in a logical manner based on the level of anaesthesia and on the changes seen in the systolic and diastolic pressure, the CVP, PAWP, and the shape of the arterial pressure wave (Fig. 1.13). Some guidelines are given in Table 1.4.

There are many drugs available. Know the properties of a few. A reasonable armoury would be halothane, isoflurane, atropine, hydralazine, methoxamine, ephedrine, propranolol, labetalol, glyceryl trinitrate, sodium nitroprusside, dopamine, isoprenaline and calcium.

Postoperative phase

It is vitally important to continue good monitoring and management into the postoperative period. Depending on the severity of pre-

Table 1.4. Guide to logical treatment of cardiovascular abnormalities.

Abnormality	Cause	Treatment
Tachycardia	Hypovolaemia	Check CVP, test infusion of fluid. Give blood.
	Light anaesthesia	Deepen anaesthesia
	Vasodilatation	Vasoconstrictors
	Above excluded, therefore, sympathetic overactivity	Beta-adrenoceptor blockade
Hypertension	Light anaesthesia	Deepen anaesthesia
	Vasoconstriction	Vasodilate
	High contractility	Reduce with halothane
	Hypercarbia	Increase ventilation
Hypotension	Vasodilatation – especially epidural or spinal	Vasoconstrict
	Fluid overload	Check CVP, vasodilate
	Poor contractility	Inotropic support
Bradycardia	Hypoxia	Correct cause. 100% O_2
	Vagal stimulation	Give atropine
	Heart block	Give isoprenaline, insert pacemaker

existing disease and the magnitude of the operation this may mean 24–48 hours on the Intensive Care Unit (ICU).

One of the main dangers is the hypertensive response to arousal. It may be preferable to extubate the patient whilst still anaesthetized to minimize this. Be prepared to treat hypertension or hypotension promptly. See the section on 'hypertension' for detailed management but always check whether pain or bladder distension is the problem.

Ensure good oxygenation at all times. See Chapter 2 for the pulmonary response to anaesthesia. Make arrangements for the usual drug therapy to be given parenterally if unable to be taken orally. Do *not* forget about urine output.

PART II. INDIVIDUAL CONDITIONS

It is assumed that the basic history, examination and investigation covered in the general section is completed. In addition to the general principles of management already described the important points for specific conditions are highlighted here. It is intended that both sections of the chapter should be used together in determining the optimum plan for any given patient.

Ischaemic heart disease

In England and Wales, ischaemic heart disease is responsible for 27% (160 000 per year) of all deaths and affects about 20% of the male population aged less than 60 years.

Definitions

Angina is the pain felt when the oxygen supply to the myocardium is insufficient for its demands.

Hypertrophy is a physiological response of the ventricle to an increased work load. It is detectable electrocardiographically but cannot be seen *per se* on a CXR. The increased muscle mass increases the overall oxygen demand and can thus precipitate features of coronary insufficiency.

Ventricular dilatation occurs when the ventricle, because of intrinsic weakness or excessive work load, is unable to produce an adequate stroke volume without allowing an increase in end diastolic volume. The ejection fraction is reduced and ventricular output depends heavily on adequate ventricular filling. It is seen by an increase in size of the cardiac shadow on CXR and is usually accompanied by the ECG changes of ventricular hypertrophy.

Ventricular failure is difficult to define, but can be described as that condition when ventricular output is able to match venous return only after a substantial increase in filling pressure has occurred.

In Western medicine, the commonest causes of LVF are hypertension and coronary artery disease: the commonest causes of RVF are secondary to LVF or pulmonary disorders (cor pulmonale).

Left ventricular ischaemia

Physiology. The distribution of the major coronary arteries has already been described (Fig. 1.12) and they arborize on the surface of the heart to form a mass of smaller epicardial arteries from which so called 'B' branches perforate directly through the myocardium to reach the endocardium. The only collateral circulation exists at sub-endocardial level and becomes of importance if there is a blockage in an epicardial vessel (Fig. 1.17). This arrangement has several consequences.

The intramural oxygen tension of the sub-endocardial muscle is normally significantly lower than that in subepicardial muscle. The 'B' perforators, because of their length, are subject to torsion and pressure during muscular contraction. As the intraventricular pressure develops during systole there is a 'tissue' pressure which by compression effectively halts flow in the sub-endocardial region. This results in the majority of useful myocardial perfusion occurring during diastole. Early diastolic relaxation is delayed if the myocardium is ischaemic.

At even low levels of activity the heart extracts approximately three quarters of the oxygen content of the blood delivered to it.

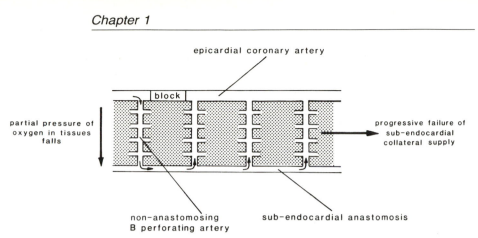

Fig. 1.17. Perfusion of the left ventricular wall. During diastole (as shown) the subendocardial vessels are patent. During systole they are compressed by ventricular cavity pressure and collateral perfusion is impossible. Also see text.

Thus, an increased demand for oxygen can only be met by increased supply rather than by increased extraction. Although the exact mechanism of this is still debated, it is thought in the healthy heart to be achieved by vasodilatation at the arteriolar and pre-capillary sphincter level.

The main determinants of the oxygen requirement are the intraventricular systolic wall tension and compression (reflected by the systemic blood pressure), the heart rate, and myocardial contractility (influenced by the patient's own sympathetic outflow and by drugs).

Those factors leading to relative ischaemia can therefore be summarized in Table 1.5.

As a measure of myocardial oxygen demand, the tension time index (TTI) was introduced and can be approximated by the product of systolic pressure (mmHg) and heart rate (beats/minute). It is also

Table 1.5. Causes of insufficient supply of oxygen to the myocardium.

Low O_2 carriage per ml of blood	Hypoxia
	Anaemia
Inability to perfuse main coronary arteries	Coronary artery thrombosis
	Hypotension
	Coronary artery spasm
Reduced coronary perfusion time	Tachycardia
Endocardial compression	Hypertension
	Aortic stenosis
Increased metabolic demand	Hypertension
	Tachycardia
	Sympathetic drive
	Sympathomimetic drugs
	Catecholamines

known as the 'rate pressure product'. Healthy adults can easily achieve levels of over 20000. Its usefulness in anaesthesia is that patients known to have exercise induced angina become symptomatic at approximately a constant value. Those who have had exercise testing (S-T segment depression of 0.1 mV is taken as significant) will have the figure recorded (or able to be calculated), in their notes. This can be taken as a guide to an acceptable upper limit during anaesthesia.

Preoperative considerations

History

Ischaemic heart disease is already well advanced when it declares itself clinically and serious underlying disease (up to 70% stenosis of a major coronary artery) *may* be totally asymptomatic. Consequently, try to identify risk factors. These are smoking, hypertension, hyperlipidaemia, diabetes mellitus and a family history of ischaemic heart disease.

Ask about angina: in particular what factors provoke it and relieve it. This may separate coronary stenosis when angina worsens with exercise (angina pectoris, common) from coronary artery spasm (Prinzmetal's variant angina, rare) where it appears at rest and disappears with exercise. The differentiation is important because patients with exercise induced angina react predictably (developing ischaemia when the myocardial work load exceeds a given limit) whereas those with Prinzmetal's angina can develop ischaemia completely without warning during or after anaesthesia. When Prinzmetal's angina occurs, beta-adrenoceptor blockers are contraindicated and coronary vasodilators such as glyceryl trinitrate or nifedipine are the drugs of choice.

Determine the degree of exercise which produces angina and how often it occurs. Remember that patients with peripheral vascular disease always have coronary artery disease but may not be able to exercise sufficiently to induce angina. Angina at rest, or on minimal exercise is a bad prognostic sign. If the angina is increasing in frequency and severity, reinfarction is a danger and any elective surgery should be delayed until the symptoms are stable.

Ask specifically if the angina is brought on by emotion because this obviously influences the way in which you explain any risks to the patient and the choice of premedication.

Record the date of any known infarction. Consider whether surgery is justified. (See 'The risks and timing of surgery', p. 20 and 'Perioperative infarction', p. 43).

41

The drug history is obviously vital and hypotensives, beta-adrenoceptor blockers, diuretics and calcium antagonists should all be continued until surgery and arrangements made for their administration in the postoperative period.

Examination

Often there are no abnormal physical signs. Exclude those of pump failure.

Investigations

ECG Changes in the ECG are not invariable and may or may not be produced or magnified by exercise. Nevertheless, in over 80% of patients with coronary artery disease the ECG is abnormal. Coronary artery disease can cause non-specific abnormalities such as those of left ventricular hypertrophy (sum of S wave in V_1 and R wave in V_5 over 40 mm), bundle branch blocks (q.v.), and disorders of A-V conduction (q.v.). Specific abnormalities are those of the S-T segment (elevation or depression over 1 mm) and the T wave (inverted or flat). These are shown in Fig. 1.18.

CXR This should be normal but check for signs of LVF and aortic and mitral valve calcification (Fig. 1.3).

Anaesthetic management

Consider whether the cardiovascular status may be improved by drug adjustments or by alleviating a pulmonary infection. Any rhythm disturbance should be treated as detailed later.

The principles of anaesthetic management have already been outlined in 'Anaesthetic considerations'. With all patients, display the ECG continuously from before induction of anaesthesia through to the postoperative period. Always look for the changes of ischaemia (S-T segments) and adjust the blood pressure and heart rate appropriately to relieve the myocardium. Non-invasive monitoring is appropriate for those patients with stable symptoms who have no evidence of right or left ventricular failure and who are undergoing short or medium length (<90 minutes) operations which do not involve major fluid shifts. On the other hand, a patient with incipient heart failure, worsening angina, evidence of left ventricular dyssynergy having an upper abdominal or thoracic operation would need arterial, central venous and pulmonary artery catheters inserted prior to induction and left in position for 24–48 hours postoperatively. Between these two extremes, there is the optimum plan for a

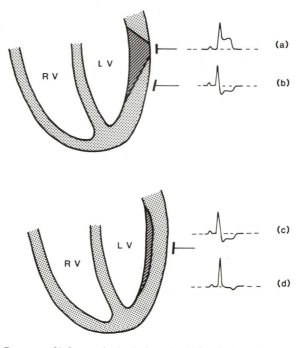

Fig. 1.18. Patterns of left ventricular ischaemia. (After C. Prys-Roberts (1981)). Electrocardiographic appearances of transmural myocardial ischaemia (above) and of sub-endocardial ischaemia (below). A wedge shaped area of ischaemia secondary to occlusion by coronary artery thrombosis (common) or spasm (rare) of a major epicardial artery may produce the characteristic elevated S–T segment in a chest lead which overlies the ischaemic area (a) or S–T segment depression in an adjacent lead overlying a marginal area of subendocardial ischaemia (b). Generalized sub-endocardial ischaemia is associated with S–T segment depression (c) and may ultimately progress to infarction in which T wave inversions occur (d).

given patient. The great advantage of invasive, beat by beat monitoring is that it allows early trends to be treated before they do any harm, and one can immediately see the effect of drug treatment on rapid changes which have occurred unexpectedly.

Perioperative infarction

Established infarction

The associated risk with surgery has already been mentioned in 'The risks and timing of surgery', p. 20. Approximately one third of patients who undergo surgery within three months of a myocardial infarct develop a reinfarction in the first postoperative week and half of these die. The incidence of reinfarction is higher after long operations, after thoracic and upper abdominal operations and in patients who had complications at the time of their original infarction (LVF, hypertension, dysrhythmias, high blood urea). There is now very good evidence to suggest that the reinfarction rate increases in those patients who have preoperative congestive heart failure, or *who experience intraoperative hypertension, tachycardia or hypotension*. Thus careful preoperative preparation, aggressive, invasive cardiovascular monitoring and the prompt treatment of haemodynamic abnormalities are all important in optimizing the welfare of these exacting patients. It is therefore a reasonable plan to postpone elective surgery for 6 months, to accept that there is nothing to be gained by further delay and to do one's best as appropriate to the patient's problems at that time, provided their symptoms are stable.

If surgery has to proceed urgently, the patient should be treated as outlined in 'left ventricular ischaemia'. The maximum incidence of reinfarction occurs on the third postoperative day. Whether postoperatively they should spend a week on ICU, or indeed whether this is beneficial, is debatable. Wherever they go they should, however, have good nursing care, no episodes of hypoxia, stable cardiovascular parameters and adequate analgesia.

The diagnosis of postoperative infarction

The diagnosis of infarction depends upon three things.

● *Clinical picture*. This is characteristic but can occasionally be difficult to identify after thoracic and upper abdominal surgery. However, the nature (constant, gripping, crushing) and radiation of the pain, the perspiration and the mental anguish contrast with the sharp pain, accentuated by movement and coughing which is secondary to surgical incisions.
● *Cardiac Enzymes*. Creatine phosphokinase (CPK) is increased within a few hours, is maximum at 24 hours and returns to normal in 3 days.

Aspartate transaminase (AST) in increased within 12 hours, is maximum at 24–36 hours and returns to normal in 4 days.

Lactic dehydrogenase (LDH) is increased within 12–48 hours, is maximum at 3–6 days and returns to normal by 8–14 days.

These enzymes are usually elevated postoperatively in all patients because of surgical trauma. Isoenzyme measurements (CPK-MB, LDH-1) are needed but these are not universally available. Nevertheless, serial samples may support the diagnosis of myocardial infarction because of a typical time course.
● *ECG changes*. These are found in over 95% of patients, usually soon after the onset of pain. Serial ECGs with sequential changes are more helpful than an isolated one. The hardest evidence of infarction

in the postoperative period are new and persisting Q waves and altered R wave progression in the precordial leads. A preoperative ECG is, under these circumstances, invaluable for comparison. The Q waves result from an infarcted 'ventricular window' failing to obscure septal depolarization, and the R wave reduces in size because of a loss of active muscle beneath the electrode.

The non-specific changes of pyrexia, leucocytosis and raised ESR which normally accompany myocardial infarction are all abnormal after surgery anyway.

The care of such a patient is similar to that of a person on the coronary care unit who has not just had surgery.

Right ventricular-ischaemia

The right ventricle is a thin walled chamber which receives its blood supply in both diastole and systole. Because it usually only generates low pressures it has a lower oxygen demand than the left ventricle.

When right ventricular ischaemia does occur, the ischaemic pain is not distinguishable from that of left ventricular ischaemia. The clinical picture may resemble that of a pulmonary embolus or constrictive pericarditis and requires invasive monitoring for diagnosis. Characteristically, the CVP is raised, LAP or PAWP is normal or low, PA pressures are low and the cardiac output is low. The ECG most commonly shows changes of inferior infarction (inferoposterior wall of the right ventricle) in leads II, III and aVF.

Although right ventricular disease is comparatively rare, it is now receiving more attention from cardiologists. The anaesthetic literature is scanty compared to that which considers the haemodynamically more important left ventricle. The principles of management are as set out in the general section.

Cor pulmonale

Definitions

Cor pulmonale (chronic) is right ventricular hypertrophy secondary to longstanding disease of the lung which affects its vascular resistance. Right ventricular malfunction secondary to LVF, or congenital or acquired heart disease is not included under the term cor pulmonale, even if the malfunction is due to the effects of heart disease on the lungs.

The conditions causing cor pulmonale can be divided into three:
• Disease affecting the pulmonary vessels—primary pulmonary hypertension, multiple pulmonary embolism (rare).

● Diseases affecting movements of rib cage and diaphragm, e.g. severe kyphoscoliosis, neuromuscular disorders.

● Diseases affecting lung parenchyma—chronic bronchitis and emphysema (commonest), chronic asthma (not rare), pulmonary fibrosis of many aetiologies (primary, sarcoidosis, pneumonitis, radiation etc., rare).

Acute cor pulmonale is a rarely used and rather ill defined term employed to describe a sudden change in right ventricular function secondary to an acute event in the pulmonary vasculature or airways which increases the impedance to pulmonary blood flow (e.g. large pulmonary embolus occluding a pulmonary artery, very severe asthma, acute bronchitis and pneumonia). Usually there is no evidence of previous right ventricular hypertrophy.

Right ventricular failure (RVF). In response to an increased afterload, the right ventricle changes from its normal crescent shape to being more ellipsoidal, and there is a long period of hypertrophic compensation before signs of RVF development. RVF is directly analagous to LVF. The right ventricle is unable to pump away the venous return without an increase in ventricular filling pressure, an increase in ventricular volume and a fall in the ejection fraction. Right ventricular function is severely compromised if there is a stiff interventricular septum secondary to previous infarction. RVF has several aetiologies, the commonest being secondary to LVF. When this occurs, in addition to a high right ventricular outflow impedance, there is often an element of functional tricuspid incompetence due to a stretched valve ring (see Fig. 1.14(c)). Both resolve when the LVF is treated. Other causes are end stage cor pulmonale, ischaemic heart disease, acquired valvular disease and congenital heart disease.

Pathophysiology of cor pulmonale

The normal pulmonary circulation is an elastic, low resistance, low pressure system. The increased pulmonary vascular resistance resulting in cor pulmonale may be due to anatomical or vasoconstrictor mechanisms, the latter having, at least theoretically, potential for pharmacological reversal.

The majority of cases of cor pulmonale result from chronic obstructive airways disease. Secondary to alveolar hypoventilation producing alveolar hypoxia, there is a generalized constriction of pulmonary arterioles and pre-capillary sphincters. If sustained over a period of years hypertrophy of the vascular smooth muscle occurs and with it an irreversible elevation of pulmonary vascular resistance. Acidosis (respiratory from a raised $PaCO_2$ or metabolic from tissue hypoxia) acts synergistically with alveolar hypoxia in intensifying the degree of vasoconstriction. By definition therefore, these patients are always hypoxic, usually are cyanosed, and frequently have secondary polycythaemia. Some rely on a hypoxic ventilatory drive and require care with the inspired oxygen concentration.

Right ventricular function is often inadequate to survive a superimposed acute chest infection, an episode of asthma or LVF.

Preoperative considerations

History

In cor pulmonale the history is dominated by the symptoms of the underlying chest disease (see Chapter 2). From the hypoxaemia (cyanosis) and low cardiac output there may be mental confusion. The peripheral oedema of RVF is usually mentioned spontaneously by the patient.

Examination

In cor pulmonale the picture is again predominantly that of chest disease. The patient is often breathless at rest with a prolonged expiration. There is usually central cyanosis, the hands and feet are warm and the pulse is of large volume due to peripheral vasodilatation. Cold peripheries are a bad sign, indicating a very low cardiac output. Because of lung tissue overlying the heart, the heart sounds are faint and the parasternal heave of right ventricular hypertrophy is not detected.

When RVF occurs, the JVP is elevated and peripheral oedema accumulates. There may be a third heart sound arising from the right ventricle.

Investigations

ECG. Surprisingly, the ECG can be normal despite right ventricular hypertrophy. In cor pulmonale, the transmission of electrical activity from the heart to the precordium is often affected by the presence of lung tissue overlying the heart. Classically, right ventricular hypertrophy is accompanied by marked right axis deviation (Fig. 1.9) with an increase in the voltage of the R wave ($>$ the S wave) in the right precordial leads (V_1, V_2). Repolarization of the right ventricle is disturbed and the T waves become inverted in V_1, V_2 and V_3. If there is accompanying right atrial hypertrophy, the P wave becomes tall and peaked (over 3 mm) in II, III and aVF (Fig. 1.38, p. 77).

CXR. This may show the evidence of lung disease. Pulmonary hypertension results in dilatation of the pulmonary artery and its main branches.

Preoperative treatment

The object of this is to reduce pulmonary vascular resistance by minimizing the effect of reversible components.

Treat a chest infection with antibiotics and physiotherapy. Carefully try to correct alveolar hypoxia by increasing the inspired oxygen concentration, always being aware of the possible onset of carbon dioxide narcosis. An increase in the PaO_2 to over 60 mmHg will reverse the majority of the pulmonary vasoconstriction possible in most patients. The ventilation may be stimulated by doxapram, the main effect of which is to reduce the respiratory acidosis. Bronchodilators, as well as dilating the airways, also relax vascular smooth muscle and can at times have a dramatic effect. Diuretics clear peripheral oedema and relieve any concomitant LVF. The use of digitalis and inotropes is controversial.

Anaesthetic management

The principles are outlined in the general section of this chapter and in Chapter 2, but the following points are relevant.
● With isolated right ventricular disease, lead II or V_2 may be better for monitoring because it is more likely to indicate right ventricular ischaemia than the CM5 lead.
● The complexity of monitoring required will reflect the severity of right heart disease and the magnitude of surgery. The worst operations are those with sudden changes in fluid load. The same principles of management apply as to left ventricular disease. The severely affected ventricle will be very sensitive to filling pressure (CVP) and afterload (pulmonary artery pressure) and these can both be monitored with a double or triple lumen pulmonary artery catheter. Not measuring the pulmonary artery pressure in a case of right ventricular disease is analagous to not measuring the systemic blood pressure in left ventricular disease.
● Compared with the effects of drugs on the peripheral circulation there is relatively little knowledge on the effects of anaesthetic agents and other drugs on pulmonary artery pressure and vascular resistance, but some general conclusions can be drawn.
● Histamine release causes both pulmonary vasoconstriction and bronchoconstriction.
● Good oxygenation and reduction of respiratory acidosis with IPPV (especially in presence of halothane) may relieve a reversible hypoxic vasoconstriction. Although this reduces pulmonary hypertension and allows an increased cardiac output it may cause a paradoxical fall in PaO_2 because of an increased virtual shunt.

48

• If inotropes are needed to maintain pulmonary artery flow, adrenaline and noradrenaline should be avoided because they increase pulmonary vascular resistance. Dopamine causes no change and dobutamine produces a slight fall in pulmonary vascular resistance.

• Right ventricular afterload can be effectively reduced by aminophylline, sodium nitroprusside (SNP), nitroglycerin, salbutamol and tolazoline.

● Nitrous oxide is regarded by many workers as being responsible for increases in pulmonary vascular resistance. Others claim that this effect can be reversed by volatile agents.

Cardiomyopathies

The definition of cardiomyopathy varies from author to author but one of the simplest is 'a primary disease of the myocardium *not* due to chest disease, hypertension, rheumatic, coronary or congenital heart disease'. It is normally subdivided into three types. All are rare in surgical patients.

Hypertrophic cardiomyopathy

This is caused by a specific abnormality of the myocardial cell which leads to progressive hypertrophy. On occasions the particular pattern of hypertrophy may lead to outflow obstruction (HOCM or hypertrophic obstructive cardiomyopathy). Consequently, the presentation and signs are variable and may mimic valve disease. Many cases are familial and it can be a cause of unexplained death in young adults.

Preoperative considerations

History

This is non-specific and includes angina, dyspnoea, syncope, and embolic episodes.

Examination

This may reveal signs of left or right ventricular hypertrophy or failure. Arrhythmias, a jerky arterial pulse and murmurs are all possible. The commonest valve lesions are aortic stenosis and mitral incompetence.

Investigations

ECG. This might be normal but may show changes of recognizable conduction defects or be bizarre.
CXR. An enlarged cardiac shadow may be seen.

Anaesthetic considerations

Physiology. The most serious complication is the development of ventricular outflow obstruction and it is important to be aware that this is not effectively fixed, as in rheumatic heart disease, but is dependent upon ventricular movement. A large ventricular end diastolic volume (EDV) distends the outflow tract and reduces the impedance to flow whereas a small EDV increases it. When there is an increased rate of rise of ventricular pressure (sympathomimetic drugs, increased sympathetic drive, tachycardia) the rapid septal contraction causes it to bulge more and further increase the obstruction. The obstruction may be so effective and the contraction so vigorous that the high ventricular pressure causes mitral incompetence.

As the disease progresses with increasingly poor myocardial function, the murmurs reduce in intensity, dysrhythmias occur and AF further reduces effective ventricular filling. The myocardial hypertrophy puts the patient at high risk of ischaemia, especially in the sub-endocardial region during ventricular contraction. Q waves on the ECG often indicate an old infarction but may purely represent septal hypertrophy.

Practical points

Many patients are now on beta-adrenoceptor blockers to reduce the heart rate and contractility, thereby reducing outflow obstruction. If AF occurs, digitalis is usually necessary but it may exacerbate the obstructive symptoms. All these patients are at risk from endocarditis and therefore need antibiotic prophylaxis.

As explained above, patients with this condition are very sensitive to small changes in ventricular volume, heart rate or blood pressure and to dysrhythmias, hypoxia and catecholamine secretion. Accordingly, at each stage of anaesthesia and in the perioperative period, care must be taken to minimize these changes, by application of the principles outlined earlier.

With HOCM, improved cardiac performance is produced by reducing the obstruction which, paradoxically, is achieved by reducing contractility (reduces the rate of rise of pressure), increasing the preload (increases EDV) and increasing the afterload (increases end systolic volume). These factors make <u>halothane</u>, beta-adrenoceptor blockers and vasoconstrictors the cornerstones of anaesthetic control.

Perioperative factors exacerbating the obstruction are preoperative anxiety, surgical stimuli, sympathomimetic drugs, low atrial pressures (hypovolaemia) and low arterial pressures (hypovolaemia, vasodilators). The drug of choice for correcting peripheral vasodilatation is <u>methoxamine</u> rather than ephedrine.

Congestive cardiomyopathy

This presents as congestive cardiac failure and is an 'exclusion diagnosis' when other diseases have been eliminated.

Although no aetiology is apparent in many cases, it is probably the end result of myocardial damage produced by a variety of toxins (alcohol, radiation, drugs and chemicals such as cobalt and phenothiazines), metabolic disorders (thiamine deficiency), infections (influenza A_2, coxsackie B, toxoplasma, diphtheria) and infiltrations (sarcoidosis, amyloid, malignancy, haemochromatosis) as well as connective tissue disorders.

Symptoms and signs are those of left and right sided systolic pump failure. The prognosis is poor, especially over the age of 55 years.

Management is as for right and left ventricular diseases as outlined above. Ventricular arrhythmias are particularly common and varying degrees of heart block are unpredictable in both onset and severity.

Obliterative or restrictive cardiomyopathy

This is very, very rare and results from fibrosis or infiltrations creating a stiff, inelastic, non contractile heart.

Hypertension

Physiology

There is no population of hypertensives. The distribution of blood pressure readings is not bimodal but is skewed towards higher values. As there is no actual division separating normality from abnormality the definition is arbitrary.

It is well established that with essential hypertension, patients have <u>cardiac outputs similar to normotensives</u>. Their increased blood pressure is therefore caused by differences in <u>vascular resistance</u>.

These are twofold. Firstly, the basic hypertensive lesion is a thickening of the arteriolar walls to such an extent that the luminar diameter is reduced, thereby increasing systemic vascular resistance (SVR). This also makes their SVR much more variable and sensitive to sympathetic stimulation, and produces a high diastolic pressure because it is 'harder' for the blood in the major arteries to 'run off' peripherally during diastole. Secondly, decreased vascular distensibility secondary to vessel wall degeneration causes an abrupt increase in aortic input impedance. This predominantly increases the systolic pressure.

Clinical features

About 20% of the caucasian adult population in Britain have blood pressures above 160/95 as measured by the Korotkoff sounds. Of these, approximately 10% have a specific aetiological factor of:
- Renal disease (chronic glomerular nephritis, chronic pyelonephritis, diabetic nephropathy, renal artery stenosis, polycystic kidney disease, polyarteritis nodosa)
- Endocrine disease (Cushing's syndrome, Conn's syndrome, phaeochromocytoma, acromegaly)
- Pregnancy (eclampsia, pre eclampsia, contraceptive pill)

or
- Coarctation of the aorta.

The patients are often symptom free. Only half have been previously diagnosed and less than half of these are on appropriate, regular treatment. When a patient does present with symptoms it indicates the presence of end organ involvement in the nervous system, heart or kidneys. Hypertension is the most significant risk factor in strokes and is as important as smoking in the aetiology of coronary artery disease. The complications of hypertension are:
- LVF.
- Strokes and hypertensive encephalopathy.
- Renal failure.
- Myocardial infarction and ischaemia.
- Retinopathy.
- Complications of treatment (postural hypotension, hypokalaemia).

The decision as to who and when to treat is constantly discussed. There seems total agreement that diastolic pressures over 100 mmHg in men and women who are under 65 years old need treatment. Below this level and above this age there is debate and personal preference but there is an increasing trend in the young for treatment to be initiated at lower levels.

After treatment, the mortality and incidence of strokes and uraemia is greatly decreased but there is a much less dramatic effect on the incidence of myocardial infarction.

Anaesthetic implications

Because so much hypertensive disease is asymptomatic, it is essential that *all* patients have their BP measured prior to anaesthesia. The question is, what if it is elevated? The only answer to this can be given in terms of guidelines: individual anaesthetists will almost certainly differ in their management of specific cases.

Considerable evidence now exists that with diastolic blood pressures of up to 110 mmHg, painstaking perioperative monitoring and precise pharmacological control of the blood pressure are probably more important than preoperative antihypertensive therapy in terms of decreasing cardiovascular complications. (The only exception to this is surgery for carotid endarterectomy.) The ideal treatment of patients with diastolic blood pressures above 110 mmHg is still the subject of some debate.

Reasonable recommendations would appear to be:

- All non-urgent cases with diastolic blood pressures over 110 mmHg should be referred for investigation and treatment.
- All non-urgent cases with diastolics up to 110 mmHg are probably acceptable, provided that there is nothing abnormal in the history (especially episodic states suggestive of phaeochromocytoma) and careful clinical examination reveals no evidence of end organ damage (especially no signs of LVF) or pregnancy (don't forget this!). In addition, the following should be normal:
- ECG (no evidence of LVH, conduction abnormalities or dysrhythmias)
- CXR (no evidence of entricular dilatation)
- FBC (no evidence of polycythaemia)
- U & E's (no evidence of renal/endocrine involvement)
- Serum glucose (not diabetic)
If there are any positive findings then the patient should be referred for investigations and treatment.
- With urgent cases, no choice is available to the anaesthetist. The only indications for a rapid reduction of blood pressure (over a period of less than one hour) are encephalopathy, acute LVF and very severe pre-eclampsia or eclampsia. Otherwise, the dangers of rapid BP reduction (blindness and cerebral episodes) are not outweighed by the benefits.

Whether or not to start antihypertensive therapy between the preoperative visit and surgery is another question with no universal answer. The prescription of an oral beta-adrenoceptor blocker is ideal for some patients, producing a modest fall in blood pressure and attenuating the hypertensive response to laryngoscopy. It is completely contraindicated in others (patients with heart failure, asthma or evidence of a conduction defect). Any treatment, if prescribed, must be logical and tailored to the individual patient.

The specific problems of a hypertensive patient are itemized below and to deal with them logically requires frequent, accurate readings of their systolic and diastolic blood pressures. This implies that for all but the very well controlled mild or moderate hypertensive undergoing minor surgery, an intra arterial pressure monitoring line is only in the patient's best interests and can prevent cardiovascular disasters. For maximum benefit, it should be placed before induction and left in position during recovery.

The approach to hypertensive episodes during and following surgery should follow logical steps (see also Table 1.4). Firstly, check that anaesthesia is not too light, that there is no hypoxia or hypercarbia and that the patient is not overtransfused. If pharmacological intervention is indicated the diastolic pressure and heart rate may influence the choice of agent. In diastolic hypertension, incremental hydralazine or infusions of diazoxide or SNP may be useful. Provided there is no evidence of conduction defects, systolic hypertension with tachycardia may be controlled by halothane or beta-adrenoceptor blockade. Alternatively, combined alpha and beta-adrenoceptor blockade (labetalol) by infusion can achieve both objectives.

The problems specific to hypertensive patients are:
• There is a greater fall in blood pressure after a normal dose of induction agent than in a normotensive patient.
• There is an exaggerated response to laryngoscopy and surgical stimulation resulting in hypertension, tachycardias, dysrhythmias and myocardial ischaemia.
• High left ventricular pressures and tachycardias can produce sub-endocardial ischaemia. This highlights the importance of continuous ECG and arterial pressure monitoring during induction.
• Patients receiving antihypertensive therapy which depletes nor-adrenaline storage in sympathetic nerve endings (e.g. guanethidine, bethanidine, debrisoquine) are very sensitive to exogenous catecholamines or direct beta-adrenoceptor stimulants.
• The commonest spontaneous dysrhythmia is the conversion from sinus to junctional rhythm (Fig. 1.24) often with an associated abrupt hypotension. This may occur more easily in the presence of hypercapnia and volatile agents.
• Atropine may cause a tachycardia leading to ischaemia. It may be

preferable to use glycopyrrolate when reversing neuromuscular blockade.

● The recovery period is very important to the hypertensive patient because the blood pressure can suddenly reach dangerously high levels. Such postoperative hypertension is more common in patients who have a previous history of severe hypertension, regardless of whether the arterial pressure was under control prior to anaesthesia. Thus, the BP needs to be monitored closely as the patient becomes more aware and pain is experienced. Firstly, if appropriate, give analgesia before embarking on vasoactive drugs.

Dysrhythmias, conduction defects and pacemakers

Dysrhythmias

CC

NB Lead V₁

all R′ with

post. MI (STA)

WPW

R heart strain,
  PE

Patients can either already have dysrhythmias preoperatively or develop them *de novo* in the perioperative period. It is important *always* to think of causes other than intrinsic cardiac malfunction since the proper treatment may not be the injection of an anti-dysrhythmic agent but the correction of a basic defect in anaesthesia. Non-cardiac anaesthetic problems which produce dysrhythmias are *hypoxia, hypercarbia,* acidosis, hypertension, hypotension, central venous, ventricular and pulmonary artery catheters, electrolyte imbalance, high levels of endogenous or exogenous catecholamines, high concentrations of volatile agents (especially halothane), and stimulating procedures (laryngoscopy, pulling on viscera etc) in the presence of light anaesthesia. Hypoxia secondary to a pneumothorax is easily overlooked until well advanced. Consequently, when a dysrhythmia arises always check the *oxygen* supply, the patient's colour, adequacy of ventilation, the concentration of volatile agents and any changes in central venous or PA readings first. It takes only a few seconds and may be life-saving.

SINUS TACHYCARDIA

The normal heart rate varies from 120 beats/minute in infancy to 70–80 beats/minute in adults (40–50 beats/minute taking trained athletes into account). Sinus tachycardia is a normal physiological event in exercise, anxiety and light anaesthesia and is frequently present in the postoperative period. It occurs as a compensatory mechanism in shock, anaemia and cardiac failure and as a toxic side effect in thyrotoxicosis and after several drugs (e.g. atropine, gallamine, ephedrine). It is only important clinically when it results in myocardial ischaemia, and the treatment should first be that of the underlying cause (e.g. deeper anaesthesia, give fluids etc) and then recourse to beta-adrenoceptor blockade. Never reduce a physiological tachycardia which is necessary for the maintenance of oxygen flux just for the sake of treating numbers. It is, however, sometimes necessary (say in severe anaemia) to reduce the heart rate to 100 beats/minute or less when reduced diastolic filling, prejudiced by a fast rate, is causing myocardial ischaemia.

Bear in the back of your mind that onset of unexplained tachycardia during surgery could be malignant hyperpyrexia.

SINUS ARRHYTHMIA

This is a normal finding in children and teenagers. Via baroreceptor control the heart rate increases during inspiration and decreases during expiration. It is markedly attenuated during all forms of general anaesthesia.

SINUS BRADYCARDIA

This is found in many healthy patients, (particularly trained athletes) but also in hypothyroidism, hypothermia and with raised intracranial pressure. When a bradycardia develops *de novo* it is often due to excessive vagal stimulation and may resolve on stopping the stimulus (e.g. carotid sinus stimulation in carotid surgery or oculocardiac reflex in eye surgery). Although the prolonged diastole which accompanies a bradycardia aids coronary perfusion, coronary blood flow still depends upon an adequate filling pressure in the aortic sinus. This in turn demands that the ventricle must be able to compensate for a reduction in rate by an increase in stroke volume. Although easy for a healthy ventricle, this may be impossible for one which is close to failure or which has been previously infarcted. Under these conditions, it is likely that a bradycardia (usually below 50 beats/minute) will result in systemic hypotension and poor coronary filling that may be sufficient to demonstrate ischaemia on the ECG. The treatment is small, incremental doses of atropine (0.1 mg steps) to return the rate to normal without overshooting to a tachycardia (unless the bradycardia occurs during carotid endarterectomy when lignocaine on the carotid sinus is the treatment of choice).

The other effect of a lengthened diastole is that it allows more time for the prepotential of automatic cells to drift (phase 4, Fig. 1.11) and reach the threshold potential thus producing ectopic activity, most frequently from a ventricular focus. Factors increasing the rate of rise of the intracellular prepotential include hypercarbia, hypoxia, catecholamines, other sympathomimetic drugs, hyperthermia and hypokalaemia. The effect of all of these is intensified with halothane.

If significant ventricular ectopic activity occurs during anaesthesia, *always* check the adequacy of ventilation (see above) and make the necessary correction. Having excluded faulty anaesthesia then treatment is again to use small doses of atropine to increase the rate. This merely shortens diastole and prevents ectopic foci from reaching their threshold potential ("pacing them out"). If this is unsuccessful and the dysrhythmia is severely affecting cardiac performance, lignocaine is the standard treatment (see 'ventricular ectopic beats').

ATRIAL ECTOPICS

These arise from a focus in the atria other than the S-A node and can be precipitated by emotion, coffee, tea and tobacco. The beat is premature, most frequently with a differently shaped P wave and altered P-R interval (Fig. 1.19). Usually the QRS complex is normal but very rarely aberrant conduction can widen the QRS complex, mimicking both left and right bundle branch block. Atrial ectopic beats predominantly occur in normal patients and do not require treatment or pose an anaesthetic hazard.

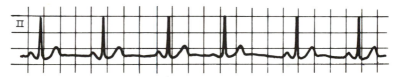

Fig. 1.19. The fourth beat is premature, preceded by an abnormal P wave and followed by a compensatory pause.

Their only significance is in patients prone to atrial tachydysrhythmias in whom they may herald the onset of an attack. They can usually be 'paced out' by atropine or the excitability of atrial tissue can be reduced by beta-adrenoceptor blockade.

WANDERING PACEMAKER

This disturbance is a form of severe atrial ectopic behaviour in which in addition to impulses from the S-A node, there are many others which originate from various foci in the atrium. As a result there is a variation in rhythm, a changing P wave shape and a changing P-R interval. The abnormalities sometimes occur in runs and a rhythm strip may be required for the presence of other pacemakers to be seen. The QRS is usually normal (apart from rare aberrant conduction as above). This dysrhythmia may occur in normal individuals but also is not uncommon following myocardial infarction, digitalis therapy and during myocarditis (especially rheumatic fever) in whom the real anaesthetic risks are those of the underlying condition.

There is little anaesthetic literature on the risks of the condition *per se* but they would appear to be very low and similar to those in the patient with atrial ectopics.

SINUS PAUSE

The term 'sinus pause' is relatively new and describes the failure of the atrium to depolarize at the expected time in a patient who is in sinus rhythm (Fig. 1.20). Two different mechanisms may initiate it. In Fig. 1.20, if y is a whole number multiple of x, then it is assumed that the S-A node is still firing but that its effect is not transmitted throughout the atrium. This is termed sinoatrial block. If there is no precise relationship between x and y, then it is assumed that the S-A node has simply ceased automatic activity, and the condition is called sinus arrest. Much debate currently exists about the exact separation, if any, of these two conditions. If the pause is sufficiently long a subsidiary pacemaker emerges (hopefully!).

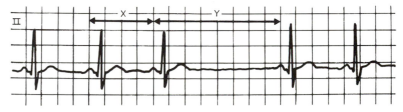

Fig. 1.20. Sinus pause. See text.

Sinus pauses can be associated with excessive vagal tone, ischaemic heart disease, digoxin, propranolol, ageing (fibrous replacement) or be a normal variant. Whether a finding is physiological or pathological is often difficult to know. It may herald the appearance of the sick sinus syndrome (see below).

From the anaesthetist's viewpoint a healthy S-A node is one which will increase the atrial rate in response to exercise or atropine, and does not allow pauses of more than 1.5 seconds on the ECG. The S-A node should be considered pathological when the pauses are recurrent, cause cerebral symptoms, co-exist with other evidence of cardiac disease or are in excess of 2.0 seconds on the ECG. Poor S-A node function may prevent a physiological tachycardia, remove the atrial contribution to ventricular filling and allow a subsidiary, slower pacemaker to emerge with a limitation on cardiac output. These cases should be treated as in sick sinus syndrome (see below).

THE SICK SINUS SYNDROME

The sick sinus syndrome is a disease of the S-A node that results in unpredictable sinus pauses (see above) and inappropriate bradycardias which at times alternate with tachycardias. It is being increasingly diagnosed in the elderly, often as a result of syncopal attacks or palpitations being investigated by a 24 hour ECG monitor. It may or may not be associated with almost any form of heart disease. Whether it is caused by the accompanying disease, or is a separate entity is not always clear. Many patients are asymptomatic, and it should be suspected in any elderly patient with an unexplained sinus bradycardia, particularly if direct questioning reveals evidence of cerebral symptoms. Frequently the bradycardia (caused by degenerative changes in S-A node) is complicated by episodes of supraventricular tachycardia (SVT). Cardiologists normally only treat the condition when it is symptomatic. When they do, a pacemaker is used to control the bradycardia and superimposed upon this are digoxin and beta-adrenoceptor blockers to suppress the tachydysrhythmias. The bradycardia may be refractory to atropine because of the disease of the S-A node.

The anaesthetic implications of pacemakers are outlined later in this chapter. The anaesthetic risk for an unpaced patient, in addition to the risks of any other underlying condition, is not known. A sensible approach is to use an anaesthetic technique which has little effect on cardiac conduction and excitability. The locality of equipment and personnel for pacing must be known. A wide bore central venous cannula *in situ* hastens emergency insertion of a temporary wire.

One unexplained feature of these patients is their propensity to pulmonary embolism so perioperative anticoagulation (if they are not chronically anticoagulated) is probably sensible. Those maintained on warfarin should be treated as described in 'mitral stenosis'.

PAROXYSMAL ATRIAL TACHYCARDIA (PAT)

PAT results from the pacemaking function of the S-A node being replaced by a focus somewhere else in the atria which discharges rapidly at a rate of 130–200 beats/minute. Conduction at the A-V node and beyond is usually normal so the QRS complex is unaffected (Fig. 1.21). In a small proportion of cases there is aberrant conduction. Each QRS is preceded by a P wave which at rates greater than 150 beats/minute is usually lost in the previous T wave.

60% of patients have no evidence of underlying heart disease. In others, it is associated with thyrotoxicosis, tobacco, caffeine,

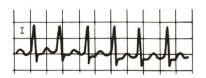

Fig. 1.21. Paroxysmal atrial tachycardia. Rate = 175 beats per minute. P waves not visible.

rheumatic mitral valve disease, coronary artery disease and the Wolff–Parkinson–White syndrome. The tachycardia starts and ends suddenly and may last any time from seconds to days. It may precipitate angina, cardiac failure, dizziness and syncope.

Initial treatment is by unilateral carotid sinus massage or the valsalva manoeuvre. Effective drugs for the acute state are practolol *or* verapamil but if refractory, direct current (DC) countershock is usually effective. Always check the serum electrolytes as a contributory cause. Patients who have recurrences are often maintained on digoxin.

If possible, PAT should always be controlled prior to anaesthesia. Underlying causes should always be suspected and treated appropriately. Refractory patients requiring urgent surgery can receive DC countershock in the presence of a cardiologist immediately after induction.

ATRIAL FLUTTER

In atrial flutter the atria are stimulated rapidly and regularly 250–400 times per minute by an ectopic atrial pacemaker. The A-V node cannot conduct at this rate and there is a varying degree of A-V block, most commonly either 2:1 or 4:1. The ECG has characteristic flutter waves interspersed with normal QRS complexes (Fig. 1.22).

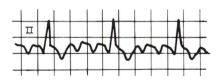

Fig. 1.22. Atrial flutter with 4:1 A–V block. When identifying flutter waves it is important to remember those coinciding with the QRS complexes and T waves.

Over 90% of cases have a basic underlying cardiac defect (rheumatic or ischaemic heart disease or atrial septal defect). Less commonly, it is associated with thyrotoxicosis, trauma to the myocardium, myocarditis and digoxin therapy. These should be excluded before surgery. Most patients find the dysrhythmia very uncomfortable and cardiac failure or angina are commonly precipitated early. Chronic control is by digoxin, verapamil or beta-adrenoceptor blockers. DC countershock is almost always effective in abolishing atrial flutter, and is the acute treatment of choice. This can be done at the induction of urgent surgery.

ATRIAL FIBRILLATION (AF)

In atrial fibrillation small areas of the atrial muscle are stimulated at different times and there is no co-ordinated contraction (Fig. 1.23). The atrial contribution to ventricular filling is lost. The ventricular rhythm is totally irregular because the majority of stimuli reaching the A-V node are either too weak to stimulate it or arrive in the refractory period. The ventricular rate is usually rapid and can precipitate angina and cardiac failure. Rarely, AF occurs as a congenital abnormality but *the majority have underlying heart disease*. Common associations are rheumatic mitral valve disease, ischaemic heart disease and thyrotoxicosis. The latter must be excluded in the elderly. Less common, acute causes of AF are pulmonary infections and infarctions, cardiothoracic surgery, cardiac trauma and myocarditis. Two important factors affecting the onset of AF are advancing age and the presence of a large atrium. On exercise, the ventricular rate increases but the cardiac output does not and this can cause distress and possible myocardial ischaemia.

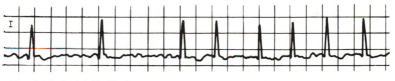

Fig. 1.23. Atrial fibrillation.

If a patient presents for surgery with AF of recent onset (it may be the cause of the admission, e.g. mesenteric infarct), any underlying condition should be elucidated and cardiological advice taken as to the wisdom of reversal of AF. It carries a high risk of embolization, and if the AF is likely to become permanent, is probably a useless manoeuvre.

Digoxin (see earlier) given IV has its onset of action at 30 minutes and peak effect at approximately 4 hours so it is only very rarely that ouabain (onset of action 10 minutes) is required for rapid drug control. Most patients presenting for surgery with chronic AF will be on digitalis (look for, and prevent, hypokalaemia).

These patients are very sensitive to changes in right and left atrial pressures because they have no atrial contractile contribution to ventricular filling and depend upon the hydrostatic pressure in the atria to fill the ventricles.

Consequently, for major surgery or where large or sudden changes in circulating blood volume are anticipated, the use of central venous and possibly PA catheters should be considered. A loading test (see earlier) prior to surgery can provide useful information about the patient's response to atrial pressure changes.

JUNCTIONAL (NODAL) RHYTHM

This is caused by an ectopic pacemaker situated close to and either above or below the A-V node. The P wave, representing atrial contraction, is therefore produced by abnormal conduction which may be retrograde. This causes the temporal relationship between atrial and ventricular contraction to be upset. Two effects follow: the P wave can precede, follow or be buried in the QRS (Fig. 1.24) and there is a diminished or absent atrial contribution to ventricular filling. Transient and permanent nodal rhythm can be found in normal people. More frequently, it follows myocardial infarction and is associated with the wide range of other organic heart diseases which produce atrial dysrhythmias. Junctional rhythm is probably the commonest dysrhythmia seen during anaesthesia and is particularly associated with halothane.

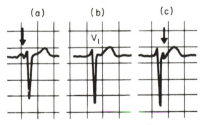

Fig. 1.24. Junctional beats. The P waves (arrowed) may precede (a). coincide with (b), or follow (c), the QRS complex.

It only needs treatment when affecting the cardiac output. With rapid rates, it may be difficult to differentiate it from PAT but both can be treated in a similar manner. If the rate is very slow, treat with atropine. During anaesthesia, in people with borderline myocardial function, the onset of junctional rhythm can cause sudden hypotension because of a reduced ejection volume. The best treatment is to remove the cause (usually halothane). If there is no response, calcium salts (calcium gluconate 250–500 mg) improve conduction and do not risk the tachycardia so often seen with atropine. Treatment is not always successful.

VENTRICULAR ECTOPIC BEATS

Ventricular ectopic beats (VE's) arise because the prepotential (see sinus bradycardia) of some automatic cells in the ventricle reaches threshold potential before the next sinus beat (phase 4, Fig. 1.11). Hence they are not preceded by a P wave. When the sinus beat does arrive, it finds the ventricles in a refractory state so there is a compensatory pause until the next one arrives. Other features are a wide and bizarre QRS complex and abnormal S-T segment and T wave (Fig. 1.25). They can occur (up to 6/minute) in normal people.

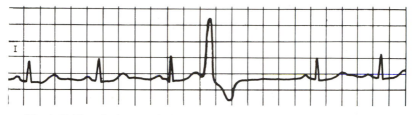

Fig. 1.25. Ventricular ectopic beat.

More than any other dysrhythmia these may be caused by faulty anaesthetic technique as outlined under 'sinus bradycardia' (p. 56). These factors should be corrected.

VE's can, however, represent underlying myocardial disease (especially after myocardial infarction) and the danger in these patients is the progression to ventricular tachycardia (VT) or ventricular fibrillation (VF). Coupled VE's are most commonly secondary to digitalis toxicity which in the perioperative period may be precipitated by hypokalaemia. Traditional criteria for treatment of VE's are if they are more than 6/minute, multifocal, occur in runs of 3 or more or show the R on T phenomenon (ectopic beat near the vulnerable period which can precipitate VF). A large body of cardiological opinion is now moving away from early treatment (especially after myocardial infarction) provided that emergency defibrillation equipment is available.

If treatment is commenced, then the standard regimen is IV lignocaine (1–1.5 mg/kg as a bolus followed by an infusion of 2–4 mg/minute).

VENTRICULAR TACHYCARDIA

Ventricular tachycardia (VT) is always life-threatening and in anaesthetic practice can be caused by anything creating ventricular ectopic behaviour. Always monitor the ECG after infiltration with adrenaline in case VT is precipitated. It is commonly associated with severe ischaemic heart disease. The pulse rate is regular and rapid (130–200/minute) leading to myocardial ischaemia and heart failure. The ECG (Fig. 1.26) can be difficult to differentiate from PAT with aberrant conduction. DC countershock is very effective but many episodes respond to IV lignocaine (1–1.5 mg/kg as a bolus followed by an infusion of 2–4 mg/minute).

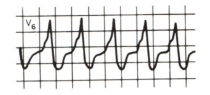

Fig. 1.26. Ventricular tachycardia. Rate = 150 beats per minute.

Conduction defects

ATRIO-VENTRICULAR BLOCK

First degree block

This is an electrocardiographic definition when the P-R interval is found to be above the upper limit of normal (0.2 seconds). It commonly occurs in the <u>absence of any organic heart disease</u> and implies a disturbance of conduction between the S-A and A-V nodes or a delay in conduction through the A-V node. It can also be caused by increased vagal tone, halothane, digitalis, ischaemia of the A-V node, almost all infective diseases, cardiomyopathy and congenital heart disease. It is of no functional significance *per se*, its importance being that of any underlying disease. If the prolonged P-R interval is due to excessive vagal tone and associated with a bradycardia, it responds to atropine.

Second degree block

Clinically, this may at times be mistaken for virtually any dysrhythmia and its diagnosis is electrocardiographic. It is a failure of some, but not all, atrial impulses to reach the ventricles because of impaired conduction. The lesion may be in the A-V node, junctional tissue, the bundle of His, or the bundle branches. When found preoperatively, the underlyng cause should be identified and, when possible, treated appropriately.

The classification of second degree block differs slightly in detail from book to book. We have described below what we think is the most logical.

• *Mobitz type I block* (Wenkebach) has a progressive lengthening of the P-R interval until there is a total failure of conduction. Then the whole cycle repeats (Fig. 1.27). Type I block is usually caused by disease of the A-V node (Fig. 1.5) but rarely, on occasions, results from conduction defects in the bundle of His or the bundle branches. When of nodal origin, it is benign and only very infrequently progresses to third degree block. When it does, a reliable high order pacemaker emerges to provide adequate ventricular rates.

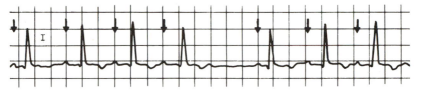

Fig. 1.27. Mobitz type I (Wenckebach) block. The P waves are arrowed.

• *Mobitz type II block* is less common than type I, but carries a much graver significance. It is characterized by a sudden failure of A-V conduction without previous lengthening of the P-R interval (Fig. 1.28). The majority of cases have widespread disease (fibrosis or infarction) of the bundle branches or fascicles (Fig. 1.5) so that if third degree block supervenes a slow, unreliable, low order ventricular pacemaker emerges. A small minority have a relatively well defined lesion in the bundle of His.

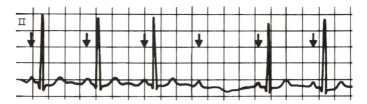

Fig. 1.28. Mobitz type II block. The P waves are arrowed.

• *'Advanced' or 'high grade' block* are terms used to describe second degree heart block with the presence of a 2:1 or greater incidence of A-V conduction failure (Fig. 1.29). In this example, because there is only one P-R interval to be examined it is impossible to classify it as Mobitz type I or type II. In the majority of cases the underlying pathology is widespread disease of the bundles and fascicles (Mobitz type II) and it frequently progresses to total block.

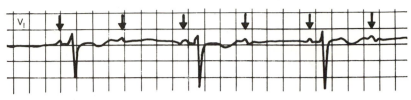

Fig. 1.29. High grade or advanced block (2:1). The P waves are arrowed.

To our knowledge, no anaesthetic literature is available which describes the effect of anaesthesia on second degree heart block. The worry is the progression to third degree block intra or postoperatively. It is sensible to:

- test the effect of atropine prior to anaesthesia;
- have an isoprenaline infusion ready;
- know the whereabouts of pacing personnel and facilities. A wide bore central venous cannula *in situ* hastens the emergency insertion of a temporary wire;
- avoid drugs known to produce or intensify A-V conduction defects (especially halothane);
- avoid periods of postoperative hypoxia, because this may intensify the block.

Third degree block

All the atrial impulses are blocked in the conducting system and the ventricular rate is controlled by a subsidiary pacemaker somewhere below the block, either in the A-V node or automatic tissue of the ventricles (Fig. 1.30). When atrial and ventricular contractions coincide there are jugular 'cannon' waves (Table 1.2). The most frequent causes in adults are fibrosis of the conducting tissue and infarction of the interventricular septum. The latter is ominous in that it indicates a wide area of damage.

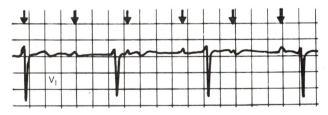

Fig. 1.30. Total (third degree) heart block. The P waves are arrowed.

When the ventricular pacemaker is near the A-V node, the heart rate is 40–55/minute with a normal width QRS complex. When the pacemaker is distant to the A-V node, the heart rate is 30–40/minute with a wide QRS.

Many patients are symptomatic with syncopal attacks, myocardial ischaemia or cardiac failure. They should have a pacemaker implanted before elective surgery. Emergency pacing may be necessary in urgent cases. The same perioperative precautions should be taken as for second degree block.

Very rarely, complete heart block is congenital in origin (1 in 20 000 live births) and one third of these have other congenital cardiac defects. Its effect on the patient is very variable. Some require pacing as children, others are able to increase their cardiac output on exercise well into adult life. As the patients age, more and more need a pacemaker.

VENTRICULAR CONDUCTION DEFECTS

The ventricular conducting system is shown in Fig. 1.5. Many texts subclassify bundle branch blocks into complete and incomplete, the latter having a normal width QRS and a less florid pattern disturbance. The distinction is arbitrary and indicates little about the potential severity of the abnormality.

Right bundle branch block (RBBB)

There is a failure of conduction of the right bundle branch (Fig. 1.5) proximally. Right ventricular depolarization is delayed because the distal right bundle branch fibres have to wait to be triggered by slow impulses passing through the septal myocardium. This results in a wide (>0.12 second) QRS complex with an RSR' pattern in leads V_1 to V_3 (Fig. 1.31). Often the T wave is inverted in all these leads but right axis deviation (Fig. 1.9) is usually only present when there is co-existing right ventricular hypertrophy.

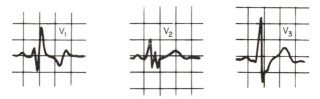

Fig. 1.31. Right bundle branch block.

Because RBBB has little effect on the lateral chest leads it is still possible to diagnose left ventricular hypertrophy and myocardial ischaemia and infarction (Fig. 1.18, p. 43) from a 12 lead ECG or a CM_5 lead.

It is a finding without underlying cause in what is variously estimated to be 1–15% of the normal adult population. Other causes are hypertensive disease, coronary artery disease, pulmonary embolism, all the causes of right ventricular hypertrophy and strain and congenital lesions, particularly those involving the septum. The treatment and prognosis is that of the underlying condition. As an isolated finding, it poses little anaesthetic risk.

Left bundle branch block (LBBB)

There is a failure of conduction of the left bundle branch (Fig. 1.5) and all impulses must pass down the right bundle branch. Septal depolarization is reversed, and the mass of the left ventricle depolarizes late and abnormally. This results in a wide (>0.12 second) QRS complex with a notched or M shape in leads V_4 to V_6 (Fig. 1.32). Abnormal left axis deviation is not a routine feature of LBBB. Because of the bizarre routes of depolarization and repolarization no further diagnostic information can be gained from examination of the QRS complex, S-T segment or T wave.

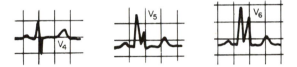

Fig. 1.32. Left bundle branch block.

It occurs almost always as a result of underlying heart disease of many types and *is almost never a normal variant*. It is associated with hypertension, coronary artery disease, cardiomyopathy, congenital lesions involving the septum, and valve disease. The anaesthetic management is that of the underlying condition and avoiding the induction of RBBB. This implies care in the passage of a PA catheter if it is indicated for major surgery. (Fig. 1.15) and taking similar precautions to those listed for 'second degree heart block' (p. 64).

Hemiblock

The left bundle branch is composed of anterior and posterior divisions (Fig. 1.5) and if only one of them is damaged, the electrical impulse passes in an abnormal manner throughout the left ventricle but the conduction is rapid. This causes an alteration in the cardiac axis but does *not* prolong the duration of the QRS.

Left anterior hemiblock causes left axis deviation and can be diagnosed if the QRS deflection is predominantly negative in lead II (Fig. 1.8) and there are no other causes of left axis deviation present (p. 14). It is by far the commonest form of hemiblock.

The posterior fascicle is more resistant to ischaemia because it is supplied by both the right and left coronary arteries. Hence, left posterior hemiblock is uncommon. It is manifested on the ECG only as mild right axis deviation (Fig. 1.34). It often appears as the upper limit of normal and is undiagnosable with right ventricular hypertrophy or after myocardial infarction.

Bifascicular blocks

These blocks are dangerous and imply that only a single conducting Channel is available to the ventricles and hence there is a high danger of total heart block.

RBBB and left anterior hemiblock is the commonest combination. It is relatively stable, only 5% of patients per year progressing to total block. It produces a broad RSR′ in V_{1-3} with left axis deviation in the frontal plane (Fig. 1.33).

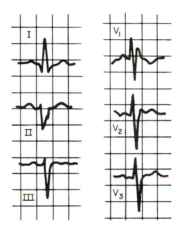

Fig. 1.33. Left anterior hemiblock with right bundle branch block.

RBBB and left posterior hemiblock is uncommon and difficult to diagnose. It is potentially more likely to progress to total heart block. It produces a RBBB pattern together with mild right axis deviation in the absence of right ventricular hypertrophy or myocardial infarction (Fig. 1.34). Compare the axis deviation in Fig. 1.34 with that normally regarded as significant in Fig. 1.9.

The optimum perioperative management of bifascicular block is both controversial and patient dependent. The major concern is the onset of total block. A reasonable approach is probably as follows. If the patient has symptoms suggesting intermittent trifascicular block (fainting episodes, absences etc.), seek the advice of a cardiologist as to the wisdom of pacing. The asymptomatic patient can be anaes-

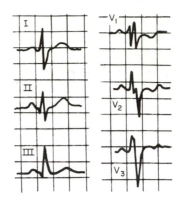

Fig. 1.34. Left posterior hemiblock with right bundle branch block.

thetized as outlined in the general section with precautions taken similar to those described for second degree heart block.

Great care is needed in the postoperative period where hypoxia may produce myocardial ischaemia and intensify the block. Patients must be monitored postoperatively in a high dependency unit.

Intermittent blocks

Various states of intermittent right and left bundle branch and hemiblocks have been described. They have occurred in association with tachycardias, hypertension, hypotension, ischaemia, hypoxia and large tidal volumes. They will be minimized by careful anaesthesia and postoperative care.

WOLFF–PARKINSON–WHITE SYNDROME

This is the commonest of the accelerated conduction syndromes with an incidence in the population of up to 0.5%. It is usually seen in individuals who show no evidence of other organic disease but occasionally it can be secondary to ischaemia of the A-V node or myocarditis. In the otherwise normal individual, it does not alter life expectancy.

The cardiac impulse travels simultaneously down the normal conduction pathway and other anomalous fibres (the bundle of Kent bypasses the A-V node). This results in a characteristically short P-R interval, wide QRS complex and an abnormally slurred upstroke (delta wave) of the R wave (Fig. 1.35).

These individuals are prone to attacks of atrial dysrhythmias, usually paroxysmal atrial tachycardia and, less frequently, atrial flutter and fibrillation.

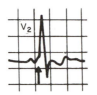

Fig. 1.35. Wolff–Parkinson–White Syndrome. The delta wave is arrowed.

Epicardial mapping can further define the anomalous pathways which can then be transected. If this is in the septum it may produce complete block.

Medical management is now predominantly with beta-adrenoceptor blockers and these should be continued to the time of surgery. Both atropine and digitalis can precipitate and intensify the dysrhythmia, as can emotional excitement.

During anaesthesia, facilities for cardioversion should be available. Light anaesthesia, catecholamines or preoperative nervousness can all produce an attack. Hence give a generous anxiolytic premedication and continue monitoring postoperatively.

Pacemakers

Pacemakers are devices which ensure that the heart beats sufficient times per minute, irrespective of the intrinsic rhythmic activity. They are inserted for different types of conduction deficit and usually only when a patient is symptomatic. Perioperative indications are discussed under individual conditions. The criteria for insertion are continuously under review by cardiologists.

Temporary pacing wires normally use the transvenous endocardial approach and rest in the right ventricle. There are some needle electrodes which can be inserted into the myocardium via the chest wall but these are for emergency use only, as in cardiac arrests. Oesophageal pacing is also possible.

Permanent pacemakers are most frequently inserted by cardiologists under local anaesthesia. The pacing wire passes via the subclavian vein and tricuspid valve to the right ventricle where it is anchored in the trabeculae by some sort of hook. A subcutaneous pocket over or close to pectoralis major is constructed for the 'pacemaker box'. They are powered by various types of battery (including nuclear devices) and the power unit can usually be felt like a 'bar of soap' beneath the skin.

Less commonly permanent pacemakers are implanted into the epicardial surface of the heart either via an epigastric incision or mini-thoracotomy. The power unit is then placed in the rectus sheath. This approach may be preferred in children as it is easy to coil up an extra length of lead to allow for growth.

The main functional division of types is between 3 modes of operation.

• *Fixed-rate* (asynchronous). These produce a fixed frequency stimulus and have the advantage of simplicity. Their rate can sometimes be altered by the use of an external magnet. A theoretical disadvantage is the possibility of the pacemaker potential doing a sort of 'R on T' phenomenon and inducing VF. The energy required to do this is, however, much greater than that delivered by the pacemaker. Nevertheless, for this reason a fixed-rate device is only inserted if the block is continuous. They are now rarely used.

• *Demand* (synchronous). These have an internal ability to suppress pacemaker activity if there is an adequate heart rate, but 'cut in' if the rate falls below a preset minimum. They remove any 'competition' between the heart and the electrode and, theoretically, remove the possibility of inducing VF. They are the most common type of permanent pacemaker.

• *Sequential*. These are the most complex models with atrial and ventricular electrodes which try to simulate physiological contraction and obtain the ventricular filling contribution of the atria. They are principally of the demand type (fired from P waves) and some can suppress ventricular pacing if the impulse from the atria is conducted normally. Others can be converted to fixed rate ventricular pacemakers by an external magnet.

Preoperative considerations

50% of patients with pacemakers have coronary artery disease, 20% are hypertensive and 10% are diabetic. They are often on several drugs with cardiovascular actions. Determine the type of pacemaker. All patients carry a 'pacemaker card' which describes its function. Often the model can be recognized from the CXR.

With demand pacemakers, slow the patient's heart rate by carotid massage or a valsalva manoeuvre to evaluate the pacemaker's ability to 'capture' the ventricle.

Note the date the pacemaker was inserted and whether the battery has been changed. Ask if there has been any recurrence of the symptoms which necessitated the pacemaker being fitted. Check on the rate of discharge of the pacemaker both by feeling the pulse and looking at the ECG. A 10% rate reduction is a sign of power failure for fixed rate models.

The ECG complexes are often abnormal during pacemaker function because of depolarization commencing from an ectopic site (Fig. 1.36).

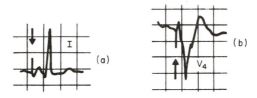

Fig. 1.36. Pacemaker ECG. (a) Atrial pacing producing a P wave and a normal QRS complex. (b) Ventricular pacing from an ectopic site. The pacemaker spikes are arrowed.

The threshold current to trigger pacing varies from person to person but is usually 1–2 milliamps. 80% of patients have stable thresholds but others have an increase in threshold annually. It is important to identify these (get the cardiologist to check the threshold) because it is possible that they have drifted close to the limits of safety. The threshold for triggering is increased by the extremes of acid-base disturbances, and hyperkalaemia and is decreased by hypercarbia and catecholamines.

Anaesthetic management

The principles are as outlined in the general section for any patient with cardiovascular disease, but it is worth stressing that good oxygenation is essential. In general any threshold changes caused by anaesthetic agents themselves are not important.

Remember that patients with pacemakers cannot produce a tachycardia to compensate for fluid loss or myocardial depression which reduces stroke volume and therefore cardiac output. For the same reason avoid sudden postural changes.

Look at the manufacturer's literature on the type of pacemaker for the recommendations concerning diathermy. Fixed rate pacemakers are resistant to external interference and usually unaffected by diathermy. Some demand pacemakers are very sensitive to interference by diathermy and it may cause VF. Alternatively, the diathermy signal can be interpreted as adequate myocardial complexes by the pacemaker with a resultant asystole. Be ready to treat VF. Do not apply the paddles over the pacemaker device.

Where possible avoid the use of diathermy. For operations where this is not possible (e.g. prostatic resection), restrict the diathermy to short bursts. Bipolar is preferable to unipolar. Place the diathermy ground plate well away from the pacemaker. Be careful to prevent earth loops with transvenous pacing wires. This might precipitate VF.

Always use a means of monitoring the pulse (oesophageal stethoscope, precordial stethoscope, peripheral pulse meter) which is not obliterated by diathermy.

Have an isoprenaline infusion available in case the pacing fails.

Valvular heart disease

For many years the commonest cause of acquired valvular heart disease has been chronic rheumatic endocarditis. Its majority position is gradually being eroded (especially in mitral incompetence) as the incidence of rheumatic fever falls and the number of survivors from myocardial infarction and congenital heart disease rises. When due to rheumatic endocarditis the mitral valve is affected in 80% of cases, the aortic valve in 45%, the tricuspid valve in 10% and the pulmonary valve in 1%. 45% of cases have mitral valve disease alone. This implies that almost all aortic valve disease co-exists with mitral valve disease.

It must be emphasized that the anaesthetic management of these cases can, on occasions, create unexpected intraoperative falls in cardiac output and episodes of myocardial ischaemia. For all but patients with minor degrees of dysfunction, *an experienced anaesthetist is needed*. It is always very helpful to discuss their management with the cardiologist in charge of the case. From catheter studies he is often able to supply important data on the resting pressures in the chambers of the heart.

Prophylaxis against endocarditis

Subacute bacterial endocarditis (SBE) occurs in people with pre-existing heart disease, especially those who have valves which are abnormal or damaged by rheumatic fever. Prosthetic heart valves, a ventricular septal defect and a patent ductus arteriosus also predispose to endocarditis but an atrial septal defect does so only rarely. The bacteraemia may arise from poor dental hygiene (refer to dentist) or from the operative site (e.g. teeth, bowel, urinary tract). There is still controversy over the best prophylactic regimen but the following are guidelines.

Patients with valvular disease: Amoxycillin (3 g orally 1 hour before and 8 hours later) or Triplopen (1 vial IM 30 minutes before). If penicillin-sensitive erythromycin stearate (1g orally 2 hours before).

Patients with prosthetic valves: Triplopen (1 vial IM) and gentamicin (80 mg IM repeated twice 8 hourly).

Patients who are penicillin sensitive or have had penicillin within 1 month could have vancomycin (1 g IV repeated after 8 hours).

Mitral stenosis

Aetiology. Over 99% of cases follow rheumatic fever. Approximately one third of cases give no history of rheumatic fever or chorea, the acute illness being mild and escaping notice. It is four times more common in women than men and the latent period from infection to presentation may be 20 years. A tiny percentage are congenital, the valve being replaced by a rudimentary perforated diaphragm.

Physiology. The basic problem in pure mitral stenosis is that the left ventricle cannot fill easily during diastole because of the progressive decrease in mitral valve area. The severity of the disease parallels the reduction in orifice size. The normal cross sectional area of the valve is over 4 cm^2. There are few symptoms until it has fallen to 2.5 cm^2, and the obstruction is severe when it is below 1.0 cm^2.

The resistance to blood flow causes a chronic increase in left atrial pressure with concomitant left atrial hypertrophy and dilatation. With progressive stenosis the left atrial pressure and therefore the pulmonary vein pressure rises. This increases pulmonary venous congestion and decreases the compliance of the lungs. The patient is now disadvantaged in three ways if required to increase his cardiac output (e.g. fever, exercise, pregnancy, excitement):
- A tachycardia reduces left ventricular filling time. The LVEDV falls and with it the stroke volume.
- The failure of ventricular filling increases left atrial pressure and when it exceeds the colloid osmotic pressure (25–30 mmHg) acute pulmonary oedema occurs.
- Because of reduced compliance secondary to venous congestion, the work of breathing increases.

With a stenotic mitral valve, left ventricular filling depends enormously on atrial contraction and the sudden onset of a dysrhythmia secondary to disorganized, stretched conducting tissue (usually AF) may be the cause of a sudden fall in cardiac output and rise in LAP.

In addition to the above changes, 25% of patients with severe mitral stenosis develop an active constriction of the pulmonary arterioles which eventually hypertrophy. Pulmonary hypertension occurs, the changes become irreversible, the right ventricle hypertrophies and there may be functional pulmonary and tricuspid valve incompetence. Congestive heart failure finally supervenes. Why only 25% of severe cases react in this way is unknown.

In severe mitral stenosis some patients also have contraction abnormalities of the left ventricle due to fusion of the chordae tendinae (when measured their ejection fraction is low) and cannot increase their stroke volume even if an induced bradycardia allows greater ventricular filling time.

Preoperative considerations

History

Symptoms result from the following features of the disease:
• Increased pulmonary venous pressure causes dyspnoea on exertion, orthopnoea, PND, haemoptysis, recurrent bronchitis.
• Atrial fibrillation (present in 40%) causes palpitations, heart failure if there is a rapid ventricular rate, symptoms of embolisation (in 10%). Patients may be on anticoagulants and/or digoxin.
• Reactive pulmonary hypertension results in a low cardiac output causing fatigue, ankle swelling, symptoms of deep vein thrombosis and pulmonary embolism.
• Bacterial endocarditis is uncommon in *pure* mitral stenosis.
• The patient may have angina.
The important feature of the history is to gauge the progression of the disease by the patient's exercise tolerance and the drugs needed to control symptoms. The onset of dyspnoea with exercise is the best guide to severity. Dyspnoea when walking slowly on the flat and episodes of PND, imply a resting LAP of 15–20 mmHg and a pressure gradient between atrium and ventricle persisting throughout diastole.

Examination

The findings depend upon whether or not there is accompanying pulmonary hypertension.

In the uncomplicated case the facies are normal, the brachial pulse is normal or rather small in amplitude, the JVP is normal and there is a tapping apex beat, sometimes with an apical diastolic thrill. The two easiest things to hear on auscultation are a loud first sound and a rumbling mid or late diastolic murmur localized to the apex (Fig. 1.37). The opening snap and pre systolic crescendo (only in sinus rhythm) are less frequently heard. The murmur can be accentuated by exercising the patient and rolling him onto his left side. If there are any signs of LVF, suspect another added problem (mitral incompetence, aortic stenosis or coronary artery disease).

With raised pulmonary vascular resistance, there are mitral facies, cool extremities, peripheral cyanosis, a small amplitude pulse, a

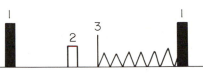

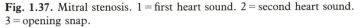

Fig. 1.37. Mitral stenosis. 1 = first heart sound. 2 = second heart sound. 3 = opening snap.

large 'a' wave on the JVP if in sinus rhythm (Table 1.2), and a parasternal heave. There may also be signs of tricuspid incompetence if the right ventricle has dilated.

Investigations

ECG. This may show P mitrale (Fig. 1.38), atrial fibrillation (Fig. 1.23), right axis deviation (Fig. 1.9) or RBBB (Fig. 1.31).

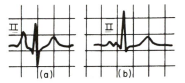

Fig. 1.38. (a) 'P' pulmonale, right atrial hypertrophy (b) 'P' mitrale, atrial asynchrony.

CXR. This shows left atrial enlargement (indents the oesophagus on an oblique film), upper venous congestion and Kerley B lines above the costophrenic angles. The mitral valve may be calcified (Fig. 1.3). The aorta is small.

Echocardiography has proved to be of outstanding value in the assessment of the state of the mitral valve by quantifying the decreased closure rate of the valve leaflets.

Cardiac catheterization records can give data about the normal PAWP and LAP.

Prothrombin time. Many patients are anticoagulated and the prothrombin ratio should be approximately twice normal.

Anaesthetic considerations

Consider whether the patient can be improved preoperatively with drug adjustments. If not digitalized confer with the patient's cardiologist as to the relative merits of prophylactic digitalization.

Those patients who are on anticoagulants must be discussed with the surgeon. There is no doubt that reducing the prothrombin time to normal increases the chance of systemic embolism. It is also true that unless it is an arterial operation or one resulting in considerable diffuse tissue damage, meticulous surgical technique can provide perfectly adequate haemostasis when the prothrombin time is two to three times normal. Thus, a reasonable way to proceed is to keep the patient on warfarin, maintain the prothrombin time at the patient's usual level, and have fresh frozen plasma (FFP) ready to return the clotting mechanism to normal if postoperative oozing or bruising becomes a problem. The half life of warfarin is prolonged by metronidazole.

If the oral route will be unavailable postoperatively, then the patient is best changed to heparin before operation.

The complications of mitral stenosis which might occur in the perioperative period are acute pulmonary oedema, RVF, atrial fibrillation, systemic embolism, SBE and bronchitis or pneumonia. In addition, pulmonary vasoconstriction is increased by hypoxia and acidosis.

Remember that the cardiac output cannot be effectively increased. It may be markedly decreased by reduced ventricular filling (tachycardia, reduced LAP, vasodilatation, hypovolaemia, myocardial depression) which should be avoided. A raised LAP can precipitate pulmonary oedema.

A sudden intraoperative fall in the cardiac output may be caused by the loss of the atrial contribution to ventricular filling from junctional rhythm (Fig. 1.24) or AF (Fig. 1.23). AF occurring *de novo* intraoperatively is probably best converted immediately by DC shock whilst under anaesthesia.

To prevent a tachycardia at induction give a sympathetic explanation (to allay anxiety) and do not use atropine. Traditionally, heavy premedication is recommended but take care to avoid ventilatory depression. Continue digoxin. Prophylaxis against SBE is essential. Induction of anaesthesia is traditionally gaseous but provided *minimal* doses of induction agent are given *slowly* this is satisfactory. Avoid ketamine and gallamine because of tachycardia.

During maintenance of anaesthesia, high concentrations of inhalational agents such as halothane or enflurane may be dangerous in patients with a severely decreased resting cardiac output. Nitrous oxide has been shown to increase pulmonary vascular resistance and since patients with mitral stenosis have an increased alveolar-arterial oxygen gradient, it is sensible to set the N_2O/O_2 ratio at $1:1$ and add an intravenous agent or a low concentration of a volatile anaesthetic to ensure hypnosis. It is a mistake to run patients at an insufficient depth of anaesthesia: adequate anaesthesia is essential to blunt the sympathetic responses to laryngoscopy and surgery all of which result in a tachycardia.

Fluid management is not easy. On the one hand, the patients require a sufficiently high circulating fluid volume to produce the necessary right and left atrial pressures. On the other hand, there is decreased compliance of the pulmonary vasculature because of existing overdistension. Consequently, the pulmonary venous pressure and the PAWP rise more than expected with a given increase in circulating fluid volume. This pulmonary fluid overload can be delivered by exogenous fluids, a head down posture or peripheral vasoconstriction. The major problems occur in the spontaneously breathing patient or on the cessation of IPPV when pulmonary oedema might quickly develop.

The problem of fluid loading can be difficult with the use of spinal or regional anaesthesia (contraindicated if on anticoagulants) when an upper limit of 1 litre should probably be set. If peripheral vasoconstriction is necessary methoxamine is the best choice, because, despite increasing pulmonary resistance, it does not increase the heart rate.

The extent of invasive monitoring used depends upon the combination of patient and operation. With mild or moderate stenosis and no reactive pulmonary hypertension changes in the JVP will parallel changes in the LAP. With severe stenosis, advanced pulmonary hypertension and an expectation of large fluid shifts a PA catheter is invaluable. Intraoperatively it is sensible to maintain the preoperative CVP or PAWP as the minimum for adequate left ventricular filling. The problems of interpreting the PA catheter reading in mitral valve disease have already been described (p. 32).

Monitoring must be continued (invasive or not) into the postoperative period and the patient nursed in a high dependency area. Postoperatively, a PA catheter may warn of impending pulmonary oedema.

Take care not to produce a tachycardia when reversing neuromuscular blockade. Glycopyrrolate is preferable to atropine or alternatively atracurium or vecuronium could be allowed to wear off spontaneously.

Patients with mitral stenosis have decreased lung compliance, increased airways resistance, an elevated alveolar-arterial oxygen gradient and an increased work of breathing. A period of postoperative ventilation (to normocapnia) may well be required before the patient is strong enough to sustain adequate spontaneous ventilation.

Mitral incompetence

Aetiology. Approximately half of the cases are associated with rheumatic mitral stenosis. Other causes are papillary muscle dysfunction (after infarction), ventricular dilatation from LVF (not common because the valve ring is strong), and ruptured or useless chordae tendinae. Rarer causes are congenital malformations and cardiomyopathies. Functional incompetence from a dilated valve ring may disappear after LVF is treated.

Physiology. There is a regurgitant jet throughout systole and the forward flow into the aorta only represents a part of the stroke volume. This produces a large V wave on PA catheter trace (Fig. 1.16, p. 32). During diastole there is an increased flow across the valve because the regurgitated fluid is returned with the normal pulmonary venous flow. A regurgitant fraction (RF) of 0.3 or less indicates mild mitral incompetence, and an RF of over 0.6 indicates severe regurgitation.

Since the left ventricle can eject into either of two outflow paths the impedances of each will determine the ratio of volume delivery. The volume injected into the aorta is very dependent upon systemic vascular resistance and capable of manipulation by vasoconstricting and vasodilating drugs (e.g. methoxamine and sodium nitroprusside).

The left ventricle hypertrophies. The left atrium expands and dilates to accommodate the extra volume load. ('P' mitrale may be seen if in sinus rhythm, Fig. 1.38). The majority of left ventricular activity is used for fibre shortening and the tension requirements for intraventricular pressure development are little different from normal. Since myocardial oxygen consumption is related to left ventricular wall tension, heart rate and contractility and since fibre shortening itself consumes little oxygen, the energy costs of mitral incompetence are modest. Consequently, angina in patients with pure mitral incompetence is not common in the absence of co-existing coronary disease.

AF is the usual end point for severe cases. The atrial contribution to ventricular filling is, however, relatively unimportant and a deterioration from sinus rhythm to atrial fibrillation causes little change in cardiac output. The mean LAP is much lower than in mitral stenosis making pulmonary and right ventricular involvement less common. The symptom free period is longer than in mitral stenosis but the downhill course is rapid after the onset of LVF.

The exception to this sequence of events are those patients who develop acute mitral incompetence, often following myocardial infarction. They develop pulmonary oedema early because the regurgitant jet cannot be accommodated by a normally sized left atrium.

More recently a condition termed 'mitral valve prolapse', which has many possible aetiologies, has been increasingly diagnosed by cardiologists. This refers to a 'floppy valve' which leaks after leaflet closure because the ventricular pressure forces the edges of the valve apart and they 'prolapse' into the left atrium. The majority of patients are symptomless and remain stable. Others progress chronically with a course similar to rheumatic valve disease.

Preoperative considerations

History

There are no symptoms unless heart failure or other complications occur. The incidence of SBE is higher than with any other valve lesion and it has been claimed that systemic embolism is no less common than in mitral stenosis. Consequently, a proportion of these patients are maintained on warfarin, especially if there is a coincident mitral stenosis.

When LVF does occur there is usually sufficient pulmonary congestion to produce mixed symptomatology of fatigue, dyspnoea on exertion, orthopnoea, PND, haemoptysis and recurrent bronchitis.

The progression of disease is gauged on exertional dyspnoea, and the presence and onset of LVF. The symptoms of RVF occur later. Patients are often on digoxin and diuretics.

Examination

The pulse wave feels normal. The apex beat is vigorous and displaced beyond the normal limits. The murmur is pansystolic and maximal at the apex (Fig. 1.39), radiating to the axilla. A diastolic flow murmur in severe incompetence may be functional and does not necessarily imply stenosis. In serious disease AF may be present. Later there are signs of first LVF and then RVF. Arterial hypertension increases the regurgitant flow and may precipitate LVF.

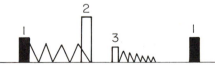

Fig. 1.39. Mitral incompetence. 1 = first heart sound. 2 = second heart sound. 3 = third heart sound and functional mitral valve flow murmur.

Investigations

ECG. This can show 'P' mitrale (Fig. 1.38), AF (Fig. 1.23) or left ventricular hypertrophy.

CXR. This shows a large left atrium and enlarged ventricles.

Echocardiography. This demonstrates an increased diastolic closure rate in contrast to the reduction found in mitral stenosis. The echocardiogram also differentiates the thickened mitral cusps of chronic rheumatic endocarditis from the thin cusps of mitral incompetence due to rupture of the chordae tendinae or from mitral valve prolapse.

Cardiac catherization. This can give data on the normal PAWP and LAP.

Anaesthetic considerations

All patients need prophylaxis against endocarditis. Those with only minor symptoms and a good exercise tolerance (e.g. can carry shopping upstairs with little discomfort) tolerate anaesthesia and surgery well.

Those on anticoagulants should be treated as described in 'mitral stenosis'.

With a symptomatic patient always consider whether or not he could be improved by manipulating his drugs. Discuss his problems with a cardiologist.

Induction can be as described in 'General principles'. Maintenance using high concentrations of halothane or enflurane is contraindicated. Patients with symptomatic mitral incompetence already have depressed contractility and the negative inotropic effects of these agents more than offsets the mild decrease in systemic vascular resistance and there is a fall in stroke volume and cardiac output.

Although bradycardias are to be avoided because there is no reserve stroke volume to compensate for the reduced heart rate, mild tachycardias are tolerated well because there is no obstruction to diastolic left ventricular filling. It is important to sustain an adequately high LAP by careful fluid management otherwise the LVEDP falls to below the 'knee' of the ventricular performance curve (Fig. 1.14(a)) causing a sudden drop in stroke work. The dilated, hypertrophied ventricle of mitral incompetence is very sensitive to this mechanism and must be maintained at a sufficient degree of 'stretch' for its optimum contractile performance.

Anything which increases systemic vascular resistance (sympathetic vasoconstriction, drugs) leads to an increased portion of stroke volume returning through the mitral valve and a consequent fall in cardiac output. This problem (outside of cardiac units) potentially occurs chiefly with light anaesthesia and the excessive use of vasoconstrictors during regional block. The solutions are to deepen anaesthesia, and to give a generous fluid load during regional block and only to give vasoconstrictors in tiny incremental doses. If the cardiac output is low because of unexplained peripheral vaso-constriction (this can occur in postoperative period), the afterload can be reduced by sodium nitroprusside in doses which do not produce a marked tachycardia.

The atrial contribution to ventricular filling is less important in patients with mitral regurgitation and loss of sinus rhythm does not have the catastrophic effect seen in mitral stenosis. Atrial tachy-dysrhythmias form part of the natural history of the disease and it is worthwhile prior to anaesthesia discussing with a cardiologist the wisdom of reversal.

As usual, the extent of invasive monitoring depends upon the particular combination of patient and operation. Because of the propensity to SBE, catheters should not be placed in the major vessels without very good reason. The features of the pulmonary artery trace in mitral incompetence have already been described (Fig. 1. 16). The advantages a PA catheter gives are the ability to maintain the PAWP at any desired level, and an indication of whether a fall in PAWP is due to hypovolaemia or RVF. It can also be used to measure the effectiveness of treatments to increase the cardiac output by inducing falls in peripheral vascular resistance. The major advantages are obviously found in those patients with moderate or severe disease who experience large fluid shifts.

If the patient has disease which is sufficiently severe and chronic to induce pulmonary vascular changes then refer to the relevant sections in the anaesthetic management of mitral stenosis.

Mixed mitral valve disease

Optimum management is by a compromise of the above depending on whether stenosis or incompetence is the dominant feature. This is ultimately decided by catheterization but if the pulse volume is small and there is no left ventricular hypertrophy (in the absence of failure), stenosis is more likely to be dominant.

Aortic stenosis

Aetiology. If the valvular stenosis is of rheumatic origin (presents <60 years of age) almost all cases are accompanied by mitral valve disease. Other causes are a congenital bicuspid valve (presents circa 60 years) and degenerative calcification (presents over 70 years). Functional, but not true, valvular stenoses at the supravalvular and subvalvular level (see cardiomyopathy) are both very rare.

Physiology. The progressive resistance to flow through the aortic valve causes the pressure in the left ventricle during systole to be higher in the left ventricle than in the aorta. The valve must be narrowed to about 25% of its normal area (approximately 3 cm^2) before there is a significant obstruction to flow across it. This results in massive hypertrophy of the left ventricle which becomes stiff and increasingly dependent upon the contribution from left atrial contraction for adequate filling. Ventricular dilatation occurs when there is associated regurgitation or when the ventricle fails. Angina may occur without significant coronary artery disease because of the precarious balance of oxygen supply and demand.

Several factors conspire to attenuate the delivery of oxygen to the sub-endocardium. The inevitably low diastolic pressure reduces the coronary artery filling pressure and, in addition, the stiff hypertrophied ventricle has impaired relaxation during early diastole. The metabolic demands of the muscle are increased because of the high intraventricular pressures, and the thickness of the ventricular wall may itself hinder an adequate oxygen flux being transported from the distributing epicardial arteries to the sub-endocardial capillaries (Fig. 1.17). It is thought that the relative failure of nitroglycerine to relieve the angina of aortic stenosis is because the coronary vessels are already maximally dilated under 'resting' conditions. Any reduction in the duration of diastole (e.g. from exercise, emotion) quickly induces angina and, on some occasions, acute LVF or VF which results in sudden death. Coronary filling is further impeded because the diseased valve distorts the aortic architecture and reduces the backflow of blood from the mainstream into the coronary sinuses. The coronary ostia can also be narrowed by calcification.

Optimum performance of the left ventricle becomes very dependent upon the correct heart rate. The rate must be low enough to allow adequate time for filling and ejection but not so slow that the end diastolic volume is excessive. There is usually a long latent period (approximately 30 years) and the disease is well advanced at presentation.

Preoperative considerations

History

There may be no symptoms or there can be angina (see above), dizziness and syncope on effort (low cardiac output) and dyspnoea (LVF). Once diagnosed, the patient is usually on digoxin and diuretics. Nitroglycerine is not as effective in relieving ischaemic pain as usual (see above) and may be harmful in reducing diastolic pressure. A sudden deterioration in exercise tolerance is often due to the onset of AF.

Examination

There is a slow rising, slow falling regular low amplitude plateau pulse (Table 1.1). AF usually indicates associated mitral valve disease. There is a sustained and heaving apex beat. Signs of LVF may be present. There may be a thrill over the aortic area (Fig. 1.2) which radiates to the neck. A loud midsystolic ejection murmur is heard in the aortic area (Fig. 1.40) which may be transmitted to the carotid arteries.

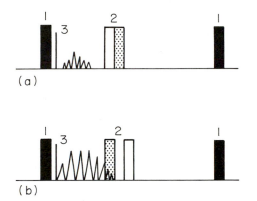

(a)

(b)

Fig. 1.40. Aortic stenosis. 1 = first heart sound. 2 = second heart sound. 3 = ejection click. In mild stenosis (a) the pulmonary component of the second sound follows the aortic. In moderate to severe stenosis (b) the aortic sound follows the pulmonary sound in expiration.

Paradoxically, in severe disease the murmur may, on occasions, become less loud because of LVF and a fall in cardiac output. The aortic component of the second sound depends upon the condition of the valve. It is normal or increased in some cases of congenital origin and soft or absent with a rigid calcified valve. The ejection click has a similar variable presence. In severe stenosis, left venticular systole is considerably prolonged and in expiration the aortic sound falls well behind the pulmonary sound — the so called reversed split (Fig. 1.40).

Investigations

ECG. This may show signs of left ventricular hypertrophy. If not present, the stenosis is not severe.
CXR. There is no increase in transverse cardiac diameter unless ventricular dilatation has occurred (see definitions, p. 39). The aorta is small but there can be post-stenotic dilatation and a calcified valve (Fig. 1.3).

Echocardiography. This demonstrates the restricted movements of the aortic valve and indicates calcification to a sufficient degree of accuracy for an accurate diagnosis to be made.

Cardiac catheterization. This is used to determine the true severity of the condition.

Anaesthetic considerations

Always prescribe prophylaxis against SBE.

Patients with a symptomatic aortic stenosis are *always serious anaesthetic risks* because the disease is advanced at presentation. If discovered incidentally during the preoperative assessment for elective surgery it is *essential* to involve a cardiologist. Valve replacement may be recommended and if so should be done first.

Possible complications during the operative and postoperative period include spontaneous VF, acute LVF, and myocardial ischaemia.

The basic approach is to preserve the baseline haemodynamic state. The single most important variable to monitor until well into the recovery period is probably the direct arterial pressure. Not only does it give beat by beat information about the diastolic pressure (which is critical for coronary perfusion) but the diastolic decay also indicates how fast the stroke volume 'runs off' peripherally (Fig. 1.13). (The stroke volume itself can also be approximated by the area under the curve up to the dicrotic notch (Fig. 1.13) but the facilities for doing this quantitatively are only found in specialized units.)

The need for a PA catheter depends upon the severity of the aortic valve disease, the magnitude of surgery and the expected changes in fluid balance. It should not be put in without good reason because its passage through the right ventricle can induce ventricular tachycardia. The problems of interpretation of the trace have already been discussed (p. 32).

Hypotension is the greatest danger to adequate coronary perfusion and may be due to peripheral vasodilatation, fluid loss, an inadequate stroke volume against a high peripheral resistance, or LVF. Combined readings from arterial and PA catheters are invaluable in identifying the cause.

Induction of anaesthesia must follow preoxygenation and be accomplished slowly. Venodilatation can lower the LVEDP enough to cause a significant fall in stroke work (Fig. 1.14(a)) which results in a drop in peak left ventricular pressure and hence a reduction in stroke volume. This in turn produces systemic hypotension and left ventricular ischaemia.

High concentrations of volatile agents, such as halothane and enflurane, not only depress contractility (with little reduction in systemic vascular resistance) with consequent systemic hypotension but also depress S-A node automaticity and may cause a junctional rhythm to emerge.

In patients with severe aortic stenosis the maintenance of sinus rhythm is paramount since the left ventricle is dependent upon a properly timed atrial systole to achieve an adequate end diastolic volume. Disturbances of rhythm should first be avoided (check the serum electrolytes and the dose of drugs, especially digoxin) and then treated by removal of the cause (e.g. switch off halothane, withdraw CVP line), before resorting to drug therapy or DC shock. Calcium is probably the drug of choice for persistent junctional rhythm. Sinus tachycardia frequently produces myocardial ischaemia and can be due to an insufficient depth of anaesthesia or insufficient circulating fluid volume. If there is no response after correction of these, then use *small* incremental doses of a beta-adrenoceptor blocker (e.g. practolol 0.5 mg, propranolol 0.25 mg). This is potentially dangerous because the patient may be depending upon endogenous beta-adrenoceptor stimulation to maintain myocardial contractility.

Severe bradycardia can also be detrimental because if the ventricle is working to its maximum possible pressure prior to the bradycardia occurring, no increase in cardiac output is possible. Heart rates of less than 45–50/minute associated with a low diastolic blood pressure and myocardial ischaemia can be treated by tiny doses of atropine but at all costs avoid the 'overshoot' to a tachycardia.

More complex dysrhythmias, unresponsive to simple measures are probably best managed by DC shock.

At the cessation of surgery either allow the neuromuscular blocking drugs time to be metabolized or use glycopyrrolate (*not* atropine) to prevent the bradycardia of neostigmine.

If cardiac arrest occurs, only *internal* cardiac massage is really effective because of the valvular stenosis.

Aortic regurgitation

Aetiology. The commonest causes are rheumatic valve disease (chronic) and infective endocarditis (acute). It may also be associated with chest trauma, connective tissue disorders (Marfan's syndrome), congenital lesions, (bicuspid valve) and aneurysms of the ascending aorta. Syphilis as a cause is now rare. The importance of hypertensive dilatation of the aortic root is disputed.

Physiology. During diastole the left ventricle is filled by blood leaking back through the aortic valve in addition to that received from the left atrium. Consequently, only a proportion of that blood ejected into the aorta actually reaches the periphery. Patients with a regurgitant fraction over 0.6 of the stroke volume have severe disease. The left ventricle dilates and hypertrophies to accommodate the increased diastolic volume. The duration of ventricular systole is normal and hence there is a rapid forward flow causing a functional systolic murmur.

The determinants of the regurgitant volume are the valve area available for backflow, the diastolic pressure gradient from aorta to left ventricle and the time available. Thus, the regurgitant fraction is increased by a high systemic vascular resistance, a compliant left ventricle and a bradycardia. The influence of heart rate on controlling regurgitation is said to explain the clinical observation that patients with aortic regurgitation often tolerate exercise well but may develop symptoms of pulmonary congestion at rest.

Mild or moderate degrees of back flow are tolerated well and compatible with a normal life. If the disease progresses, LVF or ischaemic heart disease occurs which leads to death in 1–3 years.

Preoperative considerations

History

The patient may be completely symptomless until features of LVF (dyspnoea on exertion, orthopnoea, PND) or angina occur. Sudden death is rare. They are often on digoxin and diuretics. RVF secondary to LVF is a late event.

Examination

The pulse is regular, of large amplitude (high systolic, low diastolic) and collapsing (Table 1.1). If AF is present suspect mitral involvement. The left ventricle is large and the apex beat hyperdynamic and displaced beyond the normal limits.

There is abrupt distension and collapse of the carotid arteries (Corrigan's sign) and there is said to be capillary pulsation in the nail beds.

Aortic regurgitation may be difficult to detect on auscultation. Classically, there is a blowing, high pitched murmur beginning immediately after the second sound loudest at the third and fourth left intercostal spaces close to the sternum (Fig. 1.41). Sometimes it can only be elicited at the end of expiration when the patient leans forward. There is almost always a functional systolic ejection murmur in the aortic area (Fig. 1.2) which is usually transmitted to the carotids.

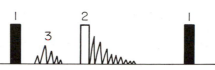
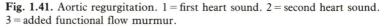

Fig. 1.41. Aortic regurgitation. 1 = first heart sound. 2 = second heart sound. 3 = added functional flow murmur.

Investigations

ECG. Left ventricular hypertrophy may be present.
CXR. The heart may be enlarged and the aortic root dilated.
Echocardiography. This will detect the movement of the aortic valve leaflets and eliminate or confirm co-existent mitral involvement.

Anaesthetic considerations

All patients need prophylaxis against SBE. Those with minor degrees of regurgitation and a good exercise tolerance, tolerate anaesthesia and surgery well.

The management of a more serious case should always be discussed with a cardiologist. There may be an improvement in medication possible or valve replacement might be offered prior to elective major surgery.

Induction can be as described in 'General principles'. Maintenance using high concentrations of halothane or enflurane is contraindicated. The dilated, hypertrophied myocardium already has depressed contractility and the negative inotropic effects of these agents can produce a marked drop in stroke volume and cardiac output.

As in mitral regurgitation, the atrial contribution to left ventricular filling is relatively unimportant provided that the left ventricular end diastolic volume is maintained. The dilated left ventricle is very sensitive to fibre length and if it falls below the 'knee' of the ventricular performance curve (Fig. 1.14(a)) there may be a sudden drop in stroke work. Some patients are exquisitively sensitive to venodilatation because of this mechanism. In cases in which large fluid shifts are expected a PA catheter can be invaluable in maintaining the optimal PAWP. There are problems in interpretation of the reading in the rare and severe cases with early mitral valve closure (p. 33).

When adverse changes in cardiac output occur, the combination of direct arterial monitoring and PA catheter can be invaluable in evaluating the cause.

Cardiac output is a balance between heart rate, stroke volume, contractility and systemic vascular resistance. Anything which increases systemic vascular resistance (sympathetic vasoconstriction, drugs) leads to an increased portion of the stroke volume returning through the aortic valve and a consequent fall in cardiac output. This potential problem (outside cardiac units) occurs chiefly with light anaesthesia and the excessive use of vasoconstrictors during regional block. The solutions are to deepen anaesthesia, and to give a generous fluid load during regional block and only to give vasoconstrictors in tiny incremental doses.

Although a fall in systemic vascular resistance reduces regurgitant flow, it also induces hypotension and may lead to an inadequate coronary artery filling pressure. Vasodilators, when employed to reduce left ventricular afterload must be used carefully to prevent this happening.

A mild tachycardia is permissible provided that it does not prejudice left ventricular filling. Bradycardia is poorly tolerated because of the increased regurgitant flow (see above) and should be corrected by small doses of atropine or prevented by the use of a vagolytic muscle relaxant such as pancuronium.

Mixed aortic valve disease

The dominance of stenosis or incompetence is indicated clinically by the deviation of a normal pulse to either plateau or collapsing. The true contribution of each is only possible by catheterization.

Tricuspid stenosis

Organic tricuspid valve disease only very rarely occurs in isolation and *the cardiac picture is usually dominated by other associated abnormalities*.

Almost all cases of tricuspid stenosis are of rheumatic origin with mitral involvement. Very rare isolated lesions occur in the carcinoid syndrome, systemic lupus erythematosus and as congenital abnormalities. There is invariably a regurgitant component.

Tricuspid stenosis produces a low cardiac output state with a high right atrial pressure. This in turn may lead to throbbing headaches and a pulsating liver which can progress to mild chronic jaundice and cirrhosis (q.v.) There is fatigue and peripheral oedema. Large 'a' waves are seen in the JVP (Table 1.2). The murmur of tricuspid stenosis is similar in timing to that of mitral stenosis, maximal in the tricuspid area (Fig. 1.2) and accentuated during inspiration. A pansystolic murmur of tricuspid incompetence is usually also present. 'P' pulmonale may be seen on the ECG (Fig. 1.38). The enlarged right atrium is prominent on the right heart border of the

CXR. Management is by diuretic therapy and low physical exertion. Anaesthetic considerations are analagous to those for mitral stenosis with LA = RA, LV = RV and systemic vascular resistance = pulmonary vascular resistance. Fluid overload in tricuspid stenosis does not lead to early pulmonary oedema.

Tricuspid incompetence

The majority of cases are rheumatic in origin with co-existent mitral involvement. Congenital lesions are Ebstein's anomaly and endocardial cushion defects. An increasing, but still rare, cause is acute bacterial endocarditis in mainlining drug addicts. Dilatation of the relatively weak valve ring in RVF may produce a serious regurgitant state. This usually responds well to medical treatment. Symptoms are similar to those of tricuspid stenosis but there are jugular 'v' waves (Table 1.2) and signs of right ventricular hypertrophy. A pansystolic murmur louder in inspiration is heard at the lower end of the sternum. The ECG shows right ventricular hypertrophy, and the CXR has an enlarged cardiac shadow.

The physiological consequences of tricuspid incompetence *per se* are very well tolerated because of the highly distensible systemic venous system and even complete removal of the valve is possible. However, this equilibrium is easily upset by an increased right ventricular load secondary to pulmonary hypertension or LVF. In extreme cases, low right ventricular output and massive regurgitation can result in a CVP which is higher than the LAP.

Anaesthetic considerations are as for valve disease in general. The optimum care of the right ventricle is produced by meticulous attention to left ventricular function and by avoiding drugs which appreciably increase pulmonary vascular resistance.

Pulmonary valve disease

The majority of cases are congenital stenotic lesions and account for 10% of all cases of congenital heart disease. 90% are valvular and 10% infundibular. 10% of cases have an associated atrial septal defect, and infundibular lesions are usually accompanied by a ventricular septal defect. Rheumatic and carcinoid causes are very rare.

Symptoms may be absent but severe stenoses produce fatigue, angina (ischaemic right ventricle) and syncope. There is usually a thrill in the pulmonary area (Fig. 1.2) with a systolic or continuous murmur. The other physical signs and positive findings on investigation are those secondary to right ventricular hypertrophy and/or

91

failure. The most important haemodynamic disturbance of marked stenosis is a low cardiac output. Anaesthetic considerations are analogous to those for aortic stenosis. There is, in severe cases, a sufficient gradient across the pulmonary valve such that changes in pulmonary vascular resistance have little effect on cardiac output.

Very rarely the pulmonary valve is absent. This has little haemodynamic effect on the heart but dilatation of the pulmonary artery can compress the trachea or left main bronchus causing airway obstruction.

Patients with prosthetic valves

Although a prosthetic valve corrects the direction and ease of blood flow it does not immediately correct the consequent left or right ventricular hypertrophy that has occurred. Replacement of a diseased valve does, however, produce an early improvement in 90% of surviving patients and over a period of 2 to 5 years radiological signs of cardiomegaly and pulmonary arterial hypertension gradually decrease. Management is that of the residual ventricular condition. On auscultation, the prosthetic valve can be heard clicking.

Patients are often on anticoagulants to prevent embolization. Treat them as described in mitral stenosis. Antibiotic prophylaxis (q.v.) is essential. Unless there are strong indications do not use a PA catheter because of the increased risk of SBE.

Congenital heart disease

The overall incidence is approximately one case per 200 live births. An increasing percentage now survive to adulthood because of improved methods of treatment. The majority are discovered at birth because of routine physical examination. Diagnosis and treatment recommendations are a specialist's prerogative. Almost all cases have been well investigated prior to being seen by the anaesthetist for non-cardiac surgery.

Congenital heart disease may present as an isolated cardiac abnormality or as part of a more generalized systemic syndrome. The cardiac abnormality can be single or a combination of lesions. Well over a hundred conditions have been described but less than ten occur commonly. These can be divided into left to right shunts, right to left shunts and outflow obstructions. The management of these will be discussed in general terms so that the conclusions can be applied to other, rarer syndromes. It must be emphasized that *it is an area in which things can go unpredictably wrong* and that for all but the simplest cases, *experienced help is needed.*

All patients need antibiotic prophylaxis (q.v.). If anomalous murmurs and signs are discovered *de novo* during the preoperative visit it is always best to get a cardiological opinion.

Left to right shunts

Irrespective of their exact site, these lesions all produce an increased pulmonary blood flow. The magnitude of this is a function both of the size of the hole and the pressures on either side of it. These pressures are themselves partly dependent upon systemic and pulmonary vascular resistances. Thus, variations in these resistances indirectly influence the magnitude of the shunt. Theoretically, drugs which decrease pulmonary vascular resistance or increase systemic resistance will increase the shunt.

If the flow is high enough, some patients will develop reactive pulmonary hypertension with right ventricular hypertrophy. Ultimately this progresses to a reversal of the shunt (Eisenmenger syndrome) and to right and left ventricular failure. The philosophy of medical treatment is to prevent pulmonary hypertension occurring by closure of the defect at a sufficiently early stage. The Eisenmenger syndrome is rare, difficult to manage and not considered further.

ATRIAL SEPTAL DEFECT

Atrial septal defects (ASD) comprise 15% of all congenital heart disease. 95% of these are ostium secundum and 5% ostium primum defects.

Ostium secundum This defect is usually well tolerated by the child and untreated often does not present until the 2nd or 3rd decade when there is irreversible pulmonary hypertension. It is often discovered incidentally or because of repeated chest infections.

Ostium primum This defect is embryologically different and often involves the A-V valves. Symptoms present more floridly and earlier than in the secundum defect reflecting a bigger and more complex lesion.

Examination

The pulse volume is normal and when the pulmonary blood flow exceeds the aortic blood flow by approximately 3:1 there is a loss of sinus arrhythmia. The defect itself produces no murmur but because of the increased blood flow through the lungs there is a pulmonary ejection systolic murmur in the pulmonary area (Fig. 1.2) and there may on occasions be a diastolic tricuspid murmur (Fig. 1.42). The murmurs are louder on inspiration and the second sound has a fixed split. There are often signs of a hypertrophied hyperkinetic right ventricle.

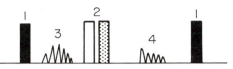

Fig. 1.42. Atrial septal defect. 1 = first heart sound. 2 = second heart sound with fixed split, pulmonary valve closure coming late. 3 = pulmonary valve flow murmur. 4 = tricuspid valve flow murmur.

Investigations

ECG. Right bundle branch block and right axis deviation are common.
CXR. This may be normal or may show large pulmonary vessels and an enlarged right atrium.

Anaesthesia

Defects with left to right shunts and no evidence of ventricular failure pose few problems. Otherwise apply the concepts developed in 'General principles'. Theoretically, because of increased pulmonary blood flow the uptake of gaseous agents is more rapid and the effect of IV agents is slower in onset. Although systemic air embolism is theoretically unlikely from a left to right shunt, it is good practice to be meticulous in removing air from syringes and cannulae before use. By effects on the pulmonary and systemic vascular beds, IPPV and volatile agents tend to reduce the shunt. Postoperative chest infections are common so vigorous physiotherapy and early mobilization are vital.

VENTRICULAR SEPTAL DEFECT

Ventricular septal defects (VSD) comprise 30% of congenital heart disease. The presentation and clinical manifestations depend upon the size of the lesion. Small defects are haemodynamically unimportant but may have a loud murmur and 20–30% close spontaneously. They are compatible with a normal life. Large defects can present with failure to thrive, tachypnoea and heart failure within a month of life. Between these extremes the magnitude of the shunt is assessed by ECG evidence of left ventricular hypertrophy, increased cardiac diameter on CXR, signs of pulmonary hypertension, and ultimately cardiac catheterization.

Examination

Often the patient is symptomless but if symptoms occur they are those of any significant left to right shunt (frequent bronchitis, dyspnoea). The pulse is of normal volume and with significant lesions there is an abrupt and forceful apex beat (volume overload of the left and to a lesser extent the right ventricles).

The murmur of the defect is a harsh pansystolic murmur in the 3rd or 4th intercostal space at the left sternal edge which intensifies on expiration. Superimposed upon this are the flow murmurs of the pulmonary valve and mitral valve (Fig. 1.43).

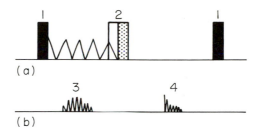

Fig. 1.43. Ventricular septal defect. 1 = first heart sound. 2 = second heart sound, pulmonary valve closes later than aortic. (a) sounds of the defect. (b) added sounds. 3 = pulmonary flow murmur. 4 = mitral flow murmur.

Investigations

ECG. This may be normal or show the voltage changes of left ventricular hypertrophy.
CXR. This may be normal or show large pulmonary vessels, a large left atrium and biventricular enlargement.

Anaesthetic considerations are similar to those of ASD.

PATENT DUCTUS ARTERIOSUS

Patent ductus arteriosus (PDA) comprises 10% of congenital heart lesions. In a PDA the shunt is from the aorta into the pulmonary artery. The majority are asymptomatic and discovered incidentally. It may be part of the rubella syndrome. If there is a large shunt, recurrent bronchitis and dyspnoea on exertion occur. Untreated, heart failure and pulmonary hypertension appear in the teens.

Examination

The pulse volume is normal when the defect is small but becomes high volume and collapsing (Table 1.1) as it increases in size. There is an abrupt forceful apex beat from a dilated and hypertrophied left ventricle which has an abnormally large stroke volume. Blood flows through the ductus throughout the cardiac cycle and produces a continuous murmur, maximal at the first left intercostal space which is loudest towards the end of systole and on expiration (Fig. 1.44). In addition, there may be superimposed aortic and mitral flow murmurs (but these are usually obscured) from the excessive flow of blood through these valves.

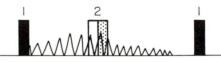

Fig. 1.44. Patent ductus arteriosus. 1 = first heart sound. 2 = second heart sound. Normally the pulmonary valve closes last but with a large defect there is a reversed split with aortic closure falling appreciably after pulmonary valve closure during expiration.

Investigations

ECG. This may be normal or show changes of left ventricular hypertrophy.
CXR. This may be normal or may show enlargement of pulmonary vessels, ascending aorta, aortic knuckle, left atrium and ventricles.

Anaesthetic considerations are similar to those of ASD.

Right to left shunts

A right to left shunt needs a communication between the systemic and pulmonary circulations and an imbalance in ventricular pressures (there may be a common ventricle) such that venous blood can enter the aorta by bypassing the lungs. There is usually reduced pulmonary blood flow. *Air embolism from intravenous injection is a great danger.*

The only commonly occurring defect is Fallot's tetralogy which comprises 10% of all congenital heart disease and 65% of cyanotic heart disease.

FALLOT'S TETRALOGY

Physiology. There is a large VSD (functionally a common ventricle) in which the shunt is from right to left because of pulmonary stenosis (infundibular and/or valvular and/or in the pulmonary artery). There is an accompanying over-riding of the aorta which sits over the septal defect. The load on the right ventricle results in right ventricular hypertrophy completing the tetralogy.

Alteration of the relative resistance of the pulmonary and aortic outflow tracts changes the magnitude of the shunt. Although the resistance of a pulmonary artery or valve defect is effectively fixed, that of the infundibulum, which is dependent upon tone, can be increased by emotional crises, catecholamines or sympathetic activity from light anaesthesia and reduced by halothane, beta-adrenoceptor blockers and deep anaesthesia. There is no resistance to flow into the aorta and the aortic impedance is controlled by the systemic vascular resistance, a fall in this increasing the right to left shunt and the cyanosis.

History

Failure to thrive, growth retardation, dyspnoea, syncope and squatting (thought to increase systemic vascular resistance by kinking major blood vessels) are common.

Examination

Cyanosis and finger clubbing (over 6 months) are obvious. Considering the gravity of the defect, auscultation is disappointing. The murmur of pulmonary stenosis is heard in the pulmonary area (Fig. 1.2) but there is no VSD murmur because it is so large (Fig. 1.45). Heart failure is rare in infancy.

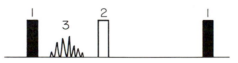

Fig. 1.45. Fallot's tetralogy. 1 = first heart sound. 2 = second heart sound. 3 = pulmonary stenosis.

Complications include emboli, strokes, epilepsy, endocarditis, cerebral abscesses and most important of all cyanotic and syncopal attacks (which can be fatal).

Investigations

FBC. Polycythaemia is usual.
ECG. Right axis deviation is usual.
CXR. The aorta is large (right sided in 25% of cases) and the pulmonary vasculature only shows faintly.
Blood gases. The $PaCO_2$ is normal or low and hypoxia and metabolic acidosis are evident.
Treatment is now definitive total correction at 4–6 years which may or may not be preceded by a palliative operation to increase pulmonary

blood flow. Many children with cyanotic attacks are now on propranolol to control infundibular obstruction.

Anaesthesia

Often the children are not used to and frightened of hospitals. Do
not allow them to become dehydrated through prolonged withhold-
ing of fluids. A generous premedication (oral followed by IM) should
ensure a sedated child at induction. Crying and fighting at induction
can lead to a cyanotic attack.

The overall principle in the uncorrected case is to prevent the
complications of the condition and not to increase the shunt and
thereby intensify the hypoxia. Venous access is usually easy and IV
(or IM) induction with a small dose of the agent is preferred.
Theoretically, its effect will be quicker than usual.

Optimum haemodynamic management can be achieved in several
ways. Some anaesthetists concentrate on maintaining the systemic
vascular resistance with ketamine and pancuronium whilst others concentrate on reducing infundibular spasm with halothane and beta-
adrenoceptor blockers. The best management of any case is obviously
that tailored to the individual, but in those patients with marked infundibular obstruction, the magnitude of the resistance is dynamic
(see above), and must not be allowed to increase during anaesthesia.
Maintenance is usually with a nitrous oxide/oxygen mixture and a
relaxant ± other agents. IPPV with normal inflation pressures has
little effect in reducing pulmonary blood flow because the resistance
of the pulmonary outflow tract is already so great. Keep the child
well hydrated to maintain the blood pressure.

These patients can be difficult to handle and should only be anaesthetized in the presence of an experienced anaesthetist.

Outflow obstructions

Aortic stenosis (comprises 7% of total) and pulmonary stenosis
(comprises 10% of total) are as outlined under valvular disease.

COARCTATION OF AORTA

Coarctation of the aorta comprises 5% of all congenital heart disease. It
can occur alone or in association with a bicuspid aortic valve, VSD,
PDA, cerebral artery aneurysms, and Marfan's and Turner's syndromes. The two types are pre-ductal and post-ductal.

Pre-ductal (2%). This is the most florid form presenting within the first
first weeks of life and is frequently associated with other cardiac

defects and severe biventricular failure. Medical treatment is with digoxin and diuretics and early (often semi-emergency) surgical correction. They rarely present untreated for any other operation than correction itself.

Post-ductal (98%). This is a much less severe form which may not present until adulthood when it may only be a chance finding. It is less frequently associated with other major defects but 20–50% have a bicuspid aortic valve. Untreated the majority die in the 3rd or 4th decade from endocarditis, cerebrovascular accident or LVF.

History

60% are asymptomatic. 40% have symptoms of hypertension, cerebrovascular accidents, endocarditis or intermittent claudication.

Examination

Proximal hypertension is common. The BP is higher in the arms than in the legs and there is frequently a difference in BP between the right and left arms. The radial pulse is felt before the femoral. Occasionally there are visible, palpable or audible scapular collaterals. A loud, rough systolic murmur is heard at the apex of the left lung. There is a forceful apex beat often displaced beyond the normal limits.

Investigations

ECG. This shows signs of left ventricular hypertrophy.
CXR. This may reveal a double aortic knuckle, a small descending aorta, rib notching, and increased cardiac size.

Anaesthesia

If not in LVF (which should be treated) these patients are effectively normal except that those parts of the body supplied by the collateral circulation are at risk of ischaemia. This can produce damage to both the spinal cord and kidneys and is disastrous when it happens.

A good plan is to measure the BP in *both arms and legs* preoperatively and to maintain these values throughout surgery. This requires careful attention to fluid balance and may necessitate the use of vasoactive drugs. Some texts suggest that the mean BP in the legs should not fall below 50 mmHg. A good convenient, non invasive measurement of leg blood pressure is obtained from an oscillometric or oscillotonometric cuff applied to the calf. It is, however, desirable to use the same cuff and measuring system preoperatively as intraoperatively because there are considerable inter-instrument variations.

FURTHER READING

ABC of Hypertension (1981) A collection of articles published by the *Br. Med. Ass.*

Asiddao, C.B., Donegan, J.H., Whitesell, R.C. *et al.* (1982) Factors associated with perioperative complications during carotid endarterectomy. *Anesth. Analg.*, **61**, 631–7.

Beeley, L. (1984) Drug interactions and beta-blockers. *Br. Med. J.*, **289**, 1330–31.

Chambers, D.A. (1979) Acquired valvular heart disease. *In*: Kaplan, J.A. (ed.), *Cardiac Anaesthesia* Grune & Stratton, New York. 197–240.

Cobbe, S.M. (1983) Congenital complete heart block. *Br. Med. J.*, **286**, 1769–70.

Cullen, B.F. & Miller, M.G. (1979) Drug interactions and anesthesia: a review. *Anesth. Analg.*, **58**, 413–23.

De Bono, D. (1982) Echocardiography in adult heart disease. *Hospital Update*, **8**, 265–77.

Evans, D.W. (1984) Atrioventricular block. *Br. J. Hosp. Med.*, **31**, 328–35.

Foex, P. (1981) Preoperative assessment of the patient with cardiovascular disease. *Br. J. Anaesth.*, **53**, 731–44.

Foex, P. (1984) Alpha and beta adrenoceptor antagonists. *Br. J. Anaesth.*, **56**, 751–65.

George, R.J.D. & Banks, R.A. (1983) Bedside measurement of pulmonary capillary wedge pressure. *Br. J. Hosp. Med.*, **29**, 286–91.

Goldman, L., Caldera, D.L., Nussbaum, S.R. *et al.* (1977) Multifactorial index of cardiac risk in non-cardiac surgical procedures. *N. Engl. J. Med.*, **297**, 845–50.

Horgan, J.H. (1984) Cardiac pacing. *Br. Med. J.*, **288**, 1942–4.

Howard, P. (1983) Drugs or oxygen for hypoxic cor pulmonale? *Br. Med. J.*, **287**, 1159–60.

Hutchinson, S. & Lorimer, A.R. (1984) Bundle branch block. *Br. J. Hosp. Med.*, **31**, 331–40.

Hutton, P., Dye, J. & Prys-Roberts, C. (1984) An assessment of the Dinamap 845. *Anaesthesia*, **39**, 261–7.

Hutton, P. & Prys-Roberts, C. (1982) The oscillotonometer in theory and practice. *Br. J. Anaesth.*, **54**, 581–91.

Oakley, C.M. (1984) Mitral valve prolapse: harbinger of death or variant of normal? *Br. Med. J.*, **288**, 1853–4.

Opie, L.H. (1980) Drugs and the heart. A collection of papers published by *The Lancet*.

Pereira, E., Prys-Roberts, C., Dagnino, J. *et al.* (1985) Auscultatory measurement of arterial pressure during anaesthesia. A reassessment of Korotkow sounds. *Eur. J. Anaesth.*, **2**, 11–20.

Prys-Roberts, C. (1981) Cardiovascular monitoring in patients with vascular disease. *Br. J. Anaesth.*, **53**, 767–76.

Prys-Roberts, C. (1984) Anaesthesia and hypertension. *Br. J. Anaesth.*, **56**, 711–24.

Rao, T.L.K., Jacobs, K.H. & El-Etr, A.A. (1983) Reinfarction following anaesthesia in patients with myocardial infarction. *Anesthesiology*, **59**, 499–505.

Rees, J. (1984) Treatment of pulmonary hypertension in chronic bronchitis and emphysema. *Br. Med. J.*, **289**, 1398–9.

Reid, D.S. (1984) Sick sinus syndrome. *Br. J. Hosp. Med.*, **31**, 341–52.

Slogoff, S., Keats, A.S. & Arland, G. (1983) On the safety of radial artery cannulation. *Anesthesiology*, **59**, 42–7.

Waller, J.L. & Kaplan, J.A. (1981) Anaesthesia for patients with coronary heart disease. *Br. J. Anaesth.*, **53**, 757–65.

Zaidan, J.R. (1984) Pacemakers. *Anesthesiology*, **60**, 319–34.

2/Pulmonary function, chest disease and anaesthesia

Part 1: Lung function and assessment in the perioperative period
Preoperative considerations
  History
  Examination
  Investigations
  Preoperative preparation
Peroperative phase
  Minimal interference techniques
  Maximal support techniques
Postoperative phase
  The normal response to anaesthesia
  Assessment and initial management
  Management after extubation

Part 2: Problems of specific conditions
Obstructive airways disease
  Chronic bronchitis and emphysema
  Asthma
Restrictive airways disease
Pneumothorax, bullous conditions and bronchopleural fistula
Cystic fibrosis
Bronchiectasis and infections
Sarcoidosis
Carcinoma of the bronchus
Pulmonary effusions

Chronic airflow limitation is common in all urban communities. In Britain, chronic bronchitis and emphysema cause the loss of over 30 million working days and 25000 deaths each year. Asthmatics number 2–3% of the population but only 1200 die annually from their disease. With this prevalence of morbidity it is inevitable that many patients present for surgery with compromised pulmonary function.

For patients with any form of pulmonary dysfunction, the key to successful anaesthesia lies in the preoperative assessment and preparation, and in the postoperative management. In order to prevent repetition, the general principles of perioperative care in chronic chest disease and the response of normal lungs to anaesthesia are discussed first and the features and any additional points relevant to individual conditions are itemized later.

PART 1. LUNG FUNCTION AND ASSESSMENT IN THE PERIOPERATIVE PERIOD

Preoperative considerations

Functional assessment compares the patient with a healthy peer. The main objectives are to identify and minimize risk factors and to predict postoperative problems. Elective surgery need only be delayed if the patient's condition can be improved. In emergencies, even those with severe pulmonary disease will, with appropriate management, survive the operation. Their greatest danger is in the postoperative period.

History

The six cardinal symptoms of chest disease are cough, sputum, dyspnoea, wheeze, chest pain and haemoptysis. Remember that some of these may occur without parenchymal lung disease (e.g. a recurrent dry cough in neurosis). Frequently, people with chronic lung disease, because of its insidious onset, come to regard their own state as 'normal', so it is essential to ask leading questions about coughing, sputum, breathlessness, smoking and the limitations of physical activity. If there are positive replies to any of these questions, determine whether or not this is an acute exacerbation which could be improved with treatment before surgery, or whether this is his normal condition, making a delay unnecessary. Whilst patients are not always good predictors of their own state, do not ignore complaints of being worse than usual.

The subjective sensation of dyspnoea has still not been adequately explained in physiological terms and is most frequently regarded as an 'inappropriateness' between the amount of breathing the patient feels is required for his needs and the amount he in fact has produce. Dyspnoea can be caused by an increase in the work of breathing (all the causes of airways obstruction, decreased pulmonary compliance, restricted chest expansion), by increased pulmonary ventilation (compensatory for any cause of increased physiological dead space), by hysteria, by hyperventilation to reduce the $PaCO_2$ in compensation for a metabolic acidosis, by a weakness of the muscles of ventilation (neuromuscular defects) or when the chest expansion is limited by pain.

The variability of symptoms and the severity of exertional dyspnoea are particularly important. Variable symptoms tend to be caused by reversible airways disease. Bronchospasm may be precipitated by drugs (especially beta-adrenoceptor blockers and histamine-releasing agents) or endotracheal intubation and may be relieved by bronchodilators or halothane. The symptoms might be worse at a particular time of day.

The degree of exertional dyspnoea gives an index of the patient's compromised pulmonary function. Chest physicians often use a five point scale of the type given below.

Grade 1. Normal.
Grade 2. Able to walk with normal people of his own age and sex on the level but unable to keep up on hills and stairs.

Grade 3. Unable to keep up with normal people on the level but can walk long distances at his own pace.

Grade 4. Unable to walk more than 100 yards on the level before being stopped by breathlessness.

Grade 5. Unable to walk more than a few steps without dyspnoea, and becomes breathless on washing and dressing.

Ask about coughing and whether it is productive. A dry cough indicates bronchial irritation, pulmonary congestion or, rarely, distortion of the trachea or bronchi. Establish whether the sputum is purulent or mucoid and what volume is produced daily. These factors are particularly important in deciding the optimum condition likely to be attained. Check on the amount and duration of smoking and the desire to give up (encourage strongly!).

Assess the patient's mental state. Mild confusion is not uncommon in the elderly who have pulmonary disease. If necessary, take the history from the relatives. The patient may be a chronic dement or his mental confusion may date from the onset of illness. In the case of the latter he may well have CO_2 retention, hypoxia, electrolyte imbalance, hypoglycaemia, or have suffered a cerebrovascular accident secondary to his primary pathology. It is important to identify the cause of confusion (see Chapter 10) because it may well be reversible. Initially CO₂ retention gives rise to disturbed sleep and early morning headaches but as the $PaCO_2$ rises further it causes poor concentration, drowsiness and confusion.

Note the patient's medication, especially bronchodilators, antibiotics and steroids. Determine the effects of previous anaesthetics, and where possible look at the anaesthetic record for clues as to the best management. Chronic chest disease can eventually lead to cor pulmonale (see Chapter 1) and its presence should always be suspected. It will not be considered further in this chapter.

If the patient is on intermittent oxygen therapy, record the fractional inspired oxygen concentration (F_IO_2) which is known not to suppress the ventilatory drive.

Examination

General. Get a good view of the chest from the end of the bed and observe any asymmetry of movement. Diminished movement means pathology on that side of the chest. Note the use of the accessory muscles of respiration. The patient may be unable to finish a sentence without taking a breath, and may be leaning forward propped up on a pillow or on his hands. Facial anxiety, pursed lips (providing a physiological PEEP to prevent airway closure) and clubbed, warm, blue hands (central cyanosis) complete the picture of severe pulmonary disease. A tracheal tug may be present.

Restrictive lung disease tends to produce rapid, shallow breathing. Always look for tobacco-stained fingers and the ominous signs of weight loss.

Chest. Inspection, palpation, percussion and auscultation will reveal localizing signs the significance of which are outlined in Table 2.1. Think now whether this will influence intraoperative positioning or the use of endobronchial tubes.

The three clinical signs of chronic obstructive airways disease (COAD) are hyperinflation, prolongation of the expiratory phase and expiratory rhonchi. Hyperinflation causes the chest wall to be held permanently in the almost inflated position, the ventilatory excursion being provided by the diaphragm and the accessory muscles of respiration (which lift the whole rib cage vertically). In patients with COAD, there is usually sufficient hyperinflated lung between the heart and the chest wall to cause loss of cardiac dullness to percussion, and to make the heart sounds difficult to hear.

Prolongation of the expiratory phase may be obvious. In borderline cases, problems of expiration can be unmasked by asking the patient to breathe out from a maximal inspiration. In patients without COAD the expiration should be complete within 5 seconds and the patient should be capable of extinguishing a lighted match with an open mouth from 15 cm (Snider match test). Listening over the trachea during a forced expiration one ought not to hear any added rhonchi, and the initial coarse, rapid expiratory sounds should die away within 2 seconds.

Expiratory rhonchi are frequently regarded as the *sine qua non* of COAD. There are various theories explaining their production, the most popular being the presence of high velocity air passing through narrow or partially collapsed airways. In severe cases they are audible from the end of the bed. In mild cases they can be produced if the patient does a series of deep breaths and forced expirations.

The presence of sputum is usually obvious from a productive cough. Sputum is retained when the expulsive movements of coughing are so compromised by expiratory resistance or lack of muscle power that the airways are not cleared by the rapid exhalation of dead space and alveolar air. If there are coarse moist sounds at the lung bases which clear on deliberate coughing it is likely that there is no serious inability to expel sputum. The only rider to this is that very severe sputum retention may cause a silent area on auscultation because there is insufficient movement in the small air passages to produce either crepitations or rhonchi.

Table 2.1. Clinical findings in chest disease

Pathology	Chest Wall Movement	Mediastinal Displacement	Tactile Vocal Fremitus	Percussion Note	Breath Sounds	Added Sounds
Consolidation (e.g. lobar pneumonia, extensive pulmonary infarction, pneumonic tuberculosis)	Reduced on affected side	None	Increased	Dull	Bronchial	Fine crepitations early, coarse later
Massive collapse (e.g. obstruction by carcinoma, foreign body)	Reduced on affected side	Towards lesion	Absent	Dull	Decreased	None
Large pleural effusion	Reduced on affected side	Towards opposite side	Absent	Stony dull	Absent	Absent or pleural rub
Large pneumothorax	Reduced on affected side	Towards opposite side	Decreased	Hyperresonant	Decreased	None
Fibrosis	Reduced slightly on affected side	Towards lesion	Increased	Dull	Bronchial	Coarse crepitations
Emphysema	Reduced bilaterally (Barrel chest)	None	Decreased	Hyperresonant	Decreased	Absent
Bronchitis	Reduced bilaterally	None	Normal	Normal	Prolonged expiration	Rhonchi Coarse crepitations
Asthma	Reduced bilaterally	None	Normal or decreased	Normal	Prolonged expiration	High-pitched expiratory rhonchi

CVS. Look for the signs of cor pulmonale (see Chapter 1). Chronic hypercapnia is associated with poor handling of salt and water, so there is often peripheral oedema and a raised JVP. The dilated vascular bed results in a rapid, high volume, bounding pulse, and because the cardiac output is frequently increased, the BP may be raised. Pulsus paradoxus (Table 1.1) is seen in COAD and its degree is a reflection of the severity of obstruction. A difference between the systolic blood pressure in inspiration and expiration of 40 mmHg may be reached in severe disease.

Abdomen. There may be excessively strenuous movements to aid expiration in both obstructive and restrictive lung disease.

NS. Hypercapnia may be revealed by a coarse tremor or irregular twitching of the outstretched dorsiflexed hands.

Investigations

U & E's, LFT's. These should all be normal. If the urea is elevated check the nephrotoxicity of antibiotics and the dose of diuretics. Abnormalities of serum potassium are usually due to diuretics or steroids. Persistent cor pulmonale with a raised JVP can be produce altered liver function tests.

FBC. If polycythaemia is present suspect chronic hypoxia. An increased white cell count may indicate a chest infection.

Arterial blood gases. The physical signs of hypoxia and CO_2 retention are variable and need to be quantified by arterial blood gas estimations. Although not a routine investigation, they may be indicated if abnormalities are found on physical examination and are essential in patients with severely compromised ventilatory reserve. Baseline values (essential for severe respiratory cripples) can be invaluable in diagnosing and predicting postoperative problems. There are some points to remember in their interpretation:
• The PaO_2 varies throughout life, decreasing from a peak in young adulthood. Several regression equations are available but none have an upper limit of over 75 years. Consequently PaO_2 values for ages above this are all reached by unreliable extrapolation.
• The increased pulmonary venous admixture secondary to airway closure in dependent lung zones (an effect which increases with age), causes a reduction in PaO_2 of over 7.5 mmHg (1.0 kPa) from the sitting to the supine position. Hence, the position of the patient should always be recorded with the blood gas results. A useful

regression equation predicting the PaO_2 between the ages of 15 and 75 years for a patient sitting propped to 75° with the legs horizontal is that of Mellemgaard:

$$PaO_2 \text{ (mmHg)} = 104–0.27 \text{ (age in years)}.$$
$$PaO_2 \text{ (kPa)} = 13.8–0.036 \text{ (age in years)}.$$

The marked effect that venous admixture has on the PaO_2 occurs because of the nonlinearity of the oxygen dissociation curve. It causes little change in the $PaCO_2$ which remains constant throughout life.

● It is essential to relate the blood gas results to the inspired oxygen concentration. For a patient breathing air, or one who is intubated, this is easy. In order to ensure a constant F_IO_2 in a patient breathing oxygen enriched air from a facemask, the gas flow rate must exceed the peak inspiratory flow. This implies the need for a high flow rate from an oxygen/air mixer (30 litres/minute) into a well fitting facemask, or the use of a fixed performance device such as a Ventimask.

The patterns of blood gas derangement fall into three main subdivisions; hyperventilation, alveolar hypoventilation and a shunt or gas transfer defect. Often the latter two categories are mixed.

● In hyperventilation the PaO_2 is normal or elevated and the $PaCO_2$ is reduced. It is almost invariably due to anxious overventilation on the part of the patient and merely indicates healthy lungs. It is usually of no clinical importance. Exceptions are the hyperventilation of cerebral origin and the low $PaCO_2$ which is compensating for a metabolic acidosis.

● Alveolar hypoventilation can result from COAD, impaired mechanical ventilation (acute airways obstruction, stiff lungs, flail chest, pneumothorax), muscular weakness (myopathy, neuropathy) or central depression from drugs. In essence there is insufficient alveolar ventilation to both oxygenate the blood and to wash out the CO_2 so the $PaCO_2$ is elevated and the PaO_2 is reduced. It is important to recognize the presence of alveolar hypoventilation because the PaO_2 (but not the $PaCO_2$) can be greatly improved by increasing the F_IO_2. If the failure of alveolar ventilation is secondary to chronic abnormal neuromuscular function the patient often shows little clinical distress, but if it is secondary to a mechanical problem he will make vigorous efforts to increase his tidal and minute volumes.

● Shunt or gas transfer defects describe those situations in which there is no airways obstruction and the lungs are expanded normally, but there is imperfect interfacing of pulmonary blood and alveolar air. This can arise from both generalized parenchymal conditions

108

(sarcoidosis, fibrosing alveolitis, shock lung) and localized problems (pulmonary embolus, lobar collapse, lobar pneumonia). This collection of circumstances results in a situation where the $PaCO_2$ is normal (because hyperventilation can wash out CO_2 adequately from the normal lung tissue) but, because of the necessary mixing of blood with varying oxygen tensions in the pulmonary veins and because of the shape of the oxygen dissociation curve, the PaO_2 is reduced. In the presence of a shunt of 50% of the cardiac output, there is very little to be gained from increasing the F_IO_2 to very high levels. This merely increases the risk of pulmonary oxygen toxicity without improving the PaO_2.

CXR. This is an unnecessary investigation in fit asymptomatic people under 40 years old. For others, it is a useful, but expensive, screen to reveal localized disease of the thorax. In asymptomatic patients over 70 years old, over a third have abnormal findings. Nevertheless, it is often a poor indicator of the efficiency of the lungs as a gas exchanger.

Read a chest X-ray systematically and know the criteria of normality in a standard posterior-anterior (P-A) film. The following notes may help:
• Check the name and date.
• Check that there is no rotation. When correct the medial ends of the clavicles lie equally on either side of the spinous processes.
• With correct exposure the posterior ribs are just visible behind the cardiac shadow.
• On an inspiratory film the level of the diaphragm should be at, or below, the anterior part of the sixth rib and the posterior part of the tenth rib.
Then on a P-A film look at the individual structures:
• Diaphragm. Both the right and the left domes should be well defined. The right side is 2 cm above the left. Loss of costophrenic angles indicates pleural fluid.
• Ribs, pleura and bones. Compare right and left. Examine the rib edges. Look for pleural thickening. Look at the shoulder joints, clavicles, scapulae and visible vertebral bodies.
• Mediastinum. This should be centrally situated with a cardiothoracic ratio of less than 50%. The cardiac outline is illustrated in Chapter 1 (Fig. 1.3).
• Hila. These are made up of pulmonary arteries and upper lobe veins, concave on their lateral aspect with the left 1-2 cm higher than the right.
• Trachea. This should be central. The carina is at the lower border of the body of T4.

- Horizontal fissure. This goes from the right hilum to meet the 6th rib in the axilla.
- Lungs. Both lung fields should be of equal 'greyness' (due to blood in the pulmonary vasculature) with markings extending to the peripheries.
- Other. Look at the soft tissues surrounding the chest and below the diaphragm.

On a lateral film:

- One can localize lesions seen on a P-A film.
- The oblique fissure runs from T5 to the angle between the diaphragm and the anterior chest wall.
- Look at the dorsal vertebrae.
- Pay particular attention to the area below the lip of the diaphragm which is hidden on P-A view.
- Retrosternal and retrocardiac shadows should be approximately equal.

On an anteroposterior (A-P) film:

- The heart shadow is bigger.
- It is often difficult to tell whether it is A-P or P-A.

ECG. This should be normal but may show signs of right ventricular strain and cor pulmonale (see Chapter 1).

Lung function tests. The object of lung function tests is to put a numerical index on a given physiological variable so that the patient can be compared with a normal peer, the effect of treatment can be monitored, or the progress of disease or recovery from anaesthesia and other insults can be assessed. Their value as predictors of post-operative complications is the subject of some discussion (see later). Lung function tests need to be related to age, sex and height in standard tables. There is a wide range of normal va... the 95% confidence limits being approximately 20% either side of the mean. The three most useful and commonly measured variables are the vital capacity (VC or forced vital capacity, FVC), the forced expiratory volume in the first second of expiration (FEV_1) and the peak expiratory flow rate (PEFR). They can all be carried out at the bedside and depend upon the patient's co-operation. The three most commonly used instruments are the Wright's respirometer, the Vitalograph and a peak flow meter.

All lung function tests should be repeated at least three times and the best values taken. They can be done before and after bronchodilator treatment to assess the influence of reversible airways obstruction.

The Wright's respirometer is a miniature air-driven turbine which directly indicates the number of litres which have passed between two successive readings. Its factory calibration (which is grossly non-linear) is done with steady flows and it must be accurate to plus or minus 2% at 16.0 litres/minute and over read between +5 and +10% at 60 litres/minute. With intermittent flows its accuracy is adequate for clinical monitoring. Its greatest precision is at mean flow rates of 4–6 litres/minute and only during gross underventilation and moderate hyperventilation will its error exceed 10% of the scale reading. Even then, the error is such that it exaggerates the departure from normality and very importantly, underventilation is highlighted. It may be used to measure both the resting tidal ventilation (V_T) which is best averaged over several breaths, and the minute ventilation (by timing over a fixed period). Following a vital capacity manoeuvre (full inspiration to full expiration) the V_T/VC ratio can be calculated. This is an estimation of the lung's reserve capacity. Less conveniently, but more precisely, these measurements could be made with a wet spirometer or an integrating pneumotachograph. The most common instrument in clinical use for measuring the VC accurately is the Vitalograph.

The Vitalograph is a book bellows which moves after 100 cc of expired air has entered. It produces a trace as shown in Fig. 2.1. Note that the horizontal axis is calibrated up to only 6 seconds and that the vertical axes read expired volume corrected to both ATPS and BTPS. The VC is measured by asking the patient to exhale fully from a maximal inspiration. In healthy subjects fast or slow exhalation produces the same VC, but in those with airways obstruction a forced expiration causes alveolar air trapping and the 'slow VC' is larger. A problem with the Vitalograph is that the chart stops moving after 6 seconds. This may be insufficient for an expiration to residual volume in severe airways obstruction (which can take up to 30 seconds). The marker will, however, continue to record the expired volume by a vertical line (see Fig. 2.1). Some causes of a reduced vital capacity are given in Table 2.2.

The FEV_1 is reduced by both obstructive and restrictive defects. It is normally over 80% of the vital capacity. In obstructive defects the FEV_1 is proportionately much more reduced than the VC so the FEV_1/VC ratio decreases. In restrictive defects proportionality between FEV_1 and VC tends to be maintained (see Fig. 2.1).

An additional measurement which can be made from the Vitalograph trace is that of the mean rate of air flow over the middle half of the VC (i.e. between 25 and 75% of the VC). This is called the midexpiratory flow and is used because it is little affected by the resolve of the patient, thereby providing an 'effort independent' index of airways obstruction. The PEFR cannot be estimated from the Vitalo-

111

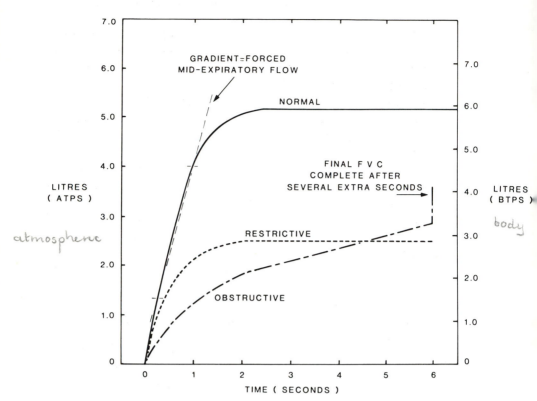

atmospheric

body

Fig. 2.1. Typical traces obtained from a Vitalograph in normals and in those with restrictive and obstructive lung disease. See text for further details.

Table 2.2. Some causes of a reduced vital capacity.

Reduced lung volume	Pulmonary fibrosis and infiltrations
	Large pleural effusions
	Collapsed or absent lobes or lung
	Pulmonary oedema
	Skeletal abnormalities
Inability to expand lungs	Limitation by pain
	Obesity
	Splinted diaphragm
Severe airways obstruction (because of premature airways closure)	Asthma
	Emphysema
	Chronic bronchitis
Muscular weakness	Neuromuscular blocking drugs
	Myopathies
	Neuropathies
	Myasthenia gravis

graph trace because of starting artefacts, and therefore has to be measured with a peak flow meter.

The PEFR (normal range in healthy adults is 450–650 litres/ minute) is a reproducible estimate of airways obstruction but it is extremely effort dependent and the value is low whenever the vital capacity is reduced (see Table 2.2). It is useful for following the progress of asthma and neuromuscular disorders. One of its most important uses is serial measurements in the same patient to assess the response to the treatment of airways obstruction. A genuine PEFR of under 120 litres/minute indicates severe obstruction. An artificially high PEFR can be obtained by the patient doing a sort of trick cough. An artificially low PEFR can be obtained from failing to expire from a maximal inspiration.

To our knowledge, there is no study employing large numbers of patients which relates the results of preoperative lung function tests to postoperative complications and eventual outcome (apart from those assessing the feasibility of pneumonectomy). Some general deductions can, however, be made. If the V_T is close to the VC, then there is little 'ventilatory reserve' and the adequacy of postoperative ventilation easily deteriorates with opioids and residual neuromuscular block (including that provided by a thoracic epidural). Irrespective of the cause, perhaps the most important feature of low values of FEV_1 and PEFR is an indication that the patient cannot expel air rapidly. Although these tests are not a direct measure of the 'power' of a cough, they are closely related to the ability to expel sputum. An FEV_1 of less than 2 litres or an FEV_1/VC ratio of less than 50% are sometimes quoted as values which define serious disease. The lower the value recorded, the more important it is to optimize the patient's state preoperatively, to monitor them closely in the postoperative period, and to subject them to vigorous and frequent physiotherapy. When lung function tests reveal abnormal results it is obviously important to combine them with a blood gas estimation. It is only this that demonstrates the effect which the ventilatory defect has on the efficacy of gas exchange.

Other pulmonary function tests must be carried out in a specialized laboratory and tend only to be done on highly selected cases. They are used primarily to follow the progress of chronic disease and are not usually helpful in preoperative assessment. For absolute lung volumes, a measurement involving residual volume must be done, usually by helium dilution. The single breath carbon monoxide test is used for measuring the barrier to the diffusion of gases, and tests of regional lung function require the use of radioisotopes. A single breath nitrogen test estimates the closing capacity and more recently the response to rebreathing carbon

113

dioxide has been used as an index of the sensitivity of the respiratory centre to a change in the $PaCO_2$.

Over the past few years there has been a trend amongst chest physicians to combine the results from a forced vital capacity manoeuvre (integrated electronically) with a measurement of residual volume by helium dilution to produce flow volume loops. Ideally they should show the difference between airways obstruction and restrictive lung disease (see Fig. 2.2) but because of the variations between normal subjects and patients they have as yet added little to the anaesthetic assessment of preoperative lung function.

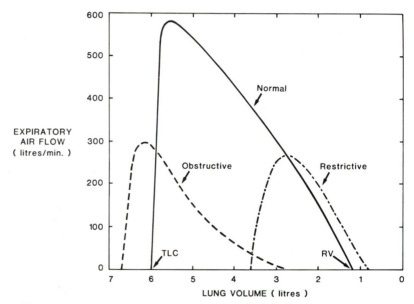

Fig. 2.2. Flow volume loops in normals and in patients with obstructive and restrictive lung disease. TLC = total lung capacity, RV = residual volume.

Preoperative preparation

As a result of preoperative assessment the degree of pulmonary incapacity will be apparent. The objective is to optimize pulmonary function prior to surgery. In emergencies this may be impossible.

Patients for elective operations with chronic lung disorders need to be admitted several days before surgery and at a time of year when their condition is not exacerbated. If there is a reversible component to their airways obstruction, bronchodilator therapy (e.g. nebulized salbutamol) ought to be started. Sputum should be collected for culture and sensitivity and antibiotics prescribed on the advice of the microbiologist. Many hospitals have prescribing policies for antibiotics to try and prevent the emergence of resistant bacterial strains. This is particularly relevant to the ICU.

The physiotherapist and patient should meet as early as possible to establish rapport. This enables postural drainage, percussion, coughing and breathing exercises to be practised preoperatively. Incentive spirometry has also been used with success in patients with COAD, but its exact position and benefits are as yet undetermined.

It is important during this period to assess the patient's ability to breathe when lying flat especially if local, regional or facemask techniques are envisaged. Outline the problems of postoperative analgesia to the patient and discuss the acceptability of various techniques.

Two of the most severe aggravators of postoperative pulmonary function, obesity and smoking, are very refractory to advice, but both should be reduced if at all possible. There is now evidence that there is a substantial reduction in postoperative pulmonary complications if patients have stopped smoking for at least 8 weeks before surgery. This implies that anaesthetists have to educate their surgeons to encourage patients to lose weight and stop smoking at the outpatient appointment. If this has been unsuccessful, as a bare minimum try to prevent smoking in the 24 hours before surgery in order to reduce the carboxyhaemoglobin content of the blood and hence improve oxygen transport. There are, however, some badly addicted patients who, if they have co-existing heart disease, may have angina induced in the stressful preoperative period because they are unable to experience the relaxing effects of a pipe or cigarette. With them, discretion must be exercised. One solution is to allow smoking to continue; another is to prescribe an anxiolytic.

For premedication it is sensible to avoid ventilatory depressant drugs. If an anxiolytic is required, a small dose of a short acting benzodiazepine is suitable (e.g. Temazepam 10–20 mg).

Peroperative phase

Opinions differ widely as to the best method of anaesthetizing patients with pulmonary disease. Views vary from those who would use a local or regional technique at all costs to those who recommend IPPV on all occasions. The pros and cons of each technique are described below. In practise the optimum management is a reasoned decision based on the site and length of operation, and the wishes of the patient, anaesthetist and surgeon.

Minimal interference techniques

The logic of this philosophy is to use local or regional blocks to provide adequate anaesthesia and to keep the patient conscious or only

115

mildly sedated whilst breathing spontaneously and retaining the ability to cough. It is most applicable to fairly short operations on the limbs and lower abdomen.

Advantages are that it avoids upsetting the patient's ventilatory control and the problems of weaning from the ventilator. If the patient's ventilation is barely adequate, it does not reduce the patient's functional residual capacity (FRC) or increase the physiological dead space as does a general anaesthetic. There is no reversal of physiological intrathoracic pressure swings which might put emphysematous bullae at risk. It also avoids residual neuro-muscular block. Another advantage is that the patient can use his nebulizer if bronchodilation proves necessary.

Disadvantages are that an awake patient must be acceptable to the surgeon, and the theatre staff must be careful with their comments. The patient may have to lie still for long periods in an embarrassing position resulting in both mental and physical discomfort. The postural change may worsen compromised ventilatory function to a distressing level, but this can often be overcome by operating with the patient semi-recumbent. Long procedures are likely to be punctuated by coughing, making the operation longer if not im-possible (e.g. tendon suturing, hernia repair, prostatic resection). The patient needs to have a robust personality because the treatment of intraoperative anxiety with intravenous sedatives, although often successful, can be harmful. They can reduce the conscious level, suppress ventilation, cause confusion and create problems with the airway. Similar problems surround the use of sedative premedica-tions. Nitrous oxide/oxygen/air mixtures given through a lightly applied facemask are often well tolerated. With patients who rely on a hypoxic drive, the F_IO_2 must not be allowed to rise to a level which suppresses ventilation.

It is most important not to minimize the potential dangers of regional techniques. A pneumothorax from a supraclavicular block or an intravenous injection during a brachial plexus block can be disastrous in the presence of a compromised cardio-pulmonary sys-tem. When using spinal or epidural blockade beware of fluid over-load which may later cause pulmonary oedema. A reasonable upper limit of fluid load is 500 ml of 0.9% saline in addition to the intra-operative losses. Hypotension caused through sympathetic blockade not responding to this is best treated with vasoconstrictors.

An awake patient is no excuse for inadequate monitoring but the ex-tent will depend on the individual case. If it is felt necessary to have an arterial line purely for sampling intraoperative blood gases then mini-mal interference is probably the wrong technique to choose since the blood gas status can only be corrected by manual manoeuvres.

Maximal support techniques

In fit, healthy, anaesthetized patients breathing spontaneously there is a reduction in the FRC. The physiological dead space (V_D) to tidal volume (V_T) ratio (including apparatus dead space) is approximately 0.5 when intubated and 0.65 when breathing from a mask. It is not uncommon for the alveolar ventilation to fall to below 2 litres/minute and for the $PaCO_2$ to rise to 70 mmHg (9.3 kPa) after one hour. Consequently, in patients with pulmonary disease, spontaneously breathing techniques are really only suitable for short procedures (e.g. check cystoscopy).

For longer operations, particularly those on the upper abdomen, there is an increasing tendency to use a balanced technique with paralysis, analgesia and ventilation. Once this decision has been made, there is usually no intraoperative problem in maintaining the PaO_2 and $PaCO_2$ at any desired level and the anaesthetist has effectively transferred the majority of his difficulties to the postoperative period. A combination of general and local anaesthesia can have the advantage of minimizing the dose of muscle relaxant needed (and hence the likelihood of postoperative muscle weakness) and avoiding ventilatory depression from narcotics.

The extent of invasive monitoring is an individual decision and may be determined by the type of surgery but in most of the severe 'respiratory cripples' an arterial line for the measurement of blood gases proves invaluable.

In the fit, healthy patient having a general anaesthetic there is a virtual shunt of 10% of the cardiac output producing an alveolar-arterial PCO_2 gradient of only 0.6 mmHg (0.08 kPa). There is also a well-defined alveolar plateau when the expired CO_2 is recorded (see Fig. 2.3) which therefore represents an accurate measure of $PaCO_2$. In the patient with pulmonary disease there is frequently not only an increased virtual shunt but also a wide variation in the efficiency of

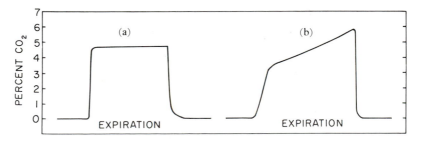

Fig. 2.3. Expiratory CO_2 traces. (a) Normal. (b) Patient with obstructive lung disease.

alveolar gas exchange causing a slope in the expired CO_2 trace (see Fig. 2.3). Under these conditions, the $PaCO_2$ cannot be estimated accurately from the end-tidal PCO_2 and arterial blood samples are needed.

There are good theoretical reasons for maintaining the intraoperative $PaCO_2$ at the preoperative level. This continues the previous steady-state acid-base homeostasis and prevents shifts in CSF bicarbonate which would take time to recover later. With high tidal and minute volumes this often necessitates the addition of CO_2 to the fresh gas flow or the use of a partial rebreathing circuit. Many workers, however, report success ventilating patients who are normally hypercapnic to a $PaCO_2$ of 40 mmHg (5.3 kPa) and then allowing the $PaCO_2$ to rise at the end of the operation. Doing this, spontaneous ventilation, if it resumes, is usually triggered at a $PaCO_2$ below the preoperative level. A prolonged period of hyperventilation inevitably produces a net loss of CO_2 from the body. In the postoperative period this implies that there will be an obligatory period of hypoventilation whilst the deficit is repaid.

There is little hard evidence available that certain ventilatory patterns are preferable to others. However, it is logical to supply large tidal volumes (12–15 ml/kg) and a sufficient inspiratory time (either with a slow rate or an inspiratory hold) to maximize the equality of ventilation between fast and slow alveoli. Similarly, the expiratory phase should be long enough for a full exhalation. Avoid excessively high inflation pressures because of the dangers of bursting an emphysematous bulla.

Patients with copious secretions or focal sepsis may benefit from appropriate positioning to keep the affected lung dependent, or endobronchial intubation to isolate the good lung from the bad lung. Frequent aspiration should be carried out to prevent soiling of the good lung.

Intraoperative fluid balance is important. Dehydration makes secretions more viscous and difficult to suck out and overhydration risks postoperative pulmonary oedema. In the presence of normal renal function the latter can, provided that it is recognized, be treated effectively with diuretics.

Postoperative phase

The normal response to anaesthesia

In all patients who have been anaesthetized with nitrous oxide there is an unimportant, transient decrease in the PaO_2 of up to 10 mmHg (1.3 kPa) which lasts for 10 minutes when they resume breathing air.

118

It can be prevented by giving 100% oxygen for 2 minutes at the end of the operation.

The major effects of anaesthesia on pulmonary gas exchange in the postoperative period depend upon the site of surgery. In the operative and immediate postoperative period the FRC is reduced with alveolar gas trapping and there is an increased right to left shunt. The cause is unknown but it can produce falls in PaO_2 of up to 30 mmHg (4.0 kPa) when breathing air and compared with the preoperative level. It is easily corrected by giving 30–40% oxygen on a facemask. After the first hour or two those patients who have undergone limb or superficial body surgery reverse these changes and effectively return to their normal preoperative state. However, when patients with previously healthy lungs undergo abdominal or thoracic surgery this reduction in oxygenation continues for at least 48 hours and may extend for up to 5 days. This effect is worst with upper abdominal, thoracic and paramedian incisions and least with lower abdominal incisions. Factors known to exacerbate these effects are wound pain (prevents deep breathing, can reduce vital capacity by up to 50%, reduces expiratory force), abdominal distension (splints the diaphragm), the supine position (when the relationship of FRC to closing volume is least favourable) and over transfusion (tendency to pulmonary oedema).

All the above changes are intensified in patients with poor preoperative lung function, cigarette smokers, the obese and the aged. They are also the groups most at risk from infection and segmental collapse secondary to sputum retention.

Assessment and initial management

After reversal of neuromuscular block some patients will make ventilatory movements which are obviously adequate on clinical grounds alone, and they can be extubated immediately. In others it is preferable to make a more formal assessment of the ventilatory state before extubation. Some anaesthetists do this purely on clinical grounds, principally by assessing distress, ventilatory rate, tachycardia and adequacy of tissue oxygenation. Others apply numerical values such as a ventilation rate below 30 breaths/minute, a PaO_2 over 70 mmHg on 40% FIO_2, a vital capacity of over 12–15 ml/kg and an inspiratory force of over 30 cm H_2O.

Once the patient is extubated it can be very difficult to make an accurate visual assessment of the adequacy of ventilation, or to measure tidal or minute volumes. Other measurements such as VC and PEFR are dependent on the co-operation of the patient and may indicate low values because of sedation, pain or residual neuro-

119

muscular block and may not reflect the adequacy or otherwise of ventilation. *If there is any doubt it is best to measure the blood gases on a known F_IO_2.*

If ventilation is absent or obviously inadequate continue IPPV while the cause is being identified. Once muscular weakness has been excluded by peripheral nerve stimulation the major factors influencing apnoea are the $PaCO_2$, the level of sedation and drug-induced ventilatory depression. Gradually let the $PaCO_2$ rise to the preoperative value and allow a sufficient time for the elimination of volatile agents. If the pupils are small, consider opioid reversal with naloxone, the dose being titrated so as not to aggravate postoperative pain. Once spontaneous ventilation recommences keep the endotracheal tube in place. This allows accurate control of the inspired gas mixture and ease of aspiration of secretions until ventilation is established as satisfactory.

Further measures which can improve borderline ventilation are continuous positive airway pressure (CPAP) and nursing the patient in the sitting or semirecumbent position. Both of these measures improve the FRC. Another possiblity is to 'drive' ventilation with the stimulant drug doxapram. There is a wide variation in the infusion rate required and it must be adjusted to give adequate ventilation without an unpleasant level of nausea, mental anxiety and peripheral tremor.

Occasionally, in that minority of patients who are on hypoxic drive (they normally have a preoperative PaO_2 of below 50 mmHg) it will be necessary to lower the F_IO_2 to stimulate ventilation. It is pertinent here to stress the dangers of uncontrolled oxygen therapy to these patients. Initially the PaO_2 is maintained but the $PaCO_2$ rises and ultimately leads to coma, cessation of breathing and hypoxia. Once they are extubated, use fixed performance masks (such as a Ventimask) with either 24% or 28% O_2.

If there is still clinical and objective evidence of ventilatory failure IPPV must be continued. This may only be a short-term requirement to allow for further metabolism of drugs.

Management after extubation

After extubation, the patient should ideally go to a 24 hour recovery unit. If this is not available, in borderline cases, an overnight stay on ICU is the safest recourse, despite the possibly unnecessary use of expensive resources.

Posture. Provided the surgical procedure allows it, minimize the factors reducing the FRC by sitting the patient up.

120

Oxygen therapy. After upper abdominal and thoracic operations hypoxia persists for several days. Oxygen therapy is universally advocated but the desirable amount and duration are poorly established. A sensible approach is to supply an F_IO_2 (by mask or nasal prongs) sufficient to maintain adequate oxygenation, usually for 24 hours. Reassess at this time if it needs to be continued. Always identify and treat any cause of alveolar hypoventilation (narcotics, pneumothorax, pain, sputum retention).

Analgesia. Good pain relief allows maximal ventilatory activity. When using narcotics this represents a balance between pain reduction and the depression of ventilation and the conscious level. There is enormous individual variation in the response to opioids and it is often better to give the initial dose gradually IV and titrate it against ventilatory depression (this is usually maximal from 5–10 minutes after injection).

The reduction of pain of upper abdominal incisions by regional blockade has frequently been quoted as optimizing postoperative lung function. Thoracic epidurals have the facility for easy top-ups and can certainly provide excellent analgesia. Epidural analgesia can be with a local anaesthetic or opioid, given intermittently, or by continuous infusion. Remind the nursing staff of the dangers of hypotension, especially in the sitting position. A problem occasionally encountered in severe restrictive lung disease is a deterioration in gas exchange as a result of paralysis of intercostal and abdominal musculature. Intercostal blockade, although effective, is not easy to repeat and can cause a pneumothorax.

Secretions. The ability to cough and remove secretions is of paramount importance and a 'fruity' cough with no sputum production is a bad prognostic sign. Try to remove secretions by postural drainage and physiotherapy. This is not always possible because of the surgical procedure. The best results are obtained if the peak action of both the analgesia and the physiotherapist coincide.

A portable chest X-ray will help to identify any localized problems such as lobar collapse. Fibreoptic bronchoscopy under local anaesthesia by a skilled user can sometimes remove a plug of mucus without recourse to intubation.

Obstructive apnoea. Although the magnitude of the problem is not yet defined, sleep apnoea has, over the past few years, been regarded with increasing suspicion as a cause of postoperative hypoxia. It has been shown that sleep, and most probably anaesthesia, causes a reduction in the muscle tone of the tongue and pharynx, thus allowing these structures to collapse inwards and occlude the airway.

121

These changes may possibly persist up to 12 hours after anaesthesia and are more common when parenteral opioids are used.

Apnoeic periods occur almost entirely during sleep and are associated with oxygen desaturation. When patients with obstructive airways disease fall asleep they may develop severe hypoxia associated with obstructive apnoea.

The loss of muscular tone is also apparent in the intercostals (but not the diaphragm which has little spindle control) and these have a poor compensatory response to partial or complete obstruction of the airway.

PART II. PROBLEMS OF SPECIFIC CONDITIONS

Only the features relevant to individual conditions are described in this section. It is assumed that the overall management of the patient will, for the most part, follow the principles outlined in Part I.

Obstructive airways disease

This is caused by the narrowing of the peripheral parts of the bronchial tree by muscular activity, oedema or mucus and presents as chronic bronchitis, emphysema or asthma. The interrelationship between the three conditions is shown in the Venn diagram of Fig. 2.4. They may occur singly or in combination in any patient. The airway narrowing associated with chronic bronchitis and emphysema is largely irreversible. There is, however, a degree of overlap with asthma because some asthmatics have a productive cough and patients with chronic bronchitis and emphysema may have a component of reversible airway constriction.

Chronic bronchitis and emphysema

Chronic bronchitis is defined clinically as a persistent cough with sputum production for more than 3 months of each year for three consecutive years. Emphysema is defined purely pathologically as dilatation of air spaces distal to the terminal bronchioles, with destruction of their walls. Its extent can only be determined post mortem. A tiny minority of patients have pure emphysema. The rest have mixed disease which is related to cigarette smoking, urban pollution and low social class. Chronic bronchitis causes airway obstruction by mucus in the lumen and inflammation in the walls of the bronchioles. Emphysema causes obstruction by loss of elastic tissue and airway collapse on expiration.

They present with any degree of ventilatory disablement. Exacerbations are often due to superimposed infection by Haemophilus-

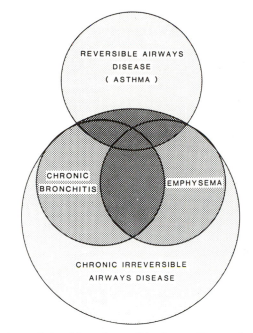

REVERSIBLE AIRWAYS
DISEASE
(ASTHMA)

CHRONIC
BRONCHITIS

EMPHYSEMA

CHRONIC IRREVERSIBLE
AIRWAYS DISEASE

Fig. 2.4. The interrelationships of reversible airways disease, chronic bronchitis and emphysema.

Influenzae and Streptococcus Pneumoniae and these should be treated prior to surgery. Even at their best these patients have excess bronchial mucus predisposing to infection and distal collapse from blocked airways. Clinically they are represented by a continuous spectrum ranging from the 'pink puffer' to the 'blue bloater'. The underlying cause for these two distinct entities is not known. Although at autopsy the 'pink puffer' always has extensive emphysema, it can also be found to a similar extent in 'blue bloaters', so the exact underlying physiological and pathological processes are still unclear. The two syndromes are contrasted in Table 2.3.

The degree of reversible airways obstruction is assessed by a trial of the effects of bronchodilators and/or steroids on the results of lung function tests, (usually the PEFR and FEV_1). Those using steroid sprays may develop oral moniliasis and this can be transmitted to the chest by intubation.

ANAESTHETIC CONSIDERATIONS

Two classes of drug to prescribe with great care are sedatives and beta-adrenoceptor blockers. Oversedation can precipitate ventilatory failure. Beta-adrenoceptor blockers cause bronchoconstriction by $beta_2$ blockade, thus, if they are needed a cardioselective type (e.g.

123

Table 2.3. The clinical and investigative findings in the 'pink buffer' and the 'blue bloater'.

	'Pink Puffer'	'Blue Bloater'
Clinical Features	Pink, breathless Not cyanosed Thin, wasted Signs of cardiac failure and fluid retention rare.	Warm blue hands Central cyanosis Obese No dyspnoea Signs of cor pulmonale common.
ECG	Normal	Changes of cor pulmonale
FBC	Hb normal	Polycythaemia
CXR	Normal in mild-moderate disease Later, marked hyperinflation with long small heart Large retrosternal window on lateral view	Normal in mild-moderate disease Later, normal sized lung fields with cardiomegaly and upper lobe blood diversion
Lung FT's	Obstructive pattern Total lung capacity increased VC reduced	Obstructive pattern Normal lung capacity VC reduced
Gases	Normal at rest, rapid onset of hypoxia with exercise	Hypoxaemic with raised $PaCO_2$
Asleep	Maintain a normal PaO_2	May have frequent spells of oxygen desaturation.

acebutalol, atenolol, metoprolol) should be used, but only in very small doses. Even then it may cause a rapid deterioration in effective ventilation.

All patients with chronic airflow limitation and especially those with overdistended lungs are at risk of developing a pneumothorax. This should always be suspected if there is a sudden onset of breathlessness (especially if it is associated with sudden pleuritic chest pain) in the perioperative period. It is a particular risk during anaesthesia when high ventilation pressures are required and the location of a chest drain should always be known.

Hypotension in these patients can be dangerous for three reasons. Firstly, collapsed lung segments are often poorly perfused because of compensation by hypoxic pulmonary vasoconstriction. The use of sodium nitroprusside and other vasodilating agents reduces this compensation, thus increasing the shunt and reducing the PaO_2. Secondly, hypotension always causes an increase in the physiological dead space with consequent deterioration in CO_2 removal and the PaO_2. Thirdly, the use of ganglion and beta-adrenoceptor blockers as part of the technique may precipitate or intensify the broncho-constrictive component of airways obstruction. Posturing and sub-cutaneous injections of local anaesthetics with adrenaline are really the only safe methods of assisting haemostasis.

Asthma

Asthma is difficult to define accurately but an adequate description is 'a clinical syndrome of multifactorial origin, the predominant symptoms of which are dyspnoea and wheeze of fluctuating severity and in which reversibility of airflow obstruction can be demonstrated by objective measures'. There are two main clinical groups.

Extrinsic asthma (childhood, allergic, atopic asthma) begins in childhood and there is usually a family history of atopy and asthma. Acute attacks tend to be precipitated by specific circumstances, e.g. pollens, house dust, cats, various foods, exercise, excitement, cold air or pulmonary infection. Other precipitants are certain contacts and occupations (animals, farming, pharmaceutical and plastics laboratories) and drugs (aspirin, paracetamol, phenylbutazone and indomethacin). There are often positive skin sensitivity tests, blood eosinophilia, and a good response to sympathomimetic aerosols or sodium cromoglycate.

Approximately 70% of asthmatic children will outgrow their asthma by the age of 12 years. Very few need steroid treatment. The severity of the condition is assessed by the frequency of attacks, time off school, their growth rate and the number of hospital admissions. Pigeon chest deformities are now very rare because of effective treatments. Attacks may occur abruptly and be brief in duration (a few hours), or may last intermittently for a week or more. In acute episodes the PEFR and FEV_1 are reduced, but are normal at other times. Status asthmaticus is defined as an asthma attack of over 24 hours duration.

Treatment of the acute attack is by sympathomimetic inhalers or nebulisers and intravenous salbutamol or aminophylline. Chronic control is by sympathomimetic or steroid inhalers, oral salbutamol or theophylline or by sodium cromoglycate. The latter is a mast cell stabilizer taken regularly as a preventative measure.

Intrinsic asthma (late onset, non atopic asthma) begins in adult life and there is usually no allergic or family history and no demonstrable skin sensitivities. There is blood and sputum eosinophilia and attacks are less responsive to therapy than they are in extrinsic asthma. Subnormal figures for PEFR and FEV_1 may be recorded for weeks, months or years with acute deteriorations during exacerbations, which are often associated with infection.

The diagnosis of late onset asthma can be very difficult and is often confirmed by the reversibility of lung function tests after bronchodilator or steroid therapy combined with the exclusion of other con-

125

ditions. Its differential diagnosis includes chronic bronchitis (with which it may co-exist), polyarteritis nodosa, extrinsic alveolitis (farmer's lung etc) aspergillosis and the carcinoid syndrome.

These patients often need to take steroids indefinitely, either orally or by inhalation in addition to using sympathomimetics or theophylline derivatives.

The margin between the 'extrinsic' and 'intrinsic' patients is, nevertheless, very blurred and they should only be thought of as representing the ends of a spectrum.

The anaesthetist becomes involved with asthmatic patients in two ways: in anaesthetizing an asthmatic who is on treatment or in remission and in the treatment of very severe asthma on the ICU.

ANAESTHETIC CONSIDERATIONS

When taking the history, ask about the frequency and severity of attacks, what drugs the patient takes and what has successfully aborted an exacerbation in the past. The most sensitive indices of bronchial tone are the PEFR and FEV_1. Ideally, the patient should be at their best for surgery but this is not always possible in emergencies. Allow them to continue their normal medication up to the time of operation and bring their inhaler to theatre with them. In severe asthmatics prophylactic antibiotic therapy is indicated. All patients need a chest X-ray, both as a baseline and to show the presence of bullae and hyperinflation.

Despite its prevalence in the community, there are very few articles dealing with anaesthesia for asthmatics. However, the three most commonly quoted problems are bronchospasm on intubation or during gas induction, the possibilities of a pneumothorax when on IPPV, and bronchospasm secondary to thiopentone or other histamine-releasing drugs (curare, suxamethonium, morphine, etc.).

Adequate premedication is important because an attack can be precipitated by fear. An antihistamine such as promethazine can be particularly useful both in preventing bronchospasm and in producing general sedation. If analgesia is also desired with the premedication, then pethidine is preferred because it does not release histamine. Alternatively, benzodiazepines are satisfactory. Methohexitone, etomidate and ketamine are all suitable induction agents but thiopentone is to be avoided.

Bronchospasm after intubation can be minimized by spraying the cords and trachea with local anaesthetic first, and by not intubating in a light plane of anaesthesia. During intubation only sufficient endotracheal tube should be passed for the upper part of the cuff to be just below, but not touching the cords. This ensures that the carina is not irritated.

If bronchospasm does occur after intubation (readily recognized by raised inflation pressure or wheezing), check the position of the tube and if necessary pull it back, then manage the episode as an ordinary acute asthmatic attack.

There are four possible therapeutic approaches.

• The use of a sympathomimetic agent to relax the bronchioles by an agonist action on beta$_2$ adrenoceptors. This stimulates the action of intracellular adenyl cyclase which converts ATP to cyclic AMP. The standard drug is salbutamol (2–4 µg/kg IV over 15 minutes). Although much smaller doses can be effective when the drug is inhaled by a conscious person experiencing an asthmatic attack, aerosols are extremely difficult to use on an unconscious person.

• The use of a theophylline derivative which, by inhibiting phosphodiesterase, prevents the breakdown of cyclic AMP and thereby increases its intracellular concentration. This results in relaxation of bronchial muscle. IV aminophylline (up to 7 mg/kg over 15 minutes) is the most commonly recommended regimen. It is probably the drug of choice for use during anaesthesia since it does not have the same degree of generalized sympathomimetic activity that beta$_2$ agonists possess.

• Direct relaxation of bronchial muscle at a cellular level by volatile anaesthetic agents. Traditionally ether has the reputation of being the supreme bronchodilator but halothane or isoflurane will break most episodes of spasm. It may be dangerous to follow sympathomimetic bronchodilators with halothane because of the reduced threshold for dysrhythmias.

• The prophylactic use of steroids at this stage is controversial.

If these measures fail, and cyanosis continues with high inflation pressures, always suspect a pneumothorax. Preferential ventilation or air trapping can cause an emphysematous bulla to burst and a large pneumothorax quickly develops. This may well become a tension pneumothorax and on time and volume cycled ventilators the inflation pressure will continue to rise. The situation then requires urgent treatment to prevent a fatality. Clinically, there is increasing cyanosis and a low blood pressure with the classical physical signs of a pneumothorax (see Table 2.1). At the least suspicion insert a wide bore cannula (a large IV needle will do in emergencies) and immediately follow it with a chest drain. This should always be put on to free drainage to an underwater seal because suction pumps cannot deal with the gas transmission into the pneumothorax during IPPV.

The response of asthmatics to histamine-releasing drugs is unpredictable. It is therefore sensible only to use suxamethonium in emergencies, to use pancuronium as the muscle relaxant of choice and to use pethidine or fentanyl as the analgesic.

After operation if the patient cannot immediately resume his maintenance therapy, rectal aminophylline or an IV infusion of aminophylline both work well.

Hypotensive anaesthesia can pose problems. There is no evidence, if there is normal preoperative lung function, that it is in any way harmful. However, bronchospasm under hypotensive anaesthesia (which invariably increases physiological dead space) can be disastrous, so beta-adrenoceptor blockers, ganglion blockers and trimetaphan should never be used as part of the technique. Safer methods include regional block, SNP and halothane.

Intraoperative dysrhythmias, if they need treating (and are not due to hypoxia or a raised PaCO$_2$) are better treated with lignocaine, verapamil or disopyramide rather than beta-adrenoceptor blockers.

THE TREATMENT OF SEVERE ASTHMA

The changes in lung volumes during an asthmatic attack are shown in Fig. 2.5. Note the greatly increased residual volume and functional residual capacity, the prolonged inspiratory and expiratory time, and the reduced vital capacity and inspiratory reserve volume. Apart from the degree of ventilatory distress and inability to speak the following clinical features strongly suggest that the attack is severe.

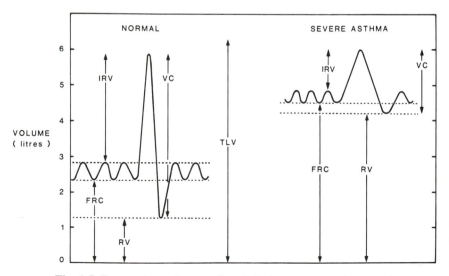

Fig. 2.5. Lung volumes in normals and during a severe asthma attack. TLV = total lung volume. VC = vital capacity. IRV = inspiratory reserve volume. RV = residual volume. FRC = functional residual capacity.

128

- Tachycardia over 120 beats/minute (slows in profound hypoxia).
- Marked pulsus paradoxus (systolic BP more than 20 mmHg lower in inspiration than expiration). Later hypotension occurs from hypoxia.
- Indrawing of the intercostal muscles as well as the use of accessory muscles.
- Mental and physical tiredness.
- Confusion, drowsiness, central cyanosis and so little air entry that there is a 'silent chest' are particularly ominous.

Inability to talk implies inability to drink and the patients usually require aggressive rehydration.

Investigations

Always do a chest X-ray to exclude a pneumothorax, pneumomediastinum, atelectasis or infiltration. Arterial blood gases are essential and a low PaO_2 combined with a rising $PaCO_2$ is evidence that the patient's ventilation is failing. Lung function tests are impossible to perform in a severe attack.

Management

Usually there is a trial of conservative therapy the results of which decide whether or not to ventilate. Death from severe acute asthma is due to hypoxic cardiac arrest. Since these patients do not retain CO_2 (unless there is co-existing chronic bronchitis) oxygen can and should be given in high concentrations. Often the mask distresses the patient and it is better to use high flows on a loose fitting mask, or to employ nasal prongs. In very serious cases where ventilation is probably necessary in the immediate future put the concentration up to 100% oxygen.

In severe attacks the patient ceases to show any response to bronchodilator aerosols, because the ventilation is so poor that insufficient quantities of drug reach the lungs. Therefore, persistence with this line of treatment is futile.

The drug of choice is probably aminophylline, up to 7 mg/kg IV loading dose over 10–15 minutes followed by an infusion of up to 0.9 mg/kg/hour. By working on cyclic AMP via inhibition of phosphodiesterase this does not have the pronounced cardiac side effects of salbutamol which are more dangerous in the presence of hypoxia and hypercarbia. Give a loading dose of 200 mg hydrocortisone followed by 1000 mg in divided doses in the first 24 hours.

Rehydrate aggressively. Check the potassium every 2 hours when steroids and/or salbutamol are used. The use of sodium bicarbonate to correct a severe metabolic acidosis is controversial.

[handwritten margin note: pokalaemia / high circulating catecholamines]

129

The majority of the patients, if they are going to do so, respond rapidly to treatment. Indications for ventilation are:
- Intolerable respiratory, physical and mental distress.
- Bradycardia and hypotension.
- $PaCO_2$ over 50 mmHg and rising, despite treatment.
- PaO_2 below 50 mmHg and falling, despite treatment.

Intubating and ventilating an asthmatic patient is a difficult process and should not be undertaken by an inexperienced anaesthetist working alone. Always obtain reliable nursing or ODA assistance. Take the head of the bed off. Preoxygenate the patient with 100% oxygen in his most comfortable position, usually sitting forward. Induce anaesthesia with methohexitone (or ketamine or etomidate) followed by atropine and suxamethonium. Either intubate sitting or lower him to the horizontal, an assistant supporting the back of his neck with one hand and applying cricoid pressure with the other. Intubate with a sterile, low pressure, cuffed tube.

When setting the ventilator, start with 50% oxygen and ensure a long expiratory phase. Use a slow ventilatory rate and adjust the inspiratory flow to try and keep the inflation pressure below 50 mmHg. Always be alert to the possibility of a pneumothorax. Use sedatives and relaxants as required and monitor the progress of the asthma by blood gas estimations, keeping the F_IO_2 and inflation pressures as low as possible. If there is no improvement over the first few hours, halothane or ether will 'break' most episodes of bronchospasm. Extubation should be undertaken when the lung compliance has returned to normal and the patient has breathed spontaneously for several hours without distress.

Restrictive pulmonary disease

A restrictive expiratory pattern on a spirometer trace (see Fig. 2.1) has many aetiologies caused by both lung disease (intrinsic) and other conditions (extrinsic). All are characterized by an increased work of breathing necessary to overcome a low total compliance and a rapid, shallow pattern of ventilation is characteristic. Blood gas tensions (especially the $PaCO_2$) are well preserved until the disease is well advanced. Lung function tests reveal a decrease in total lung capacity and all its subdivisions (V_T, IRV, FRC, RV, VC, ERV), with a high V_D/V_T ratio.

The importance of restrictive lung disease for the anaesthetist is that considerable effort is required to expand the lungs (hence requiring good reversal of relaxants) and the reduction in vital capacity may so reduce the FEV_1 and PEFR *pari passu* that effective expectoration of sputum and secretions is impossible.

Causes of *extrinsic* restrictive disease are deformities or rigidity of the thoracic cage, e.g. kyphoscoliosis, obesity, ascites, mesothelioma and pregnancy. A similar condition is also produced by neuromuscular disorders. In extrinsic restrictive disease, the function of the lung parenchyma is absolutely normal, the problem being that the bellows function of the lung presents an inadequate fresh gas supply to the alveoli. The chest X-ray, apart from being of low volume, is effectively normal.

Causes of *intrinsic* restrictive disease are cryptogenic fibrosing alveolitis, fibrosing alveolitis associated with systemic disorders (connective tissue disorders, haemosiderosis, coeliac disease, cirrhosis, chronic active hepatitis, chronically high left atrial pressure, sarcoidosis) and pulmonary fibrosis and alveolitis resulting from external insults (organic dusts, asbestos, silica, busulphan, cyclophosphamide, paraquat, mercury, radiation damage, ARDS, aspiration pneumonia).

Symptoms can vary from very mild to very severe and often correlate poorly with the X-ray changes of fibrosis. As the disease progresses, there is an increasing excess of perfusion relative to ventilation causing persistent hypoxaemia which is difficult to correct by increasing the F_IO_2. Many patients are on steroids.

Perioperative care is by application of the principles outlined in Part 1. There is little reversible airways obstruction and if IPPV is used the ventilator should be adjusted to give the lowest inflation pressure compatible with adequate blood gas exchange to minimize the risk of pneumothorax and the side effects of raised intrathoracic pressure. This often results in a ventilatory pattern similar to that seen in life: a high ventilatory rate with a low tidal volume. A period of postoperative IPPV may well be necessary to offset the problems of neuromuscular blocking drugs, blood transfusion, recumbency and pain.

Pneumothorax, bullous conditions and bronchopleural fistula

The majority of pneumothoraces occur spontaneously with the sudden onset of one-sided pleuritic pain. In people with existing chest disease the only evidence may be a sudden deterioration in their ventilatory status. Conditions predisposing to pneumothorax include ruptured emphysematous bullae, asthma, tuberculosis, chest trauma, pneumonia, carcinoma of the bronchus and IPPV, especially with PEEP.

Rapid diagnosis depends upon a high index of suspicion in 'at risk' situations, the elicitation of physical signs (Table 2.1), which is not always easy, and confirmation by chest X-ray (there is not always time for this in life-threatening situations). Specific treatment by chest tube is indicated in a tension pneumothorax, if there is marked breathlessness, if there are bilateral pneumothoraces, if there is a co-existing pleural effusion, if it complicates a pulmonary infection, if it is very large, and if the patient might need IPPV.

On CXR the pneumothorax is best seen in an erect subject, with the diaphragm in maximal expiration, as a strip of radiolucency devoid of vascular markings. In the supine position the air lies anteriorly to the lung and A-P or P-A films may not reveal it. If the patient must be horizontal it is best seen by lying the patient on their side with the suspect lung uppermost and taking an A-P or P-A film in this position.

Many patients with a pneumothorax have a suction pump attached to the chest drain. This must always be removed prior to IPPV and a simple underwater seal attached, because the reversal in pulmonary pressures and the high gas flow rate may well expand a pneumothorax faster than the pump can clear it.

If any patient on IPPV is suspected of having a pneumothorax it is better to needle the chest because the alternative of 'wait and see' can be fatal. In addition to the normal physical signs (Table 2.1) there is an increasing ventilation pressure and unremitting cyanosis.

Bullae and lung cysts (often undetectable clinically but seen on chest X-ray) can be congenital or acquired, large or small. They share a hazard with a pneumothorax in that they can expand insidiously during N_2O anaesthesia. In the case of a pneumothorax this danger is completely overcome by a chest tube.

The fact that a cyst remains inflated implies a communication with the bronchial tree, and the object is to prevent overdistension or rupture during general anaesthesia (always consider regional anaesthesia as an alternative). Possibilities include spontaneous ventilation with oxygen enriched air combined with an intravenous technique, IPPV as normal if the bulla is small, or, in severe cases, endobronchial intubation to isolate the affected side. Whatever technique is chosen a large needle should *always* be available to relieve an expanding cyst if it occurs. This creates a bronchopleural-cutaneous fistula and a large minute volume may be necessary to compensate for gas losses by this route.

Patients sometimes present for various types of surgery with an acute or chronic bronchopleural fistula. If there is an associated abscess or effusion this should be drained first under local anaesthesia. There are basically two approaches to the problem, both of which commence with an induction with the affected lung in the dependent position so that the rest of the bronchial tree is not flooded by infected fluids. The first is to maintain spontaneous ventilation throughout, intubate the patient with an endotracheal tube, keep the fistula dependent and use frequent suction. The second is to isolate the fistula by means of endobronchial (or double lumen) intubation and use IPPV, after which the patient can adopt any position. This manoeuvre, even when double lumen tubes are used, can lead to a reduction in the PaO_2 if the majority of the tidal volume enters the fistula. The PaO_2 needs to be checked periodically during surgery. Acute bronchopleural fistulae are much more dangerous than chronic ones. The latter have a fibrous, non-valvular communication which is often stable, even during IPPV.

Cystic fibrosis

This is a hereditary, recessive disorder occurring equally in males and females which usually presents in childhood with repeated pulmonary infections. These are secondary to obstruction from viscous bronchial secretions and can cause secondary bronchiectasis (q.v.) or abscesses. There is also pancreatic malabsorption with steatorrhoea and weight loss.

A vicious cycle of bronchial obstruction, chronic infection, tissue destruction, bronchiectasis, fibrosis and increasing A-V shunts develops. Modern treatment and the use of antibiotics have greatly increased the quality and expectancy of life. Lung function tests show a mixture of restrictive and obstructive features. The chest X-ray findings are variable but frequently show bronchiectasis.

If regional anaesthesia cannot be used, the individual pulmonary problems should be treated as described in general principles. Facemask ventilation is suitable for only short operations because it allows no facility for aspirating secretions. Anticholinergic premedication is probably contraindicated because of the effect on mucus viscosity. Humidified gases are usually recommended.

An unexpected complication is excessive salt loss from sweating leading to circulatory collapse which may occur if the patient is pyrexial. This requires careful prescription of replacement IV fluids.

Bronchiectasis and infections

Chest infections, whenever possible, should be treated prior to anaesthesia. An occult infection still found occasionally in tramps, immigrants, the Irish, the immunosuppressed and the elderly is pulmonary tuberculosis. There can be fibrosis, pleural effusions, cavitation and secondary infection.

In any infective lung condition it is important to use an anaesthetic circuit which can be autoclaved and a disposable endotracheal tube.

Bronchiectasis means dilatation of the airways. It is now rare. It becomes significant when very extensive or when infected. The cavities house a wide variety of pathogens and sputum culture is essential for the prescription of antibiotics. Lung function tests present a mixed obstructive and restrictive picture and are of little help. The mainstay of treatment is postural drainage and physiotherapy. If regional anaesthesia is not indicated, the object during general anaesthesia is to prevent the transfer of infected secretions. This can be done by posture and frequent suction, or if the bronchiectasis is extensive and unilateral, by the use of a double lumen tube.

Sarcoidosis

This is a disease of unknown aetiology thought for many years to be a variant of tuberculosis. It manifests itself as a systemic granulomatous reaction which may involve any tissue but which most commonly affects the lungs, mediastinal lymph nodes and skin. It presents as an acute syndrome in young people (20–40 years) with fever, malaise, erythema nodosum, and polyarthralgia. Hilar nodes are invariably present on chest X-ray and may be found incidentally. This form of the disease has little effect on lung function and requires no special anaesthetic management.

Less commonly, and more seriously, the disease can present insidiously with a cough and progressive dyspnoea. Hypercalcaemia may occur. The chest X-ray shows parenchymal mottling or diffuse fibrosis. The gas transfer test shows reduced diffusing capacity and later the spirogram demonstrates a restrictive pattern (q.v.). The patients may also be on steroids. In severe cases they have a reduced PaO_2 on air.

Carcinoma of the bronchus

This causes 35 000 deaths per year in the UK and is sufficiently common to be discovered occasionally as an incidental finding in patients presenting for unrelated surgery. Its presence is suggested by cough, haemoptysis, superior vena caval (SVC) obstruction, Horner's syndrome, Pancoast syndrome, hoarseness, cervical glands, dysphagia, cardiac arrhythmias and clubbing. Confirmation is by chest X-ray, sputum cytology or bronchoscopy.

Pulmonary disability secondary to carcinoma can be minimal or severe and should be managed as in general principles described above. Of particular importance to the anaesthetist is the occurrence of mixed sensory or motor peripheral neuropathies, proximal myopathies and the relatively rare myasthenic (Eaton–Lambert) syndrome (see Chapter 3) which may make the patient very sensitive to non-depolarizing neuromuscular blocking drugs. With SVC obstruction inject drugs in leg veins for a reliable circulation time.

Pulmonary effusions

To be detectable clinically (Table 2.1) at least 500 mls of fluid must be present. Radiologically, the first sign is loss of the costophrenic angle and, depending upon the position, up to 300 mls is needed to see a marked fluid shadow. The fluid surface is only level if there is free gas above it. Of itself, an effusion only produces breathlessness if it is very large (over 1000 cc with normal lungs) but often there is an associated fever or toxaemia. Symptoms such as pleuritic pain, cough and haemoptysis usually arise from the underlying pathology and many small effusions are symptomless. Causes are carcinoma (primary or secondary), cardiac failure, pulmonary embolus and infarction, tuberculosis, pneumonia and the connective tissue disorders. Thoracentesis is used for diagnosis and relief of symptoms. Large effusions should be aspirated in stages (500–1000 cc) otherwise pulmonary oedema may be precipitated.

To the anaesthetist the significance is that of the underlying disease and of a restrictive pattern of breathing if the effusion is large. Drainage should be accomplished prior to anaesthesia unless the effusion is small, or the operation very short, since pulmonary function may well deteriorate postoperatively.

FURTHER READING

Altose, M.D. (1979) The physiological basis of pulmonary function testing. *Clinical Symposia*, **31**, No. 2, CIBA Pharmaceutical Co.

Anonymous (1980) Centrally acting drugs in chronic airways obstruction. *Br. Med. J.*, **281**, 1232–63.

Bartlett, R.H., Gazzaniga, A.B., Tamar, R. *et al.* (1973) Respiratory manoeuvres to prevent postoperative pulmonary complications. *J. Am. Med. Ass.*, **224**, 1017–21.

Browne, D.R.G. (1984) Weaning patients from mechanical ventilation. *Int. Care Med.*, **10**, 55–8.

Coombs, D.W. (1983) Aspiration pneumonia prophylaxis. *Anesth. Analg.*, **62**, 1055–8.

Craig, D.B. (1981) Postoperative recovery of pulmonary function. *Anesth. Analg.*, **60**, 46–52.

Deneke, S.M. & Fanburg, B.L. (1982) Oxygen toxicity of the lung: an update. *Br. J. Anaesth.*, **54**, 737–49.

Gold, M.I., Schwann, S.J. & Goldberg, M. (1983) Chronic obstructive pulmonary disease and respiratory complications. *Anesth. Analg.*, **62**, 975–81.

Hill, S.L., Barnes, P.K., Holloway, T. *et al.* (1984) Fixed performance oxygen masks: an evaluation. *Br. Med. J.*, **288**, 1261–3.

Jones, J.G. (1984) Pulmonary complications following general anaesthesia. In: Kaufman, L. (ed.), *Anaesthesia Review 2*. Churchill Livingstone. 22–38.

Kafer, E.R. (1980) Respiratory and cardiovascular functions in scoliosis and the principles of anesthetic management. *Anesthesiology*, **52**, 339–51.

Lauckner, M.E., Beggs, I. & Armstrong, R.F. (1983). The radiological characteristics of bronchopleural fistulae following pneumonectomy. *Anaesthesia*, **38**, 452–6.

Milledge, J.S. & Nunn, J.F. (1975) Criteria of fitness for anaesthesia in patients with chronic obstructive lung disease. *Br. Med. J.*, **3**, 670–3.

Nunn, J.F. & Ezi-Ashi, T.I. (1962) The accuracy of the respirometer and ventigrator. *Br. J. Anaesth.*, **34**, 422–32.

Pearce, A.C. & Jones, R.M. (1984) Smoking and Anesthesia: Preoperative abstinence and Perioperative Morbidity. *Anesthesiology*, **61**, 576–84.

Rigg, J.R.A. & Jones, N.L. (1978) Clinical assessment of respiratory function. *Br. J. Anaesth.*, **50**, 3–13.

Robinson, D.A. & Branthwaite, M.A. (1984) Pleural surgery in patients with cystic fibrosis. *Anaesthesia*, **39**, 655–9.

Slavin, G., Nunn, J.F., Crow, J. *et al.* (1982) Bronchiolectasis — a complication of artificial ventilation. *Br. Med. J.*, **285**, 931–4.

Tattersfield, A.E. (1979) Airway pharmacology. *Br. J. Anaesth.*, **51**, 681–91.

Vickers, M.D. (1982) Postoperative pneumonias. *Br. Med. J.*, **284**, 292.

Warner, M.A., Divertie, M.B. & Tinker, J.H. (1984) Preoperative cessation of smoking and pulmonary complications in coronary artery bypass patients. *Anesthesiology*, **60**, 380–3.

3/Disorders of nerve and muscle

CNS
Epilepsy
Cerebrovascular disease
Parkinsonism
Multiple sclerosis
Injuries to the spinal cord
   The acute spinal cord injury
   The longstanding spinal cord injury
   Non-traumatic spinal cord lesions
Head injuries
Motor neurone disease
The hereditary ataxias
Neurofibromatosis

Peripheral NS
Peripheral neuropathy
Guillain–Barré syndrome

Neuromuscular junction
Denervation hypersensitivity
Myasthenia gravis
The myasthenic syndrome

Muscles
The muscular dystrophies
Myotonia
Malignant hyperpyrexia

Infections
Poliomyelitis
Tetanus

CENTRAL NERVOUS SYSTEM

Epilepsy

This term represents a group of disorders (incidence 1 in 200 people) characterized by local or general seizure activity, or temporary absences. The causes are:
- Unknown (idiopathic epilepsy).
- Intrinsic brain disease: tumour, abscess, post trauma, malaria.
- An abnormality external to, but affecting brain cell function:
  Faints (vasovagal, micturition, emotion)
  Intra and extracerebral vascular disease
  Insufficient cardiac output (Stokes Adams attacks, heart block)
  Hypotension (often postural) due to drugs (especially in the elderly)
  Metabolic insults (hypoglycaemia, renal failure, hepatic failure, water intoxication, drug overdose).

CLINICAL MANIFESTATIONS

Petit mal epilepsy. Brief absences (up to 30 seconds) may be accompanied by muscular jerks. This almost always disappears at adolescence but can be succeeded by grand mal fits.

137

Temporal lobe epilepsy. Altered consciousness is accompanied by déjà vu or visual, gustatory or olfactory hallucinations. There is often a sense of oppression or depersonalization. On occasions automatism follows the aura.

Jacksonian or focal epilepsy. These fits commence in one localized part of the body and gradually increase to involve more of that side. Ultimately they may spread to the whole body and be followed by Todd's paralysis (lasts from several minutes to hours).

Grand mal epilepsy. This is the most common form. The fit is often preceded by an aura. Tonic and clonic phases are followed by a deep sleep. During the fit, cyanosis usually occurs as a result of combined high oxygen consumption and brief ventilatory arrest. Tongue biting and incontinence of urine and faeces can occur. Bilateral upgoing plantar reflexes may be elicited.

PREOPERATIVE CONSIDERATIONS

Assess the severity of epilepsy by the frequency of fits. Ask if they are increasing or decreasing in frequency. Find out when they last had a fit.

The age of onset may give a clue to the underlying aetiology. Young children are prone to febrile convulsions which they usually grow out of. Fits in adolescence are usually idiopathic or follow trauma. Onset between 30–50 years is due to brain tumours in 30%. Over the age of 50 years cerebrovascular disease is the most frequent cause. Enquire whether there are any precipitating factors, e.g. fever, hypoglycaemia, flashing lights.

Ask about drug therapy and whether the dosage has been modified because of increasing fits. In grand mal and temporal lobe epilepsy the most commonly used drugs (alone or in combination) are phenobarbitone and phenytoin. Ethosuximide and valproic acid are used for petit mal.

There are no abnormal findings on examination in idiopathic epilepsy. Any abnormalities may indicate another underlying cause.

Investigations

Although the electroencephalogram (EEG) is the most important test in evaluation and follow up, it is unnecessary in the routine preparation for surgery.

FBC. This is indicated because phenobarbitone and phenytoin may cause a macrocytosis accompanied by a mild anaemia. Treatment with ethosuximide and valproic acid on rare occasions results in thrombocytopenia and aplastic anaemia.

ANAESTHETIC CONSIDERATIONS

Unless there are any other diseases present, the main problems are those of the effects of maintenance therapy and the prevention of a fit in the perioperative period. This is important, not only because of potential airway problems but also because epileptics are only allowed to hold a driving licence if they have not had a daytime fit for three years.

Premedication. Continue anticonvulsant medication on the day of surgery to prevent a withdrawal fit. Fits can be induced by extreme nervousness, so a sedative premedication is advisable. Diazepam has the same metabolic pathway of phenytoin and may precipitate phenytoin toxicity (dizziness, diplopia, nystagmus, ataxia, confusion and coma). Cholinergic drugs and phenothiazines can also evoke convulsions and are best avoided.

Induction. It is sensible to avoid agents which produce extraneous movements and may trigger off a fit, e.g. methohexitone, ketamine or etomidate. The anticonvulsant properties of thiopentone make it an obvious choice. Patients on phenobarbitone are sometimes resistant to thiopentone and need an increased dose.

Maintenance. Enflurane increases EEG activity and may be potentially epileptogenic. It is therefore sensible not to use it. Phenobarbitone, being a classic microsomal enzyme inducer, often makes the effective half lives of drugs shorter and the concentration of metabolites (which may be toxic) higher. There is likely to be an increased danger from repeated halothane administration in patients on phenobarbitone, especially if breakdown occurs via a reductive pathway (see Chapter 4, halothane hepatitis). Do not hyperventilate because hypocarbia lowers the convulsive threshold.

Postoperative care. Especially during emergence from general anaesthesia, avoid photic or auditory stimulation. This might produce a seizure. Do not misinterpret the 'halothane shakes' as a fit and ensure that they are not recorded as such on the chart because of the legal implications for the patient. Continue anticonvulsant therapy, if necessary parenterally.

When prescribing drugs for reasons unrelated to epilepsy, use alternatives to those agents that interact with phenytoin and phenobarbitone and compete for plasma protein-binding sites (e.g. salicylates, warfarin, sulphonamides).

Status epilepticus

This is the rapid repetitive recurrence of any type of seizure without recovery between attacks. The patient has tonic and clonic seizures, disturbed breathing, a high blood pressure and is often incontinent. It can occur spontaneously, but most often follows sudden withdrawal from anticonvulsant medication and it requires urgent treatment. The seizure activity invokes a high cerebral oxygen consumption and risks brain damage. The mortality of untreated status epilepticus is over 10% and a further 10–30% have permanent neurological damage.

Treatment. Protect the airway and ensure good oxygenation. Prevent trauma to the patient's head and body from surrounding objects. Start anticonvulsant treatment with phenytoin (13–18 mg/kg diluted in saline *not* dextrose, at a rate of up to 50 mg/minute) or diazepam (10 mg, or more, is effective but may cause ventilatory depression). If thiopentone is more readily available this can be used. IV glucose may help even in the absence of hypoglycaemia.

If it is necessary to paralyse and intubate the patient to gain airway control continue to give adequate anticonvulsant therapy. Brain damage can still result even though the fits are masked by peripheral neuromuscular blockade.

Cerebrovascular disease

Transient ischaemic attacks are brief episodes of focal neurological disturbance with an abrupt onset and, usually, full recovery within a few minutes. Most authors accept 'transient' as a duration of symptoms and signs for up to a maximum of 24 hours. They are often associated with amaurosis fugax and are caused by small emboli from the carotid (listen for a bruit) or vertebral arteries. The patients are sometimes maintained on antiplatelet therapy (e.g. aspirin). If the frequency of attacks increases it can indicate a pre-stroke syndrome.

A stroke or cerebrovascular accident (CVA) implies an area of permanent brain damage resulting from a circulatory disturbance. As symptoms develop it is called a stroke in evolution and once they are stationary it is called a completed stroke. It can result from thrombosis, embolism or haemorrhage. Clinical differentiation between these causes is impossible except that embolism is more likely if there is atrial fibrillation, after myocardial infarction or in endocarditis. Haemorrhage is more common in hypertensives, and thrombotic episodes tend to have a slower, more protracted evolution. Definitive diagnosis can usually be made by computerized axial tomography. In Britain over 100000 people are living with the permanent effects of strokes.

PREOPERATIVE CONSIDERATIONS

Look for any cause for the stroke (hypertension, heart disease) and treat it appropriately (q.v.). Otherwise, the extent of the stroke must be recorded carefully both for baseline data and for medicolegal reasons. If there has been an accurate diagnosis of thrombo-embolic disease the patient may be on anticoagulant or antiplatelet drugs. Many patients have expressive rather than receptive problems, so ask questions in a manner which allows the patient to answer 'yes' or 'no' rather than with a full sentence. Emotional lability is common and dementia may occur. Taking a history can be impossible or unreliable. In longstanding cases look for drip sites on the non-spastic limb and position them carefully to give maximum freedom of the wrist.

PEROPERATIVE PHASE

Apart from careful positioning of the affected limbs which often have poor quality skin, the main aim is to maintain cerebral haemodynamics at their preoperative level by controlling the blood pressure and cerebral blood flow. Remember that much of the work on cerebral blood flow quoted for healthy brains does not apply to diseased brains in which there is a loss of autoregulation.

The patient should be maintained normotensive by application of the techniques described in Chapter 1. Hypotension may cause ischaemic infarction and hypertension may cause a cerebral haemorrhage. Intubation is a time of danger and a smooth technique must be the aim.

In the acute phase following a CVA, there is an area of luxury perfusion to recoverable tissue around the lesion where there is maximum vasodilatation. If the $PaCO_2$ rises (or high concentrations of volatile agents are used), blood flow to other healthy areas of the brain increases and the luxury perfusion may fall, causing an increase in neuronal death (steal syndrome). Alternatively if the $PaCO_2$ falls, blood flow to the healthy areas falls, but flow to the area around the lesion is maintained (inverse steal). It has been postulated that this may lead to further infarction of 'healthy' brain. Consequently,

141

normocapnia is essential. For all but the shortest operations this implies IPPV.

Suxamethonium can produce changes in potassium flux after an upper motor neurone injury similar to those secondary to a lower motor neurone injury (q.v.). The mechanism for this is unclear because the motor end plate is unaffected.

POSTOPERATIVE PHASE

The patient requires good recovery facilities and facemask oxygen. The blood pressure is often labile. Avoid ventilatory depression with consequent hypercarbia and hypoxia. Postoperative confusion is frequent. Treat the cause (hypoxia, hypotension, pain, full bladder, hypoglycaemia, etc.). Sedation may make matters worse. Good physiotherapy reduces atelectasis and pneumonia and prevents contractures.

Parkinsonism

This is a disease principally of the elderly with an incidence of approximately 15 per 10 000 people. Many authors claim that it is underdiagnosed. It presents as a disturbance of voluntary motor function with rigidity of the limb and trunk muscles (lead pipe or cogwheel rigidity of the elbows and knees), a shuffling gait, bradykinesia, an expressionless, unblinking face, monotonous slurred speech and a 'pill rolling' tremor (5 per second) of the hands. Often the symptoms are asymmetrical, and there is emotional lability and depression. Eventually the patient may become wheelchair bound and have difficulty swallowing.

The majority of cases are idiopathic; some are ascribed to previous encephalitis, some are associated with widespread cerebrovascular disease and some are secondary to phenothiazine or butyrophenone therapy. This latter group are represented mainly by schizophrenics and manic depressives. All cases result from the depletion of dopamine in the basal ganglia.

In the untreated patient the main anaesthetic problems are taking an adequate history, poor motivation to assist in their own recovery postoperatively and muscular weakness and rigidity. The latter can manifest itself as hypoventilation. Aspiration pneumonia may also occur. Phenothiazines or butyrophenones should not be included in the anaesthetic or be used to treat postoperative confusion.

Although the problems of Parkinsonism are often ameliorated by drug treatment, their interaction with anaesthetic agents needs to be considered. Two groups of drugs are used.

The anticholinergics (to reduce the neuronal effects of acetyl choline) benzhexol and orphenadrine, principally reduce rigidity. They have atropinic side effects of blurred vision, dry mouth and tachycardia. They pose little problem for anaesthesia but there may be a rebound of symptoms after operation if therapy is discontinued.

Levodopa is decarboxylated to dopamine in the brain. It is effective in reducing most symptoms in 75% of all patients but especially so in those with bradykinesia. Decarboxylase is widespread throughout the body and hence using levodopa is equivalent to giving a dopamine infusion. Side effects are common. Those which affect the patient most are anorexia, nausea and vomiting. Those which affect the anaesthetist are the cardiovascular effects (dysrhythmias, tachycardia, hypertension, postural hypotension, peripheral vasoconstriction and dilatation of mesenteric and renal vessels). Levodopa is often combined with carbidopa, an extracerebral decarboxylase inhibitor. This, by reducing the peripheral breakdown of levodopa, enables the effective dose of levodopa to be lowered and the peripheral side effects of nausea, vomiting and the cardiac disturbances to be minimized. Unfortunately, there is occasionally an increased incidence of abnormal involuntary movements.

The half-life of levodopa is only 4 hours. Cessation may cause rebound Parkinsonism with the difficulties of excessive salivation and chest rigidity. This can be severe enough to interfere with adequate ventilation. It should therefore be continued on the day of surgery.

The interaction between levodopa and inhalational agents is minor, but hypotension is a potential problem. Many of these patients are also on tricyclic antidepressants (q.v.).

Multiple sclerosis

This is a disease of the central nervous system in which acute episodes of neurological deficit appear irregularly in both time and site. It is principally a disorder of young adults, with an onset between 15 and 40 years and an average expectation of life of 20–30 years after the first symptoms. The incidence is high in temperate latitudes (1 per 1700 population) and low in the tropics. Certain inbred groups (e.g. Orkney Islanders) appear to have an inherited predisposition.

Pathologically, the lesions are areas of demyelination, occurring most commonly in the optic nerves, brain stem, cerebellum and dorsal and pyramidal tracts. Initially, symptoms disappear completely after the acute episode has passed, but eventually with subsequent attacks residual deficits increase. The commonest deficits are optic atrophy, diplopia, nystagmus, vertigo, cerebellar signs, paraesthesia, loss of proprioception, upper motor neurone lesions and disordered bladder function. There may be euphoria or depression. The disease process often culminates in an incontinent, wheelchair-bound spastic individual suffering from flexor spasms and bed sores. Surprisingly, despite its relatively common incidence, there is little literature available giving clear-cut advice with respect to anaesthetic management.

ANAESTHETIC CONSIDERATIONS

During the preoperative visit assess the patient's mental state, look for contractures and bed sores (think of positioning during the operation) and check the drug therapy (some are on ACTH or steroids). Of particular relevance are the presence of a bulbar palsy (making gastric reflux and inhalational pneumonia likely complications) and autonomic hyperreflexia (see spinal cord injuries). Assess the ventilatory reserve (see Chapter 2). All elective surgery should only be performed if the patient is free from infection (pulmonary or other). Record the patient's preoperative disability on the anaesthetic sheet.

It has frequently been said that pregnancy or any form of stress, emotional or surgical, can lead to a relapse or intensification of symptomatology. These effects usually abate after 10–14 days and are thought to be due to a rise in body temperature (as small as 0.5–1°C) producing a conduction block in demyelinated nerves. It is therefore logical to use sedative premedication, prophylactic antibiotics and a mild antipyretic (e.g. aspirin) postoperatively.

General anaesthesia. There is no hard evidence that any one particular technique or combination of drugs has advantages over any other. Monitor the temperature in long operations and do not allow it to rise by the over-enthusiastic use of humidified gases or warming blankets. Muscle relaxants should be used sparingly. During a period of active upper motor neurone demyelination there may be a rise in serum potassium after giving suxamethonium. In those with bulbar palsy, endotracheal intubation is indicated for most operations and especially if the patient is likely to adopt the head down position.

Regional anaesthesia. There is a reluctance to use local anaesthetics because the patient may attribute any subsequent relapse more closely with the anaesthetic if a limb has been therapeutically paralysed. There is, however, no evidence that surgery under regional blockade is any more, or less, likely to precipitate a relapse. Despite this most anaesthetists avoid it for medicolegal reasons.

144

The most common request for regional blockade is that of epidural analgesia for childbirth. In this situation the pros and cons of the procedure should be fully explained to the mother. Some anaesthetists would suggest that she ought to sign a consent form for medico-legal protection. If used, the wording should indicate that no relapse of the multiple sclerosis will be attributed to the epidural.

In all multiple sclerosis patients, the prevention of contractures is paramount. Therefore, intensive postoperative physiotherapy is vital. This can also be used to aid removal of pulmonary secretions in those with poor ventilatory function.

Injuries to the spinal cord

The classic history of spinal cord injuries was described by Marshall Hall in 1841. After the injury there is a period of 'spinal shock' which lasts from 4 to 44 days. Acute transection results in flaccid paralysis below the level of the lesion, accompanied by absent reflexes, loss of visceral and skin sensation and retention of urine and faeces. If the lesion is high enough, sympathetic control is lost with associated hypotension, dysrhythmias and bradycardia. If any recovery is going to occur it usually manifests itself within the first 24–48 hours.

In the irreversibly damaged, as spinal shock abates, it is replaced by a picture of spasticity with motor and autonomic hyperreflexia. In the fully developed 'mass reflex' (usually lesions at T_7 or above) there is a complete lack of inhibition of spinal flexor reflex arcs. Touching a foot often produces flexion of the ipsilateral ankle, knee and hip followed by a similar contraction of the opposite leg. There may be simultaneous urinary and faecal incontinence, sweating and extreme swings in blood pressure and heart rate. This 'mass reflex' also occurs in patients with transverse myelitis and advanced cases of multiple sclerosis who have effectively demyelinated the entire cross section of the cord at a given level.

Suxamethonium given between approximately 36 hours and 36 weeks following the acute injury can, on occasions, produce dangerous rises in serum potassium.

The acute spinal cord injury

A proportion of spinal injury patients have other associated injuries to the head, chest, limbs and viscera which necessitate surgery. Regional analgesia is contraindicated because it both masks the development of symptoms and may be blamed for a worsening of the condition.

145

PREOPERATIVE CONSIDERATIONS

Pay particular attention to the conscious level. If the patient was knocked unconscious get the skull X-rayed. Examine the chest closely and on a chest X-ray specifically look for a pneumothorax and broken ribs. If the first rib is broken think about the possibility of major deceleration injuries (coup and contracoup damage, torn aorta, torn viscera). Note the exact position of the cord injury on X-ray and check that the symptoms match it. There is sometimes a second, higher lesion which has been missed.

PEROPERATIVE PHASE

Operative management depends on the site of the lesion and in general terms, the higher it is, the worse it is. Whatever procedure is undertaken, careful, controlled movement of the patient is vital to prevent further cord damage.

Ventilatory and airway problems. If the fracture is below the cervical cord, the airway should be no problem. For extensive lesions at C_4 or above, because of intercostal and diaphragmatic paralysis, emergency intubation may be necessary as a life saving measure in less than optimal circumstances. The anaesthetic management of a known cervical lesion can be very difficult and anaesthesia should not be contemplated without experienced assistance.

Some of the problems encountered are:
• The patient may have a halo, tongs, or a head and/or body plaster making airway access difficult.
• There may be a full stomach. Attempts to empty it with drugs or large stomach washout tubes are ill advised. The patient will be lying on his back for spinal stability and even if he does not inhale, vomiting, straining and coughing may make the lesion worse.
• Cricoid pressure can potentially produce more cord damage.
• Direct visualization of the larynx by extension of the neck may be allowed in a flexion injury but is dangerous in an extension injury.
• The use of muscle relaxants confuses the progress of symptoms and signs.
• If there has been an associated head injury, for all but the shortest procedures, the patient needs IPPV to optimize his $PaCO_2$.

Several methods have been suggested to overcome these problems and each have their good and bad points. The correct method is the one that works for an individual patient and this is only chosen by experience. For short, minor procedures IV ketamine combined with local anaesthetic infiltration and a nasopharyngeal airway has worked well. Do not strain unnecessarily on the neck and jaw whilst maintaining the airway. In some cases, local infiltration alone will suffice. Outlined below is a plan that we have used in practice for patients requiring intubation. It is given as a *suggested* technique rather than the '*correct*' method.

Preoperatively prescribe metoclopramide 10 mg IV, gently pass a *small* nasogastric tube, aspirate what is possible and instill magnesium sulphate 30 mls. Give the patient an amethocaine lozenge to suck.

In the anaesthetic room optimize the position of the head in consultation with a senior orthopaedic or neurosurgeon. Erect a good drip and have a large bore sucker ready. Have atropine 0.6 mg IV ready to correct a reflex bradycardia if it occurs. Gently and sympathetically pass the laryngoscope down the tongue. If the majority of the epiglottis can be seen, spray below it onto the cords with 4% prilocaine and remove the laryngoscope. In this situation the chances of an easy intubation are very good and an IV induction can be used.

If the epiglottis cannot be seen and intubation looks difficult then awake intubation is probably the best. In those experienced with it, the fibreoptic laryngoscope may be useful for this, but it is not an easy device to use without practice. Blind nasal intubation whilst superficially attractive has two disadvantages. The use of CO_2 to make the patient hyperventilate is contraindicated if there has been a head injury and the inability to move the head and larynx makes alignment of the tube and trachea difficult, if not impossible to achieve.

In the most serious cases tracheostomy under local anaesthetic, or trans-tracheal jet ventilation may be necessary.

In the majority of instances IPPV is used and after the intubating dose has worn off, relaxants are only rarely necessary. Spontaneous ventilation is often inadequate because of respiratory muscle paralysis secondary to the injury.

Neurogenic pulmonary oedema can develop slowly or rapidly a few days after injury. It is usually only associated with head and cervical spine injuries and is poorly understood. It should be treated as one would treat adult respiratory distress syndrome.

Cardiovascular problems. In the acute phase only lesions above T_7 provide problems. The loss of sympathetic drive produces hypotension, dysrhythmias and (most often) a sinus bradycardia. The normal compensatory reflexes are inoperable and this makes the patient's blood pressure exquisitely sensitive to IPPV and postural changes.

It is now thought to be very important in the first 48 hours after injury to maintain normotension so as to optimize cord recovery and prevent an extension of cord ischaemia occurring secondary to hypotension.

The inability to vasoconstrict or sweat renders the patient poikilothermic. Temperature monitoring and the use of humidified gases, warming blanket, space blanket etc. are necessary. Patients can develop DVT's, pulmonary emboli and stress ulcers.

POSTOPERATIVE PHASE

Return the patient to a high dependency area. Only extubate if you are very confident all is well. Otherwise treat as in the Guillain–Barré syndrome (q.v.). Re-intubation is hazardous. Many patients have to return to theatre later for tracheostomy.

The longstanding spinal cord injury

Patients with long term dysfunction present principally for surgery on the urinary tract, anus and for orthopaedic procedures. They may not require anaesthesia because of their lack of sensation.

Many have psychiatric problems (q.v.), chronic renal disease (check Hb and U & E's), contractures making positioning difficult and poor skin with ulceration. Apart from these factors there are only three major problems (**1**, **2** and **3**, below) and two minor ones (**4** and **5** below).

1 Postural hypotension occurs frequently, so monitor the BP carefully if the patient's position is changed intraoperatively.

2 If it is a high lesion there may be weakness of the respiratory muscles to such a degree that no relaxant is required to maintain IPPV. A period of postoperative ventilation and intubated spontaneous breathing is sometimes required before extubation is advisable. Intensive physiotherapy and postural drainage is important. A measure of the patient's ventilatory reserve can be gauged from the tidal volume to vital capacity ratio. (See Guillain–Barré syndrome.) Abrupt manual pressure on the abdomen can sometimes initiate an effective artificial cough.

3 Patients with lesions above T_7 occasionally retain the mass reflex (see above). This can be triggered by skin or visceral (especially bladder) stimulation. Patients know if they possess this problem. If they do, and it is particularly troublesome, the anaesthetist is required not only to provide anaesthesia, but also to control the blood pressure. Hypertensive episodes are sufficiently intense to show ECG changes of ischaemia. Intracerebral haemorrhage is the second commonest cause of death.

Many techniques of blood pressure control have been recommended (e.g. trimetaphan, pentolinium, phentolamine, sodium

148

nitroprusside, regional block). However, the simplest and most successful ways of obtunding the mass reflex are either to produce a dense regional block of sufficient height or to give a general anaesthetic of sufficient depth to prevent the response to stimuli. Moderate hypotension is not a problem in the chronic case because cord damage is complete. The patient needs careful monitoring for several hours in the postoperative period because at this time they seem to be more 'brittle' than usual.

4 Frequent enemas can upset the serum electrolytes.

5 Osteoporosis (q.v.) can be very serious and pathological fractures are common.

Non-traumatic spinal cord lesions

The above management of acute and chronic spinal cord injuries resulting from direct trauma can also be applied to other causes of cord compression. These can be classified as neural (gliomas and ependymomas), meningeal (neurofibroma and meningioma) or extradural (prolapsed intervertebral disc, collapse of a vertebral body secondary to myeloma or metastases, Pott's disease (tuberculosis), abscess or bone marrow reticulosis). There are also a few rare cases of transverse myelitis secondary to radiotherapy.

Head injuries

This section is not intended to deal with the management of severe head injuries requiring neurosurgical intervention. It deals with the situation in which there is no focal injury, localizing signs or gross elevation in intracranial pressure (ICP) but the patient requires surgery for an associated problem (e.g. a motor cyclist knocked unconscious for a few minutes with a compound fracture of the tibia).

PREOPERATIVE CONSIDERATIONS

On the CXR look for fractured ribs and a pneumothorax. Always do the arterial blood gases unless the patient is fully conscious and alert. If there is any question at all about the patency of the airway or the adequacy of ventilatory drive, intubate early and ventilate on the ICU whilst waiting for a theatre. If breathing spontaneously prior to surgery, beware of pain relief with opioids causing ventilatory depression. The 'second insult' must be avoided at all costs. It is a nonsense to meticulously observe the signs of hypoxia and hypercarbia with the consequent rise in ICP, produce a first class set of neurological observations and end up with a brain damaged patient. It must

149

be impressed upon general and orthopaedic surgeons that they *must* make decisions early and not necessarily expect the luxury of observing the progress of symptoms.

PEROPERATIVE PHASE

Induction. The majority of patients in this category will have, or should be assumed to have, full stomachs. Consequently, they require preoxygenation and crash induction with cricoid pressure. This can be preceded by practolol up to 3 mg/kg to attenuate both the arterial pressure rise in response to laryngoscopy and the concomitant increase in ICP. Attempts to reduce the hypertensive response to intubation by hyperventilation on a facemask prior to laryngoscopy may well result in a pressurized gastric bubble and consequent reflux of stomach contents.

Maintenance. Spontaneous ventilation with halothane or other volatile agents is contraindicated because of the rise in ICP. Ventilate to normocapnia or mild hypocapnia. This is sufficiently important to warrant the use of end tidal CO_2 meter or intermittent blood gases.

Optimal fluid balance is difficult to achieve. Blood losses must obviously be replaced either with blood or clear fluids, but fluid overload aggravates cerebral oedema. It is therefore a sensible precaution to insert a urinary catheter preoperatively and give only enough fluid to maintain a urine output of 0.7 ml/kg/hour. This figure should not be adhered to rigidly if large quantities of blood have to be transfused because it could be a contributory factor in the genesis of acute renal failure. To try and prevent these conflicting requirements occurring, it is probably best to allow the Hb to fall to an estimated 10 g% before transfusing blood. By doing this, many patients will only require clear fluids or plasma expanders. When convenient, whilst anaesthetized, pass a large bore stomach tube and do a gastric washout. The surgical procedure (e.g. traction) can require the patient to be extubated supine.

POSTOPERATIVE PHASE

Whether to reverse neuromuscular block at the end of surgery is not always easy to decide. If the patient was fully alert before anaesthesia then there is no contraindication. If there was some blunting of consciousness and the operation takes place during the night, extubation the following morning with fresh ICU staff and a whole day available for careful observation may be a better plan.

After extubation, analgesia is a problem because of the danger of ventilatory depression and the effect of a raised $PaCO_2$ on ICP. The patient needs observing carefully and may require regular blood gas analysis. Regional blocks can be very useful but mask peripheral neurological signs.

Motor neurone disease

Motor neurone disease is characterized by a selective degeneration of the motor neurones of the corticospinal pathways, the brain stem, and the anterior horns of the spinal cord. There are, therefore, a mixture of upper and lower motor neurone signs. The onset is usually insidious and death occurs within 2–3 years. There are three main clinical varieties, each overlapping with the other.

* Progressive Muscular Atrophy presents with the symptoms of a lower motor neurone lesion, most commonly in the hands and arms. Fasciculation, wasting, weakness, stiffness, clumsiness and cramp-like pains occur. Gradually all muscles in the body may be affected.
* Progressive Bulbar Palsy presents with a wasted, strawberry, fibrillating tongue. Control of the tongue is poor; the muscles of the larynx and pharynx become involved. Speech suffers because of paresis of the lips, tongue and palate. Swallowing becomes increasingly difficult, food regurgitates, and inhalational pneumonia is common. Emaciation characterizes the later stages. A pseudobulbar palsy (upper motor neurone lesion) is frequently superimposed with its attendant emotional lability.
* Amyotrophic Lateral Sclerosis describes a degeneration of the upper motor neurones in the corticospinal tracts. This adds a further element of weakness, spasticity and exaggerated tendon jerks. Spasticity is usually more prominent in the legs than in the arms.

ANAESTHETIC CONSIDERATIONS

* There is usually poor airway control and a high risk of inhalational pneumonia.
* Suxamethonium may induce hyperkalaemia.
* There may be a myasthenic-like response to non-depolarizing relaxants (q.v.).
* Patients are often emaciated with poor ventilatory reserve. They need intensive postoperative physiotherapy.

There is no literature to suggest that any particular anaesthetic technique is the best.

The hereditary ataxias

This term covers a group of closely related disorders, usually hereditary or familial, which are characterized by degeneration of some or all of the following parts of the nervous system: the optic nerves, the cerebellum, the olives and the long ascending tracts of the spinal cord. The commonest (which is still rare) is Friedreich's ataxia.

Cerebellar ataxia is noted first in the legs and then in the hands between the ages of 5 and 15 years. Pyramidal tract disease produces upper motor neurone lesions of the legs with muscle weakness and spasticity. Dorsal column involvement results in absent tendon jerks. Proprioceptive changes are inconsistent. There may be a mild dementia and optic atrophy. Nystagmus and diplopia are common. There is an associated cardiomyopathy with dysrhythmias and heart failure which is usually the cause of death at 40–50 years.

There is little published data on the anaesthetic management of these cases. The considerations are those of suxamethonium during or after a demyelinating episode, the sparing use of non-depolarizing relaxants in people with muscular weakness, and the management of cardiomyopathy and dysrhythmias (q.v.). These patients present principally for elective orthopaedic procedures on the feet.

Neurofibromatosis (Von Recklinghausen's disease)

Neurofibromatosis is inherited as a Mendelian dominant with an incidence of approximately 1 in 3000. Its severity varies enormously and it has an equal sex incidence. It is usually characterized by cutaneous pigmentation and tumours on the peripheral nerves (neurofibroma) and skin (cutaneous fibroma). Blood loss from lesions in the GIT can be a problem. Less commonly, neurofibromas also form on the spinal nerve roots within the CNS (acoustic neuroma), in the autonomic nervous system and in the pharynx and larynx. Epilepsy may occur. Other rare but associated abnormalities are kyphoscoliosis, interstitial pulmonary fibrosis, phaeochromocytoma ($< 1\%$), medullary carcinoma of the thyroid and hyperparathyroidism.

Most patients live a normal span and neurofibromatosis is an unimportant condition unless symptoms arise because of the size and position of a tumour or because an associated disease develops.

Anaesthetic management is that of the individual symptoms it presents with (e.g. effective cord transection from large fibroma) and screening for and dealing with any associated disorder, especially phaeochromocytoma (q.v.). Apart from this there are no specific anaesthetic recommendations.

PERIPHERAL NERVOUS SYSTEM

Peripheral neuropathies

This heading represents a group of diseases which manifest themselves as a diffuse disorder of peripheral nerves. By convention, isolated peripheral nerve palsies (e.g. median nerve compression) are excluded.

The onset can be acute or subacute (infective or post infective) or chronic (poisoning and metabolic disorders). Usually there is symmetrical involvement of both upper and lower limbs and both sensory and motor nerves are affected. Typically, sensory symptoms appear first with numbness, tingling and paraesthesia of the hands and feet and cramp-like pains in the muscles. Weakness then follows with impairment of proprioception and clumsy, ataxic movements. Contractures develop readily, so early passive physiotherapy is important.

The disorder usually starts peripherally and works centrally giving the so called 'stocking and glove' distribution. The commonest five causes to be considered are diabetes mellitus (q.v.), vitamin B12 deficiency (q.v.), drugs and poisons, carcinoma and post infective. Only the first of these is common in general medical practice but the last is seen more frequently by anaesthetists on the ICU. Medical effort is directed at excluding carcinoma, identifying a curable or removable cause, and giving supportive treatment until spontaneous regression occurs or until the symptoms stabilize.

Anaesthetic considerations in all cases are those of the underlying disease and those of the Guillain–Barré syndrome (q.v.).

Guillain–Barré syndrome

The management of this syndrome is reviewed separately because anaesthetists not infrequently become involved in both supportive care and in anaesthetizing for a tracheostomy.

It is defined as a subacute polyneuritis of unknown aetiology which is thought to be secondary to an allergic phenomenon affecting the peripheral nerves. In many cases, in the month preceding onset, there has been an infection (viral or bacterial), an injury (traumatic or surgical) or a vaccination.

Symptoms develop over days or weeks, with 50% of patients having a maximal disability by two weeks, and 90% by four weeks. There is then a stationary phase of days or weeks followed by a slow recovery. Only a small minority have residual neurological defects. Most patients resume their occupation by six months, but full recovery may take up to two years. In addition to the characteristic peripheral sensory and motor nerve changes, autonomic nerves may be affected with bladder and cardiovascular instability.

The cornerstone of therapy is to keep the patient as well as possible until spontaneous recovery occurs. This implies good nursing (to avoid pressure sores), intensive physiotherapy (to prevent chest infection or limb contractures), some sort of urinary collection if necessary (e.g. Paul's tubing, catheterization), a cheerful, friendly, forward-looking environment (to prevent depression), and an assiduous check on ventilatory and pharyngeal musculature.

The greatest danger for these patients is ventilatory failure. Serial blood gases are useless. Abnormal results only indicate that corrective measures are being taken too late. The best way of monitoring ventilatory function is to monitor the vital capacity at least twice daily, and to plot it on a chart. If there is an inexorable downward trend, once the vital capacity is less than twice the tidal volume, artificial ventilation needs to be considered. Elective tracheostomy should be done early. If there are weak respiratory muscles, there are usually problems with swallowing and inhalational pneumonia is a very real danger. It is then best to insert a nasogastric tube for feeding. The patient seriously ill with the Guillain–Barré syndrome may not reveal his anxiety because of facial weakness. There is a high risk of DVT and pulmonary embolus and some authorities recommend routine anticoagulation.

From the patient's viewpoint this is a frightening disease because the obvious paralysis and danger to life occur in full consciousness. Therefore, constant sympathetic reassurance is vital for morale and, if possible, the patient should have some means of attracting the attention of the staff when he wants to. This often requires improvization with the positioning of a buzzer or bell pull.

Monitor the ECG and BP routinely. Abnormalities may result from a pulmonary embolus or from an autonomic neuropathy. Treat cardiovascular changes if they are symptomatic or dangerous. In those affected sufficiently to be on an ICU, a common finding is severe postural hypotension. It is important to positively look for this and to alert nurses and physiotherapists to its dangers. The patient at particular risk is the one who is 'sat out for a few minutes' whilst the bed is changed. The use of steroids in this condition is controversial.

ANAESTHETIC CONSIDERATIONS

A patient with the Guillain–Barré syndrome may require anaesthesia for tracheostomy. At this stage of the disease the patients are so weak that muscle relaxants are usually unnecessary for intubation. If they

154

are needed, <u>suxamethonium is contraindicated</u> because of the potassium efflux from muscles whose motor neurones are affected.

The major problem is the <u>instability of the cardiovascular system</u>. <u>Large falls in blood pressure</u> can be produced by <u>induction agents</u>, changes in <u>posture</u>, <u>blood loss</u> or <u>IPPV</u>. The patient should therefore be <u>preoxygenated</u>, a <u>large bore IV cannula inserted</u> and the induction drugs given <u>slowly</u>. <u>Fluid loading</u> may be necessary to maintain the blood pressure. Exercise care in the use of <u>alpha and beta stimulants</u> to produce peripheral vasoconstriction. These patients are exquisitely <u>sensitive</u> to their actions.

MANAGEMENT AFTER TRACHEOSTOMY

Ventilation. The object of management is to maintain adequate ventilatory function with minimal distress to the patient, and this is an art as much as a science. At the zenith of the disease process continuous ventilation will be required. Relaxants are unnecessary because of paralysis, and <u>lorazepam has proved a useful sedative</u>. Some patients tolerate ventilation well, others do not. If it can be achieved, night time sedation with no hypnotic drugs during the daylight hours preserves the circadian rhythm and orientation in time. Good nursing with regular turning, cardiovascular monitoring and tracheostomy care is of great importance. Physiotherapy prevents the formation of contractures and promotes the drainage of secretions.

As the patient improves, triggered ventilation and IMV are often helpful and acceptable to the patient. Later, the majority of the day can be spent off the ventilator with night time reconnection. The best indicator of ventilatory adequacy whilst off the ventilator is minute and tidal volume measurement.

Tracheostomy care

• It is very important for the tracheostomy tube to be adequately secured. Pulling and twisting from ventilator hoses erodes the edges of the wound.
• Suck out pharyngeal secretions gently and regularly.
• There now seems little evidence that periodic evacuation of a low pressure cuff is beneficial.
• All conscious patients should have a bell to hand.
• Humidification of the inspired air is essential to prevent crusting, especially in the first few weeks. Later the tracheal mucosa 'adapts'. Whilst being ventilated the inspired gases pass from the ventilator to a humidifier and then to the patient. The section of tube between the humidifier and patient is best fitted with a water trap. This tube

must be emptied regularly of condensed water and *never* be held above the patient or he may drown. When breathing spontaneously, a small mask can be put over the tracheostomy tube.

- Patients with tracheostomies cannot cough. They require physiotherapy to propel secretions from the periphery of the lung to the major bronchi and then suction to aspirate these secretions. This is unpleasant for the patient. It should not be done more than is necessary and when done it needs to be effective so that the patient has not suffered in vain.
- When changing the tube within the first two weeks, because a fibrous track may not have been formed, it must only be done when full facilities are available for rapid oral intubation.

Tracheostomy complications

- Obstruction of the tube from inspissated secretions.
- Inadvertent displacement of the tube or intubation of the right main bronchus.
- Erosion into the surrounding structures. Usually this produces bleeding from a vessel in the wound edge but in serious cases the oesophagus and carotid arteries have been breached.
- Infection is a perennial problem and thus strict asepsis in all procedures is vital.
- The trachea can ulcerate and dilate whilst the tube is in place and stenose later after removal.

NEUROMUSCULAR JUNCTION

Denervation hypersensitivity

The lower motor neurone exerts a trophic influence on the myoneural junction and any disease affecting it results in a loss of organization of the end-plate. This degeneration starts at about 24 hours, is maximal at 2–4 weeks and lasts for up to 9 months. Its effect is to make the whole of the muscle membrane (not just the end-plate region) sensitive to acetyl choline and its analogues (this applies to suxamethonium but not to non-depolarizing relaxants which are structurally dissimilar). When depolarization occurs, it does so throughout the whole muscle membrane surface with the potential for massive ionic swings. The majority of the work on this effect has been done in animal models. Evidence in man is limited to isolated case reports but these are sufficient in number to be certain that rises in serum potassium of up to 6 mmol/litre are possible after suxamethonium is given, especially if repeat doses are used. Pre-treatment with a non-depolarizing relaxant is unpredictable in reducing the level of the potassium efflux, and the best method of prevention is the avoidance of suxamethonium in the crucial period.

Although the mechanism has never been explained, similar changes in potassium flux following suxamethonium have been described in patients with hemiplegia (upper motor neurone), tetanus, and encephalitis.

Acute rises in serum potassium following suxamethonium also occur frequently in patients with burns and massive tissue damage, and rarely in patients with myopathy and myositis. The mechanism here is not, however, due to disorganization of the motor end-plate and its loss of trophic ability, but to an abnormality of the muscle membrane *per se* which 'leaks' during fasciculation.

Myasthenia gravis

'True' myasthenia is now thought to be an autoimmune disease with antibodies to acetyl choline receptors which affects the post junctional membrane. It can occur in association with a thymoma, thyrotoxicosis and other autoimmune disorders (e.g. SLE). It is rare (1 in 20 000 adults). The clinical onset is usually slow and progressive over 5 years or more but it can occasionally follow a fulminant course. There can be periods of remission of up to 3 years. Clinically it presents as a muscular weakness characterized by fatiguability after repetitive or sustained contraction. It is most marked in the face and eyes producing diplopia and ptosis. Speech and swallowing become affected and there may be a proximal upper limb weakness. The lower limbs are affected last. The greatest danger is the involvement of the ventilatory muscles and this may be very insidious. In a myasthenic crisis, ventilatory function should be monitored as in the Guillain–Barré syndrome (q.v.). Rarely, there is a cardiomyopathy.

Treatment of the neuromuscular weakness is by long acting anticholinesterases (e.g. pyridostigmine). This merely presents more acetyl choline to the post synaptic membrane. Atropine may occasionally be required to prevent bradycardia and to reduce abdominal cramps. Many patients also take ephedrine. An overdose of anticholinesterase can result in a depolarizing block (cholinergic crisis) which is difficult to distinguish clinically from a myasthenic crisis. The two can usually be separated by the lack of response to edrophonium in a cholinergic crisis. The management of both is similar to that of the Guillain–Barré syndrome (q.v.): control of the airway, suction, and if necessary artificial ventilation until medical management is effective. A change in an individual's requirements of anticholinesterase can be due to progression of the disease or to intercurrent infection.

In addition to anticholinesterases long term drug treatment is by steroids and/or azathioprine and/or thymectomy in an effort to control the progress of the autoimmune process. Also, plasmapheresis is becoming increasingly employed, particularly in the more fulminant cases.

PREOPERATIVE CONSIDERATIONS

Assess the patient carefully. Warn him of the likelihood of postoperative ventilation. Put him where he can be closely observed on the day prior to operation. Omit the dose of anticholinesterase immediately before surgery if intraoperative IPPV is planned, but continue it if spontaneous ventilation is to be used. A benzodiazepine premedication is usually safe. Where appropriate provide steroid cover.

PEROPERATIVE PHASE

Regional or general anaesthesia may be used. Lignocaine is the preferred local anaesthetic. After its use the patient requires close observation until the drug has been absorbed and metabolized. For operations on the arms, legs, lower abdomen or perineum, regional block is often the method of choice.

For general anaesthesia, only short cases in those patients with good ventilatory function (measure vital capacity) ought to be done on a mask. All others require intubation and IPPV. Thiopentone is suitable for induction. Myasthenic patients have an exaggerated response to non-depolarizing relaxants and these should be avoided. If a relaxant is required, suxamethonium is the drug of choice but the dose required is unpredictable, both 'resistance' and 'sensitivity' having been recorded. (If the patient has had a plasma exchange for a myasthenic crisis, it takes several days for the pseudocholinesterase to be replaced unless FFP is given.) The best plan is to avoid the use of muscle relaxants altogether, and deepen anaesthesia after induction by using a volatile agent. Then take over the ventilation on a facemask and intubate after spraying the vocal cords with local anaesthetic. Because of the possibility of postoperative ventilation it may be best to intubate nasally with an endotracheal tube possessing a low pressure cuff. Maintenance is by nitrous oxide, oxygen and opioid with, or without, a volatile agent.

Any cardiomyopathy should be treated appropriately (q.v.).

POSTOPERATIVE PHASE

Many well controlled or mild myasthenics will tolerate anaesthesia as described above with relatively few problems. However, after major surgery and particularly in the presence of infection the patient's anticholinesterase requirements may change. It is, therefore, often best in these cases to continue IPPV on the ICU and gradually increase the dose of anticholinesterase (given IV or down the nasogastric tube) until respiratory muscle power is satisfactory. Only extubate when the vital capacity and tidal and minute volumes are adequate and have been stable for over 24 hours in the presence of effective analgesia. This whole process can take up to 10 days in difficult cases. Problems also occur in the postoperative period because of the concomitant administration of potassium depleting diuretics and the 'micin' group of antibiotics.

The myasthenic syndrome (Eaton–Lambert syndrome)

This is a myasthenic-like condition associated with an underlying carcinoma (usually oat cell of the bronchus). It is rare, even within thoracic units. The fundamental lesion is unlike that of true myasthenia. It is caused by a prejunctional failure to release acetyl choline. This results in a poor response to anticholinesterase (negative edrophonium test), a transient increase in strength prior to fatigue, and a sensitivity to all muscle relaxants.

Management is as for myasthenia gravis. It should be thought of as a possibility in all patients having investigations and surgery for presumed carcinoma of the bronchus, particularly in the presence of non-specific, unexplained muscular weakness.

MUSCLES

The muscular dystrophies

These are a group of related disorders which are familial, primary degenerative myopathies. They are usually progressive. All are rare.

The commonest is Duchenne's (pseudohypertrophic) dystrophy which is exclusively found in males. It presents before 5 years with lower limb weakness and hypertrophied calves, but some cases are undiagnosed when they present for anaesthesia. The serum creatine phosphokinase is elevated. Associated problems are cardiac myopathy (q.v.) which can be life-threatening under anaesthesia (they usually have ECG changes), a restrictive pattern of pulmonary disease (q.v.), and an inability to cough well.

ANAESTHETIC CONSIDERATIONS

Apart from anticholinesterase therapy the principles of management of all muscular dystrophies is similar to that of myasthenia gravis and the Guillain–Barré syndrome with special attention being paid to the cardiac and ventilatory complications (q.v.). Suxamethonium is contraindicated because it releases both potassium and myoglobin from the muscles. Patients are very sensitive to non-depolarizing muscle relaxants and the myocardial depressant effects of volatile agents. In advanced cases a period of postoperative ventilation is almost inevitable after major surgery.

Myotonia

Myotonia is the inability of the muscles to relax normally after contraction. It is associated with a very rare group of diseases.

The commonest of these diseases is dystrophia myotonica. This is a hereditary disorder producing increasingly more severe symptoms and signs with time. Presenting in the second decade, there is progressive involvement of skeletal, cardiac and smooth muscle. The 'classic' case has frontal balding, ptosis, an expressionless face, cataracts, wasting of the shoulder and thigh muscles, and testicular or ovarian failure. There may be a severe cardiomyopathy (with sudden death from a dysrhythmia) and diabetes mellitus. Mental deficiency is sometimes evident. The respiratory muscles may be affected with a restrictive pattern of breathing (q.v.) and recurrent chest infections. Myotonia increases with cold, fatigue and excitement.

ANAESTHETIC CONSIDERATIONS

Apart from anticholinesterase therapy, management is as for myasthenia gravis and the Guillain-Barré syndrome with the additional problems of cardiomyopathy (q.v.), diabetes mellitus (q.v.) and restrictive lung disease (q.v.). Even in the absence of any evidence of cardiomyopathy, dysrhythmias (q.v.) must be anticipated.

Suxamethonium is totally contraindicated. As well as releasing potassium it may cause a prolonged (up to 3 minutes) generalized muscular contraction, clamping the jaw shut and making ventilation difficult or impossible. The response to non-depolarizing relaxants is prolonged.

Sensitivity to thiopentone, opioids and benzodiazepines have all been reported so give small, incremental doses and observe the effect.

Because cold can intensify the myotonia, the theatre should be warm, there should be a warming blanket on the table, the inspired gases may be heated and humidified and the patient's temperature should be monitored.

Malignant hyperpyrexia

This is a genetically determined (autosomal dominant) metabolic disease of man and swine that may result in death. It requires two components to occur; a genetic disposition and a trigger of sufficient duration and intensity. The commonest triggers in man are suxamethonium and volatile agents (especially halothane). Malignant hyperpyrexia (MH) only occurs approximately 50% of the time when MH susceptible subjects are exposed to triggers. This may be because there is an insufficient exposure or because sometimes the condition requires some additional factor (e.g. tissue damage from trauma) as a synergistic agent. Before the introduction of dantrolene the mortality from MH was 60–70%.

The incidence varies worldwide but in the UK, it occurs approximately once in 190 000 anaesthetics. It is commonest in young adult males and the incidence falls with age. Despite its rarity, because of the safety of modern anaesthesia, it potentially forms a major cause of avoidable mortality. It is seen most frequently during anaesthesia for squint, trauma, spinal deformity, torn cartilages and appendicitis. Several authors have stressed the importance of measuring temperature routinely, but in addition a high index of suspicion of any untoward events is required.

PATHOPHYSIOLOGY

During normal muscular contraction calcium released into the cytoplasm inhibits the action of troponin. This allows actin and myosin to cross link and the muscle contracts. Contraction stops when calcium has been taken up again by the sarcoplasmic reticulum and troponin is once again allowed to inhibit the interaction of actin and myosin. In MH this re-uptake of calcium does not occur and the muscle remains contracted and completely refractory to drugs acting at the neuromuscular junction.

This sustained contraction produces an enormous increase in the metabolic rate (can be up to 5 times normal basal metabolic rate) and it is the consequences of this which are so dangerous. The consequences fall into 2 main groups:
- The intense metabolic activity increases the demand for substrates which cannot be met by the normal oxygen flux. This results in intense tissue hypoxia, hypercarbia, acidosis and hyperkalaemia.
- The hypermetabolism results in an enormous production of heat as a byproduct of chemical reactions to such an extent that the temperature can rise quickly to levels incompatible with cellular (especially neuronal) function (approximately 43°C).

The acute case

Presentation is variable. If suxamethonium has been used there may be stiffness or rigidity of the jaw and skeletal muscles immediately. Defer elective surgery at this stage. More usually (and especially if suxamethonium is not used) the features appear more gradually and suspicions may not be aroused for up to an hour or more. Clinically the anaesthetist might observe muscle contractures, unexplained tachycardia, hypertension, hyperventilation (if breathing spontaneously), cyanosis and a hot, dry skin. Almost any cardiac dysrhythmia is possible and the ECG may show peaking of the 'T' wave due to hyperkalaemia (Fig. 7.1). Temperature elevation, although not invariable can be as much as 5°C per hour in fulminant cases. The key to survival for these patients is early detection and treatment, so do not wait to see the rate of rise of temperature for confirmation of the diagnosis.

Once suspicions are aroused, if you are not already doing so, monitor the temperature and ECG immediately, switch off all known triggering agents and convert to a 'safe' technique (see later). Terminate surgery and anaesthesia as quickly as possible. Take blood for U & E's and arterial blood gases. When interpreting the blood gas results apply the appropriate temperature correction. Hyperventilate (up to 3 times normal minute ventilation) with a high concentration of oxygen to increase the PaO_2 and to reduce the elevated $PaCO_2$. Commence dantrolene at 1 mg/kg increasing as required up to 10 mg/kg by rapid IV infusion (this uncouples the muscular contraction at the intracellular level via the muscle cell membrane). In severe acidaemia give sodium bicarbonate to keep the pH at 7.0. It may be counterproductive to push it higher (see O_2 dissociation curve, Chapter 9). Correct hyperkalaemia by dextrose and insulin. Treat cardiac dysrhythmias symptomatically. Insert a urinary catheter and maintain a high urine output by the administration of ice cold normal saline and mannitol. (A severe episode can destroy up to 12 kg of muscle with massive release of myoglobin leading to renal failure.) If further cooling is needed iced saline peritoneal dialysis can be used.

The patient may remain unstable for up to 48 hours and develop a rebound hypokalaemia.

The disease also presents in a less florid subacute form with a slow onset over several hours or a day with an unstable temperature for several days. Treatment is as for the more serious case with an emphasis on preventing renal failure.

Anyone who is suspected to have had MH, whether they recover or not, should have their parents, children and siblings referred for susceptibility testing.

The known case

The patient will be aware of his condition and no doubt understandably anxious. This in itself may intensify the MH response. Consequently, whatever form of anaesthesia is chosen, a diazepam premedication is safe and sensible.

It is of the utmost importance to avoid all known triggering agents. Those implicated are suxamethonium, halothane, other volatile agents (including isoflurane), cyclopropane, atropine, gallamine and curare. The amount of halothane inhaled from a machine which has not been kept 'halothane free' is unlikely to be sufficient to trigger the syndrome. Despite this, many centres keep volatile agent free anaesthetic equipment. Drugs which are considered safe in MH are thiopentone, opioids, diazepam, pancuronium and probably nitrous oxide. The exact status of various local anaesthetic agents is disputed but procaine, prilocaine and bupivacaine appear safe for both infiltration and regional block. Lignocaine and adrenaline have a bad reputation in MH.

The syndrome can be prevented by pretreatment with oral dantrolene. Its routine use is controversial. Some centres maintain volatile agent free anaesthetic equipment specifically for MH susceptible patients, only give agents known not to be triggers and have the dantrolene ready to give IV if required. Others, in addition to these precautions routinely prepare the patient with oral dantrolene. The dose extrapolated from animal studies is about 3 mg/kg, 5 hours and 1 hour before surgery. Half this dose has been used successfully. Warn the patient of the side effects of drowsiness, dizziness, nervousness and nausea.

Always monitor the BP, ECG and core temperature. Be prepared for the syndrome to develop. Have dantrolene available in theatre (it takes up to 30 minutes to dissolve), have packs of fluids kept in the fridge, and have dextrose and insulin (to treat hyperkalaemia) and cardiac arrest drugs ready.

INFECTIONS

Poliomyelitis

Since vaccination has been widespread this is now a rare condition. A small number of cases still occur and adults who suffered as children present for surgery.

163

Poliomyelitis is an acute infective disease due to three strains of virus which have a predilection for the anterior horn cells in the spinal cord and the motor nuclei of the brain stem. The virus can be cultured from the nasopharynx and stools during the active and convalescent phases.

The disease begins with a non-specific viral 'flu-like' illness followed by the onset of paralysis. The weakness usually starts, and is more severe, in the legs and there is pain and tenderness in the muscles. The progress and outcome of the disease are very variable.

ANAESTHETIC CONSIDERATIONS

During the active phase treatment is identical to that for the Guillain–Barré syndrome (q.v.). For the chronic case there are problems of positioning if there are contractures, there may be respiratory muscle weakness requiring postoperative ventilation, and depression (q.v.) and social problems.

Tetanus

Because of widespread immunization tetanus is now rare. However, anaesthetists become involved with the established case in transporting patients to regional centres, anaesthetizing them for wound debridement, and ventilating them on the ICU.

Prophylaxis. When anaesthetizing any patient with a dirty wound it is the duty of all medical staff to ensure that the patient is immunized and receives either antibiotics (benzyl penicillin) or antitetanus immunoglobulin (Humotet).

The established case. The causative organism is Clostridium tetani, a spore bearing anaerobe which enters via a wound contaminated by infected material (e.g. soil). The bacilli produce a potent toxin which is absorbed by the motor end-plate and moves centrally to the nerve cell bodies. Prediction of the severity of the attack is difficult, except that the sooner the onset of symptoms from injury (2 days is short, 3 weeks is long), the more likely the attack is to be severe. All infected patients require antibiotics, passive and active immunization and wound cleaning.

After the diagnosis, treatment is essentially supportive with close observation for the onset of complications.

Muscular problems. Traditionally patients are moved into a dark room to suppress spasms. Modern thinking supports a quiet, but well lit, room to aid the early detection of laryngeal and other muscular spasms. Mild muscle spasms respond well to diazepam. Protection of the airway is vital and if there are signs of laryngospasm it is better to intubate early. Severe laryngospasm can sometimes be induced by swallowing saliva or attempting to pass a nasogastric tube.

If there are sustained contractions of peripheral and trunk muscles, despite diazepam, therapeutic paralysis and IPPV is required.

Fluid Balance. Patients with tetanus often have a profuse production of saliva and sweat. If this happens, give enough fluid to maintain a urine output of 1–2 litres/day as the means of controlling fluid balance.

Cardiovascular. Autonomic disturbances are common. They appear usually as episodes of hypertension, tachycardia, dysrhythmias and peripheral vasoconstriction. Hypotension occasionally occurs but if persistent it is usually pre-terminal. There are grossly exaggerated responses to intubation and tracheal suction.

ANAESTHETIC CONSIDERATIONS

Because of the exaggerated responses to intubation it should be preceded by practolol. Despite disturbances of the motor end-plate, many publications recommend a thiopentone and suxamethonium induction sequence. There have been isolated incidents of hyperkalaemia. Maintenance is best done with a nitrous oxide, oxygen, relaxant, analgesic technique. Ensure a sufficient depth of anaesthesia to prevent over reaction to visceral stimuli. Careful monitoring of the BP and ECG are essential. Treat abnormalities symptomatically as described in Chapter 1.

If called upon to accompany an affected patient to another hospital, unless he is *very* well controlled, it is best to intubate prior to departure. There are many stimuli during an ambulance journey which might provoke a seizure.

FURTHER READING

Azaar I. (1984) The response of patients with neuromuscular disorders to muscle relaxants: A review. *Anesthesiology*, **61**, 173–87.

Birkinshaw, K.J. (1975) Anaesthesia in a patient with an unstable neck. *Anaesthesia*, **30**, 46–9.

Bishop, M.J., Weymuller, E.A. & Fink, R. (1984) Laryngeal effects of prolonged intubation. *Anesth. Analg.*, **63**, 335–42.

Browne, D.R.G. (1984) Weaning patients from mechanical ventilation. *Int. Care Med.*, **10**, 55–8.

Crockard, H.A. (1982) Early management of head injuries. *Br. J. Hosp. Med.*, **29**, 635–44.

Dalal, F.Y., Bennett, E.J., Raj, P.P. *et al.* (1972) Dystrophia Myotonica: a multisystem disease. *Can. Anaesth. Soc. J.*, **19**, 436–44.

Edmonson, R.S. & Flowers, M.W. (1979) Intensive care in tetanus: management, complications and mortality in 100 cases. *Br. Med. J.*, **1**, 1401–4.

Ellis, R.F. & Halsall, P.J. (1980) Malignant hyperpyrexia. *Br. J. Hosp. Med.*, **24**, 318–27.

Evans, D.E.N. (1975) Anaesthesia and the epileptic patient: a review. *Anaesthesia*, **30**, 34–45.

Fergusson, R.J., Wright, D.J., Willey, R.F. *et al.* (1981) Suxamethonium is dangerous in polyneuropathy. *Br. Med. J.*, **282**, 298–9.

Fisher, M.Mc.D. (1975) Anesthetic difficulties in neurofibromatosis. *Anaesthesia*, **30**, 648–50.

Fraser, A. & Edmonds-Seal, J. (1982) Spinal cord injuries: a review of the problems facing the anaesthetist. *Anaesthesia*, **37**, 1084–98.

Gelb, A.W., Manninen, P.H., Meyon, B.J., Lee, R.J. & Durward, Q.J. (1984) The anaesthetist and the head injured patient. *Can. Anaesth. Soc. J.*, **31**, 97–108.

John, D.A., Toby, R.E., Homer, L.D. *et al.* (1976) Onset of succinylcholine induced hyperkalaemia following denervation. *Anesthesiology*, **45**, 294–9.

Jones, R.M. & Healy, T.E.J. (1980) Anaesthesia and demyelinating disease. *Anaesthesia*, **35**, 879–84.

Kim, Y.H. & Fayos, J.V. (1981) Radiation tolerance of the cervical spinal cord. *Radiology*, **139**, 473–8.

Lambert, D.H., Deane, R.S. & Mazuzan, J.E. (1982) Anesthesia and the control of blood pressure in patients with spinal cord injury. *Anesth. Analg.*, **61**, 344–8.

Leventhal, S.R., Orkin, F.K. & Hirsh, R.A. (1980) Prediction of the need for postoperative mechanical ventilation in myasthenia gravis. *Anesthesiology*, **53**, 26–30.

Loach, A.B., Young, A.C., Spalding, J.M.K. *et al.* (1975) Postoperative management after thymectomy. *Br. Med. J.*, **1**, 309–12.

Miller, E.D., Sanders, D.B., Rowlingson, J.C. *et al.* (1978) Anesthesia induced rhabdomyolysis in a patient with Duchennes Muscular Dystrophy. *Anesthesiology*, **48**, 146–8.

Mitchell, M.M., Ali, H.H. & Savarese, J.J. (1978) Myotonia and neuromuscular blocking agents. *Anesthesiology*, **49**, 44–8.

Ngai, S.H. (1972) Parkinsonism, levodopa and anesthesia. *Anesthesiology*, **37**, 344–51.

Oakley, C.M. (1984) The heart in the Guillain–Barré Syndrome. *Br. Med. J.*, **288**, 94.

Schonwald, G., Fish, K.J. & Perkash, I. (1981) Cardiovascular complications during anesthesia in chronic spinal cord injured patients. *Anesthesiology*, **55**, 550–8.

Seay, A.R., Ziter, F.A. & Thompson, J.A. (1978) Cardiac arrest during induction of anesthesia in Duchenne muscular dystrophy. *J. Paed.*, **93**, 88–90.

Silver, J.R. (1983) Immediate management of spinal injury. *Br. J. Hosp. Med.* **29**, 412–25.

Spalding, J.M.K. (1981) The Guillain–Barré Syndrome. *Br. Med. J.*, **283**, 873–4.

Steen, P.A. & Michenfelder, J.D. (1979) Neurotoxicity of anesthetics. *Anesthesiology*, **50**, 437–53.

Wanchob, T.D., Brooks, R.J. & Harrison, K.M. (1984) Neurogenic pulmonary oedema. *Anaesthesia*, **39**, 529–34.

4/The liver

Assessment of liver function

The jaundiced patient

The patient with chronic liver
disease

Hepatitis

Drugs and the liver

Acute liver failure

The spectrum of liver disease seen by the anaesthetist is very different from that experienced by the hepatologist. The hepatologist's concern, apart from the medical management, is also the aetiology and prognosis of the underlying disorder. Although these factors should be noted by the anaesthetist, in general terms the effect of liver malfunction on the conduct of anaesthesia is broadly determined by the severity of the cellular dysfunction, irrespective of the cause.

In surgical patients in general hospitals, the commonest cause of *acutely* altered liver function is biliary tract disease which can present with, or without, jaundice. The commonest cause of *chronically* abnormal liver function is cirrhosis, the majority of which is labelled as either alcoholic or cryptogenic. Not infrequently, cirrhotic patients come to surgery for procedures related to their basic pathology.

Assessment of liver function

In terms of its biochemical capabilities the liver has a large margin of safety with considerable cellular reserves available for use in abnormal conditions. Coupled with its ability to regenerate hepatocytes, this implies two important facts. Firstly, liver disease may not become clinically apparent until it is well advanced and, secondly, liver function tests (LFTs) which reflect the spilling of intracellular contents into the circulation (e.g. AST, ALT) may be abnormal in the presence of relatively normal synthetic function (as in mild cirrhosis). Consequently, liver function tests in many cases are only crude indicators of the real hepatic state and must always be related to the clinical condition of the patient. If, however, serial tests are abnormal over a long period it is an indication that considerable

167

cellular damage is occurring. Conversely, one isolated biochemical abnormality may be of little significance.

Following acute episodes (e.g. viral hepatitis, drug-induced cholestasis, stone in the common bile duct) the return of liver function tests to normal gives good evidence of recovery but, in chronic disease (e.g. cirrhosis) abnormal levels give little guide to the severity of disease activity.

It is also important to remember that abnormal LFT's may be related to the effect of systemic diseases on the liver (e.g. congestive cardiac failure, connective tissue disorders, cystic fibrosis, granulomatous and malignant infiltrations, poisoning) which must be taken into account in the overall anaesthetic management.

The normal ranges given for LFT's differ slightly from laboratory to laboratory.

Bilirubin (normal range up to 17 μmol/litre). When the serum concentration rises above 20 μmol/litre there is usually sufficient bilirubin sequestered in the tissues to cause jaundice. This is best seen in the sclera under white light and can easily be missed on the artificially illuminated ward.

The serum bilirubin can be divided into conjugated and unconjugated fractions. These are not normally assayed separately by the laboratory. An increase in the unconjugated fraction (which cannot enter the urine and produces acholuric jaundice) results from an abnormal bilirubin load (haemolysis) or from a biochemical defect at, or proximal to, the site of conjugation on the smooth endoplasmic reticulum of the hepatocyte, The latter is typified by Gilbert's disease, a benign condition of intermittent jaundice affecting 5% of the population.

An elevation of the serum conjugated bilirubin is always evidence of liver pathology and indicates defective excretion via the normal route into the biliary tree. Once conjugated, bilirubin is water soluble and can enter the urine.

Traditional teaching suggests that disordered liver function tests, interpreted with the conjugated to unconjugated bilirubin ratio can specify whether the problem is pre, intra or post hepatic. Although neat in theory, this can rarely be done in practice because parenchymal disease ultimately possesses an obstructive component and obstructive disease produces cellular dysfunction. A more definitive diagnosis may be made with the aid of investigations such as serum virology, transhepatic cholangiography, ultrasound, liver biopsy and endoscopic retrograde cholangiopancreatography.

Aspartate transaminase (AST) (normal serum value 10–50 iU/litre) is an enzyme which facilitates transamination in the heart, skeletal muscle and the kidney as well as in the liver. Consequently it may be raised not only in liver disease but also after myocardial infarction and in the active phase of a myopathy. Therefore, the clinical presentation is important in its interpretation.

Alanine transaminase (ALT) (normal serum value 10–17 iU/litre) is more specific to the liver but this enzyme is less stable in stored serum.

Alkaline phosphatase (normal 30–85 iU/litre) is found in high concentrations in bile canaliculi, osteoblasts, small intestine and the placenta, each tissue containing different isoenzymes. Accordingly, the levels are high in liver disease (especially with cholestasis), bone disease and pregnancy. Isoenzyme determinations are not widely available and the co-existence of an elevated 5-nucleotidase (found in kidney, liver, pancreas and prostate) is often used to confirm the hepatic origin of an abnormal alkaline phosphatase.

Gamma-glutamyl transpeptidase (GGT) (normal less than 40 iU/litre) is found in liver, kidney, pancreas and prostate and is a non-specific marker. The highest levels are found in obstructive jaundice. One of its main uses is as an indication of alcohol consumption in chronic alcoholism, the levels returning to normal with cessation of alcohol intake, unless there is severe liver damage and provided that the alkaline phosphatase is normal.

Remember that all hepatic enzyme changes are indicative of cellular damage and give no guide to the functional ability of the residual cells.

Serum proteins. Serum albumin (normal 35–50 g/litre) is an indicator of the synthetic power of the liver. A level below 25 g/litre indicates extensive liver damage (provided the nephrotic syndrome and excessive protein losses in gastrointestinal disease have been excluded). Alpha$_1$ globulins (normal 1–5 g/litre) are also low in hepatocellular disease. Other globulin levels (normal serum globulin 25–30 g/litre) may increase but these changes are not diagnostic.

Prothrombin time (normal 12–13 seconds). Most clotting factors are synthesized in the liver and the synthesis of factors II, VII, IX and X are dependent on Vitamin K. Deficiency of these factors prolongs the prothrombin time. In obstructive jaundice Vitamin K is not absorbed from the intestine because bile salts are absent. Parenteral vitamin K begins to act within a few hours and usually will return the prothrombin time to normal within 24 hours. If it remains elevated ('Vitamin K resistant') this indicates cellular damage, the hepatocytes being unable to synthesize the clotting factors in the presence of active substrate.

169

The jaundiced patient

The jaundiced patient must always be taken seriously, and an accurate preoperative diagnosis of the cause is exceedingly important. Although an experienced clinician can expect to achieve a correct diagnosis in approximately 66% of cases on the basis of history and examination alone, this is increased to over 95% by the use of special investigations. An unnecessary laparotomy in a patient with severe hepatocellular failure (q.v.) may well prove fatal whereas post hepatic biliary obstruction should be relieved at the earliest opportunity. In addition, any operative procedure on a jaundiced patient carries a risk of renal failure which may be intensified if the anaesthetic is badly managed.

The content of this section concentrates on the anaesthetic management of obstructive jaundice. If the jaundice is complicated by cirrhosis or severe parenchymal failure, the additional material of the appropriate sections later in this chapter should be taken into account.

PREOPERATIVE CONSIDERATIONS

History

Most patients will have been accurately diagnosed prior to the anaesthetist's visit and the majority of those outside specialist units will have biliary obstruction. Mistakes are occasionally made, so it is always valuable to consider other causes (hereditary, haemolytic, cirrhotic, infective, toxic). Ask about a family history of jaundice, contact with jaundiced individuals, blood transfusions, tattooing, acupuncture, drug addiction, sexual orientation and contacts, foreign travel, immigration, alcohol intake (q.v.), recent drug ingestion, general health, and occupational hazards. If the answer to any of these questions is positive, it should be brought to the attention of the clinician in charge of the case. Unexplained jaundice of 4 weeks duration or longer will prove to be caused by obstruction in approximately 75% of patients.

Gall stones in the common bile duct are usually accompanied by pain and pyrexia and may present as pancreatitis, with or without jaundice. Weight loss suggests an underlying neoplasm of the bile ducts or the pancreas, and weight gain should raise the possibility of ascites secondary to cirrhosis.

Malaise, lethargy, nausea and pruritus are common and related to obstructive jaundice. Personality and mental changes are rare, unless there is severe hepatocellular failure (q.v.). The symptoms of anaemia (q.v.) may be secondary to occult or frank (haematemesis or melaena) blood loss. In the cirrhotic patient the commonest site of blood loss is oesophageal varices.

Always enquire about bruising or bleeding after minimal trauma such as at venepuncture sites (coagulation defects), oedema (cardiac failure, hypoproteinaemia with ascites), breathing difficulties (restricted diaphragm, pulmonary effusions), and recent anaesthetics (drug effects). If the patient takes medicaments regularly, note the dose and the effect on the patient: it may give a measure of the liver's metabolic capacity.

Examination

In a mildly jaundiced patient with simple biliary obstruction there are few additional physical signs and the object of the preoperative assessment is to look for features which point to hepatocellular failure (q.v.).

Hepatomegaly, whilst important to elicit, is not helpful in the differential diagnosis of jaundice. A palpable gall bladder normally indicates obstruction of the common bile duct.

Investigations

These are to confirm the type of jaundice and then to find its cause.

LFT's. See above.

FBC. A low Hb may be due to concealed blood loss or haemolysis. A raised WCC is present in cholecystitis and cholangitis.

U & E's. These should be normal. An elevated and rising urea is important and requires urgent treatment (see below).

Urine testing. Once biliary obstruction is complete bilirubin appears in the urine. Otherwise a raised bilirubin is reflected by excess urobilinogen in the urine.

Clotting studies. The prothrombin time may be prolonged.

Virology. Hepatitis B may need to be excluded.

X-rays. Chest. Both cholecystitis and hepatomegaly inhibit right-sided diaphragmatic movement thus giving a propensity for lower right chest infections and pulmonary effusions.

Abdominal. Only in a minority of cases does it show gall stones. It may have the 'ground glass' appearance of ascites.

Barium meal or endoscopy. These will reveal oesophageal varices. Distortion and fixation of the duodenum occurs in carcinoma of the pancreas.

Cholangiography. The percutaneous approach is the most effective

171

once the jaundice has resolved. Endoscopic retrograde cholangiography has a low complication rate and is effective at demonstrating the site of obstruction even when the obstruction is complete. The choice of approach depends upon the personnel available, the presence of abnormal clotting and the presence of infection.

Ultrasound and CAT. These investigations will demonstrate grossly dilated ducts. In experienced hands they also give information about the liver parenchyma, gall bladder and even the site of an obstruction.

Liver biopsy. This is dangerous in the presence of clotting abnormalities, because of the likelihood of bleeding. It does allow histological differentiation between intrinsic parenchymal disease and that secondary to biliary obstruction.

Preoperative preparation

It is imperative to make the maximum effort to avoid renal damage during surgery on jaundiced patients. Renal failure may complicate any form of jaundice but does so most commonly with obstructive jaundice, and the higher the serum bilirubin, the higher the risk. This risk is greatly increased if there is an endotoxaemia from infected bile. If there is a rising urea preoperatively, it is imperative that the biliary obstruction is relieved immediately, however ill the patient. If it is untreated the progression to irreversible renal failure approaches 100%. In extreme cases, haemodialysis has been recommended prior to surgery but this is not without problems because a period of hypotension during dialysis can intensify the renal failure. Its value is as yet unproven.

More frequently, the jaundiced patient presents for surgery with normal renal function and the object is to prevent postoperative renal failure occurring. One of the dangerous factors predisposing to renal failure in the presence of bilirubinaemia is hypovolaemia, which reduces urine production. Consequently, the patient must not be allowed to present for surgery relatively dehydrated because of the preoperative starve. A young fit patient can be given IV fluids liberally and two litres of dextrose saline (0.18% saline in 4% dextrose) in the four hours prior to surgery is reasonable. Those with borderline cardiac function need more careful handling with a fluid load titrated against a moderate to high CVP. This is best done in a high dependency area. In the pre-, intra- and postoperative periods there should be a diuresis of at least 1.0 ml/kg/hour. Urine flow needs to be monitored accurately by catheter collection but its insertion is often delayed (perhaps unwisely) until the patient is in the operating theatre.

172

If, *despite adequate hydration*, the urine flow is too low, or if the serum bilirubin is over 140 µmol/litre, 10% mannitol is the treatment of choice, 500 mls being given over approximately one hour. Some authors have also used frusemide to maintain a diuresis. It must be emphasized strongly that it is potentially disastrous to use mannitol or loop diuretics to maintain a high urine flow in the presence of a low circulating fluid volume. It is a combination which can lead to a deterioration in renal function.

As stated earlier, renal damage is more likely to occur if there is an endotoxaemia, and this can be produced during surgical manipulation of the biliary tree. Consequently, an adequate serum concentration of a suitable antibiotic (usually gentamicin or a cephalosporin) should be attained before surgery by administering it with the premedication or at induction.

Clotting studies are mandatory and if the prothrombin time is prolonged, parenteral Vitamin K is required. This takes up to 24 hours for the maximal effect to be reached and if liver function is sufficiently compromised, it may make little difference to the prothrombin time (Vitamin K resistant), see p. 169. In this case it is necessary to use fresh frozen plasma (FFP), the amount being titrated against the improvement in prothrombin time.

Postoperative chest infections are common, so preoperative physiotherapy to optimize pulmonary function and familiarize the patient with his postoperative treatment is important.

Premedication. The derangement of drug metabolism is not usually severe in obstructive jaundice, so a wide choice of oral or parenteral drugs is available, but a lower than normal dosage is advised for safety. For a narcotic, pethidine has a theoretical advantage in that it is said to constrict the sphincter of Oddi less than other agents. Whether this has any relevance to a diseased biliary tree subjected to surgical instrumentation has not been established. Avoid IM injections if the prothrombin time is prolonged.

PEROPERATIVE PHASE

Contrary to what is required, all anaesthetic techniques, both general and regional, reduce splanchnic blood flow, as do beta-adrenoreceptor blockers and ganglion blockers. Cyclopropane and methoxyflurane are usually cited as being particularly bad. Consequently, the anaesthetic technique used should aim to reduce liver and kidney blood flow as little as possible and to maintain a good urine production. Therefore, *avoid hypoxia, hypovolaemia and hypotension, maintain normocarbia, hydrate well*, and if necessary give a repeat dose of mannitol to ensure a urine output of over 1.0 ml/kg/hour.

173

Virtually all operations on people with obstructive jaundice are for the relief of jaundice and hence the incision is an upper abdominal one. This, and the possibility of clotting disorders mitigate against regional blockade as the sole anaesthetic technique. If clotting is satisfactory, think about epidural blockade for analgesia during and after the operation. Be careful to avoid hypotension with its associated reduction in liver blood flow.

The degree of monitoring above the basic requirements (ECG, BP, pulse, urine production) depends on the magnitude of the procedure and the anaesthetist's preferences. For a Whipple's operation on a sick patient an arterial line, CVP and pulmonary artery catheter may be appropriate: for the removal of a single stone in the common bile duct of a fit patient they are unnecessary.

Induction. Apart from unavoidable situations such as crash induction, pre-oxygenation should be followed with the induction agent given slowly to allow for its effects to be manifest. The choice of induction agent does not appear to be important. Hypotension during induction requires the prompt infusion of fluid, and/or a head down tilt.

Maintenance. Except for very short procedures, spontaneously breathing techniques using volatile agents are unsatisfactory because of the falls in blood pressure, cardiac output and splanchnic blood flow which occur if surgical anaesthesia is to be achieved.

Ventilation to normocapnia with end-tidal CO_2 monitoring or arterial blood gas sampling is the ideal. Pancuronium (of which approximately 11% is excreted in bile) because of its cardiovascular stability is the relaxant most commonly recommended. Atracurium, with its spontaneous breakdown by Hoffman elimination has great theoretical advantages but experience with it has not yet accumulated. Nitrous oxide is not contraindicated. Provided liver function is satisfactory there is no reason not to use parenteral analgesics (pethidine, fentanyl) and if they were given as a premedication their effects can be judged when the patient arrives in the anaesthetic room. Halothane and other volatile agents are not automatically contraindicated, but should only be used in low concentrations which do not cause cardiovascular depression.

Theoretically, the presence of hyperbilirubinaemia can augment the intrapulmonary shunt so it is often recommended to increase the inspired oxygen concentration to 40% or above. The necessity for this can easily be checked by intraoperative blood gas analysis.

The importance of fluid balance and urine flow has been emphasized above. Unless liver failure is present the choice of maintenance fluids is not important. There are good arguments for letting the haematocrit fall because this increases renal plasma flow (which is beneficial to a compromised kidney), provided that there are healthy pulmonary and cardiovascular systems to maintain a high oxygen flux (q.v.). The postoperative haemoglobin should not, however, fall below 10 g%. FFP may be needed if clotting is defective.

POSTOPERATIVE PHASE

Take the patient to a good recovery area with sufficient staff and monitoring facilities. Good reversal of neuromuscular block prior to extubation is essential. The adequacy of ventilation can usually be judged on clinical grounds (head lifting, inspiratory effort) but some anaesthetists like to see a well sustained tetanus or high train of four ratio. If there is doubt about muscle power, a period of IPPV is warranted. Re-curarization is rare but has been recorded. Once extubated, give oxygen enriched air.

Analgesia is important in the prophylaxis of lower lobe atelectasis and it can be achieved by intramuscular, intravenous or epidural opioids or by epidural or intercostal blockade with local anaesthetic. Using parenteral narcotics it can be, with upper abdominal incisions, difficult to achieve satisfactory analgesia without undue ventilatory depression. Intercostal blocks are good but need repeating every few hours. Ventilatory function often improves if the patient is sat up but it is vital to monitor the BP assiduously after topping up an epidural with local anaesthetic because of the danger of a 'sitting faint' and cerebral hypoxia. Opioid epidurals (e.g. diamorphine) work well but do not remove the sharp pain on movement and physiotherapy.

Continue to monitor the urine output and treat accordingly. Ensure that physiotherapy has been arranged. Postoperative chest infections are common, usually originating from a focus in the right lower lobe.

The use of postoperative antibiotics differs from unit to unit but it is now commonplace to continue them if infected bile was found at operation. Care must be exercised with the aminoglycosides because of their nephrotoxic effects.

The patient with chronic liver disease

The response of the liver to disease is strictly limited such that many diverse conditions have the final common pathway of cirrhosis. Cirrhosis is a pathological definition describing the end-point of the sequence cellular necrosis, fibrosis and nodular regeneration with distortion of architecture. Histologically, there are further subdivisions based on the nodule size and the location of the fibrosis but the functional result is the same. The causes of cirrhosis are summarized in Table 4.1. The activity of the cirrhotic process is assessed by clinical, biochemical and histological observations and subsequently classified as progressive, stationary or regressive.

Table 4.1. The causes of cirrhosis

Unknown or cryptogenic (30% in UK)
Alcoholic (30% in UK and rising)
Viral hepatitis, types B and non-A, non-B
Prolonged cholestasis, intra or extrahepatic obstruction
Hepatic venous outflow obstruction
Metabolic disease, e.g. haemochromatosis, Wilson's disease
                    alpha 1 antitrypsin deficiency, storage diseases
Autoimmune—primary biliary cirrhosis
               chronic active hepatitis
               'lupoid hepatitis'
Drugs, e.g. methotrexate, isoniazid, methyldopa
Intestinal bypass surgery for obesity

In many cases cirrhosis is compatible with good health and completely normal biochemical tests, the patient being totally unaware of his condition. Approximately one third of the cases of cirrhosis seen at necropsy have been unsuspected in life. This end of the clinical spectrum is termed 'latent and well compensated'. When severe, cirrhosis can run an aggressive course culminating in liver failure and death and is then termed 'active and decompensated'.

The well compensated patient can almost be regarded as normal. The following discussion of the management of cirrhosis describes the treatment of patients with serious decompensation. The optimum conduct of anaesthesia for any given patient requires a skillful clinical decision based upon where he falls between these two extremes.

Some patients admitted with apparent decompensation may previously have been well compensated and have subsequently deteriorated because of some added stress. In addition the brain of the patient with chronic liver disease is unduly sensitive to a number of insults which would not affect normals. Factors which may precipitate decompensation are diarrhoea, vomiting, haemorrhage, hypotension, paracentesis, infection, alcohol excess, portasystemic shunting, intestinal obstruction, previous surgery, myocardial infarction or drugs (antidepressants, diuretics, sedatives, opioids).

The clinical presentation of cirrhosis is either related to hepatocellular failure or to portal hypertension.

Hepatocellular failure

Hepatocellular failure is indicated by the presence of jaundice, ascites and encephalopathy. The anaesthetic implications of jaundice have already been discussed.

Jaundice. In hepatocellular failure this is due to failure of the liver cells to metabolize a normal bilirubin load and so the serum bilirubin concentration is some guide to the severity of liver cell failure.

Ascites. The two most important factors in the development of ascites are a lowered plasma oncotic pressure (because of the failure of albumin synthesis) and portal venous hypertension. When more fluid enters the peritoneal cavity than leaves it ascites develops. This results in depletion of the effective intravascular volume which causes the renal tubules to retain sodium and water. This in turn encourages further formation of ascites. Ascites may develop suddenly or insidiously over a period of months.

Encephalopathy. This neuropsychiatric syndrome may complicate liver disease of almost all types. The cause is not fully understood but is in part due to the passage of toxic substances of intestinal origin to the brain. Other metabolic events of liver failure contribute. Early clinical signs are disturbed consciousness with sleep disorders, reduced spontaneous movement, a fixed stare and apathy. Personality changes, intellectual deterioration, slurred speech and a 'flapping' tremor also occur. The clinical course fluctuates but the following gives a guide to the severity.
Grade 1. Confused. Altered mood or behaviour.
Grade 2. Drowsy. Inappropriate behaviour.
Grade 3. Stuporous but speaking and obeying simple commands. Inarticulate speech. Marked confusion.
Grade 4. Coma.
Grade 5. Deep coma with no response to painful stimuli.

Portal hypertension

In cirrhosis, the portal vascular bed is distorted and diminished and the portal blood flow is mechanically obstructed. Some of the portal venous blood is diverted into collateral venous channels and some bypasses the liver cells and is shunted directly into the hepatic vein. The normal portal venous pressure is 7 mmHg. In cirrhosis it can be raised up to 50 mmHg. The clinical features of portal hypertension are oesophageal varices, prominent collateral veins radiating from the umbilicus, dilated rectal veins and splenomegaly. Some of these may, on occasions, need surgical treatment.

177

PREOPERATIVE CONSIDERATIONS

History

Establish the likely aetiology of the cirrhosis, and check that the patient is <u>Hepatitis B negative</u>. Usual general complaints are weight loss, weakness, lethargy, anorexia and loss of libido. Weight gain and swelling of the abdomen and legs suggest fluid retention and ascites. Dyspnoea may result. Details of jaundice, hepatitis, medications, and alcohol intake are important. Bleeding and personality and mental changes are suggestive of encephalopathy.

Note the effects of any recent anaesthetics, and ask about the symptoms of <u>diabetes mellitus (q.v.) which frequently co-exists with cirrhosis.</u>

Examination

General. Look for the signs of liver malfunction; jaundice, gynaecomastia (<u>may be secondary to spironolactone</u>), spider naevi in the drainage area of the SVC, <u>white nails</u>, paper money skin, palmar erythema, dupuytren's contracture, bruising, parotid swelling, testicular atrophy and loss of secondary sexual hair.

CVS. Hepatocellular failure produces a <u>hyperkinetic circulatory state</u> with a <u>high cardiac output</u>, <u>tachycardia</u>, flushed extremities, <u>bounding pulses</u>, <u>capillary pulsation</u> and an <u>ejection systolic murmur</u>. The BP may be low and it is vital to differentiate between this state and that secondary to occult blood loss. Cyanosis is often present and hypoxia, acidosis and electrolyte disturbances may cause dysrhythmias.

RS. Approximately one third of patients with a decompensated cirrhosis have a reduced PaO_2 and are cyanosed. This is secondary to <u>intra-pulmonary shunting and pulmonary vasodilatation</u>. Chest infections are common and ascites can impair diaphragmatic movement.

GIT. Examine carefully for ascites and hepatosplenomegaly. Melaena may indicate bleeding oesophageal varices. Dilated veins suggest portal hypertension.

CNS. Look for the signs of encephalopathy and grade it accordingly (q.v.). Cerebellar ataxia and peripheral neuropathy may occur in alcoholics without encephalopathy.

Investigations

FBC. If the Hb is low look for a cause of occult blood loss. Exclude haemolysis.

178

U & E's. These should be normal. The serum potassium may be high from spironolactone therapy or low from potassium losing diuretic treatment. A low serum potassium can produce a metabolic alkalosis because of hydrogen ion excretion by the kidney which attempts to preserve potassium. If possible, correct the hypokalaemia before surgery. An elevated and rising urea and a low and falling plasma sodium indicate a poor prognosis and require urgent treatment to prevent the hepato-renal syndrome (q.v.).

Glucose. Chronic cirrhosis has an association with diabetes mellitus.

LFT's. See earlier.

ECG. This should be normal. In seriously decompensated states dysrhythmias occur. Check that electrolyte and acid-base disturbances are not the cause.

Clotting studies. See the 'jaundiced' patient.

CXR. Look for pleural effusions, pulmonary oedema and a dilated heart.

Blood gases. These are indicated in severe disease or if there is cyanosis. Usually there is a hypoxic picture with compensatory hyperventilation and a low $PaCO_2$. There may be a metabolic alkalosis secondary to chronic potassium loss or a metabolic acidosis secondary to poor tissue perfusion.

Endoscopy. If there is evidence of GI blood loss endoscopy is useful in identifying oesophageal varices, both for controlling it with sclerotherapy and for establishing the presence or absence of the commonly co-existing peptic ulcer or gastric erosions.

Liver biopsy. See earlier.

EEG. The changes are non-specific but occur early in hepatic encephalopathy. There is a slowing from the normal alpha range of 8–13 cycles/second to the delta range of less than 4 cycles/second.

CSF. No abnormality is expected.

Risks of surgery

The *principles* of management are essentially the same whether the patient is well compensated or decompensated, but the latter has a greatly reduced margin of safety. It can be helpful to grade the severity of liver disease according to a modification of Child's grouping outlined in Table 4.2. For each of the variables listed points are awarded as shown and the total calculated. Patients who score 5 or 6 points are considered to be good operative risks (Group A), those with 7, 8 or 9 points are moderate risks (Group B) and those with 10–15 points are poor operative risks (Group C). Although this grouping was introduced to estimate the risk from portasystemic shunting it can be helpful in deciding the risks of other surgery. Where possible

Table 4.2. Modified Child's grouping of the severity of liver disease. The grading of encephalopathy is outlined in the text

Clinical and biochemical measurement	Points scored		
	1	2	3
Grade of encephalopathy	Absent	1 and 2	3, 4 and 5
Bilirubin (μmol/litre)	<25	25–40	>40
Albumin (g/litre)	35	28–35	<28
Prothrombin time (seconds prolonged)	1–4	4–6	> 6
Ascites	Absent	Slight	Moderate

only patients in Group A should be considered for elective surgery and those in Group C should only be considered for surgery for life-threatening conditions.

Preoperative preparation

If the patient with cirrhosis is jaundiced it indicates an excess of liver cell necrosis over regeneration and carries a bad prognosis. *The content of this section assumes that where relevant the problem of jaundice and a prolonged prothrombin time are managed as described earlier.*

The problem of ascites, cirrhosis, fluid retention and the kidney are inextricably connected. Approximately 80% of patients seriously ill with cirrhosis, who may or may not be jaundiced, have some element of renal failure, the exact aetiology of which is not understood. The degree of renal failure is often worsened by sepsis, haemorrhage, hypotension, hypoxia and surgery.

For the anaesthetist, the presence of ascites implies abnormal binding and metabolism of drugs, abnormal excretion of electrolytes, possible poor renal function and compromised diaphragmatic movement. If the ascites is very tense and causing breathing problems, enough ascitic fluid should be removed to alleviate the symptoms and allow an adequate tidal volume and vital capacity. Do not forget that ventilatory function is worse when supine. Complete paracentesis carries a high risk of precipitating both renal and hepatic failure and encephalopathy but this total drainage is sometimes inevitable in the course of an abdominal operation.

The preoperative treatment of ascites by bed rest and diuretics to increase the sodium loss (combined with a low salt diet) must be done very gradually with careful observation of the clinical condition of the patient. Time is required to allow the fluid to shift from the ascitic to the central compartment and weight loss should not exceed 0.5 kg/day. If it does, the central circulating volume is reduced by the action of the diuretic on the kidney faster than it is replaced from the ascitic fluid and there is a high risk of developing a diuretic-induced uraemia. The organization of diuretic therapy is best done by hepatologists who will select the appropriate drugs and balance the dose against the patient's glomerular filtration rate. Occasionally, it is useful to expand the circulating fluid volume by the use of salt poor albumin. In specialist units, refractory ascites can be treated by ultrafiltration. The ascitic fluid is drained via a peritoneal dialysis cannula, passed through a dialyser with a molecular sieve (passes molecules up to 50 000 MW) and the protein concentrated fluid is returned to the patient intravenously. Weight loss is both direct and via increased urine output. Although large volumes of fluid can be lost quickly it is a complex procedure with complications of infection, pulmonary oedema, heart failure and haemorrhage.

If the patient has signs of encephalopathy the absorption of the products of bacterial degradation of protein should be reduced. Magnesium sulphate enemas, oral lactulose and/or oral neomycin are given to alter and reduce chronic bacterial flora.

For all but the most minor procedures always have blood crossmatched (as fresh as possible) and check that FFP is available.

The effect of drugs in the cirrhotic is unpredictable. Changes in albumin and globulin levels affect binding, alterations in the response at cellular level make the patient more 'sensitive', and a reduction in metabolic degradation prolongs the action of the active drug and its breakdown products. These effects are mentioned later where appropriate.

Premedication. Many premedicant drugs will themselves precipitate encephalopathy. Morphine has a particularly bad reputation for this although it is the dose, rather than the type of opioid which is important. A well tried combination is a small dose of IM promethazine combined with a *small* dose of pethidine (e.g. 0.1–0.3 mg/kg). For sedation alone, oxazepam is probably best. In some cases, if the patient is agreeable, premedication can be avoided.

If a premedication is given, observing its effects when the patient arrives in the anaesthetic room may help in assessing the response to drugs.

If the patient is on steroids increase the dose appropriately (q.v.) for the operation.

PEROPERATIVE PHASE

The maintenance of an adequate arterial blood pressure is vital in cirrhosis because the cirrhotic liver receives most of its blood supply from the hepatic artery. Hence, even a well compensated cirrhotic

181

should not be offered hypotensive anaesthesia for an elective operation (e.g. plastic or middle ear surgery). Other factors which minimize any disturbance of liver and kidney perfusion are the avoidance of hypoxia and hypovolaemia. If necessary, inotropes (at low dosage levels) can be used to maintain the arterial blood pressure once a high CVP is established.

Invasive monitoring, if it is to be used, is best put in under local anaesthetic at the outset, so that the haemodynamic effects of induction can be monitored. This is especially useful during crash induction. The necessity of arterial, central venous and pulmonary artery catheters must be judged in individual cases and their gains balanced against the risks in patients with a potential coagulation problem. They are most indicated in those patients with preoperative dysrhythmias, hypoxia and hypotension. Patients presenting with a tachycardia and a peripherally dilated vascular bed tolerate blood loss and decreases of cardiac output badly.

Induction. After preoxygenation induction agents should be given slowly to minimize reductions in cardiac output and to allow time for their effects to become apparent. In the sick patient only very small doses will be required, but in the compensated cirrhotic increased binding to globulins, or enzyme induction, may lead to an increase in requirements. Barbiturates may worsen encephalopathy. Etomidate has the theoretical advantage of cardiovascular stability.

If there has been acute GI bleeding a crash induction (or awake intubation) will be necessary with the usual precautions (preoxygenation, spare laryngoscope, cuff checked on the endotracheal tube and large capacity sucker). In extreme cases with bleeding oesophageal varices an oesophageal tamponade tube (e.g. Sengstaken) will be in place. They have up to 4 lumens: oesophageal and gastric balloons, a tube in the stomach and a fourth lumen for aspiration above the oesophageal balloon. Suck on the latter before induction. Do not remove the tamponade tube (intubation is quite possible with it *in situ*) and do not deflate the balloons. Leave it in place to minimize blood loss until the surgeon is ready either for injection sclerotherapy or oesophageal transection.

In patients with cirrhosis it has been suggested that low serum pseudocholinesterase prolongs the action of suxamethonium but there is little evidence of this being a practical problem. Patients exhibiting a prolonged response should still have their dibucaine number checked since this is the more likely cause. It should also be noted that fresh blood and FFP contain sufficient amounts of pseudocholinesterase to offset any intrinsic defect.

Maintenance. The effect of anaesthesia on splanchnic blood flow was described earlier and the importance of avoiding hypotension has already been emphasized. Careful cardiovascular monitoring is essential (pulse, BP, CVP, ECG) and always be ready to give warmed blood early, thus allowing a relatively slow transfusion and time for the adequate metabolism of citrate. This is particularly a problem in patients with bleeding oesophageal varices in whom very high levels of serum citrate have been found during multiple transfusions. With normal liver function, the risk of lowering the serum ionized calcium is small unless blood is transfused at a rate greater than one unit per five minutes or more than four units are given in total. These limits are eroded in hepatocellular failure, and calcium supplements may need to be given earlier, especially if the Q-T segment on the ECG indicates hypocalcaemia.

If non-surgical blood loss is a problem repeat the clotting screen and give fresh blood and/or FFP and platelets according to the results.

For routine maintenance fluids (apart from the replacement of a loss of circulating volume), avoid giving solutions with a high sodium content: 5% dextrose is probably the fluid of choice unless the patient is hyponatraemic. Human plasma protein fraction (HPPF) has a high sodium content of 140–160 mmol/litre.

For short procedures in fit patients where intubation is not normally required, spontaneous breathing is satisfactory provided that a volatile agent does not have to be 'pushed' to maintain adequate anaesthesia with a consequent fall in cardiac output and blood pressure. A methohexitone or etomidate infusion combined with N_2O and O_2 provides satisfactory narcosis during spontaneous or controlled ventilation.

If patients are ventilated it is good practice to maintain normocapnia because of the beneficial effect on liver blood flow. An end tidal CO_2 meter or serial blood gases are required. The F_1O_2 is best set initially at 50% to offset the possible effects of intrapulmonary shunting (this is greater than that due to simple hyperbilirubinaemia) and it can be reduced if an arterial blood gas sample shows good oxygenation. During IPPV, pethidine or fentanyl in *small* doses, can be used as adjuncts to nitrous oxide. Low concentrations of volatile agents are acceptable provided they do not depress blood pressure and cardiac output.

Cirrhotic patients have low reserves of glycogen therefore their blood glucose needs checking half hourly.

The response to non-depolarizing relaxants is not always predictable because of abnormal protein binding and possible increased sequestration in the liver. Normally, this is not a problem if the patient has adequate renal function since the kidney is the major route of excretion. Nevertheless, it is advantageous to monitor the level of neuromuscular block in prolonged procedures to ensure that only the minimum total dose is administered. As in the case of the jaundiced patient pancuronium is the relaxant most frequently recommended because of its cardiovascular stability. Atracurium has good theoretical advantages but there is, as yet, little reported experience.

Nasogastric tubes, when required, should be passed carefully if there are oesophageal varices.

Respectfully remind the surgeon, if he is working abdominally not to put packs on the hepatic artery or portal vein! Similar pressure on the IVC is probably the commonest cause of episodic intraoperative hypotension.

POSTOPERATIVE PHASE

The patient requires a good recovery area with adequate staff and monitoring facilities. He needs O_2 enriched air and his BP should be measured every few minutes. Adequate oxygenation may prevent unwanted metabolites occurring because of reductive pathway metabolism. Often patients take a long time to recover from anaesthetic drugs and can require IPPV to ensure good oxygenation until they are conscious.

Do not forget that the operation itself might cause confusion. Always eliminate hyoglycaemia as a cause of this. Conversely, remember that a diabetic state may be precipitated. Allow time for the effects of the anaesthetic drugs to wear off before giving post-operative analgesia. This can be provided with epidural local anaesthetics. Do not allow hypotension to occur. The possibility of epidural opioids (using very small doses) has attractions but has not been evaluated yet in liver failure. In the presence of portal hypertension the epidural veins are often engorged and bloody taps are not infrequent.

If using parenteral analgesics give only very small incremental doses (e.g. 0.1 mg/kg pethidine IV) until the effect has been determined. Large or 'normal' doses of any opioid can be fatal. If postoperative sedatives are required it is best to use those which are excreted renally (e.g. sodium barbitone, phenobarbitone or oxazepam).

Other problems which occur during the first few postoperative days are frequent chest infections (prescribe early and regular physiotherapy) and a deterioration in hepatic and renal function. This is especially likely if the ascites has been totally drained because of the surgical procedure. If the ascites remains, postoperative ventilatory insufficiency is common.

Hepatitis

The term hepatitis means inflammation of the liver with little or no fibrosis and nodular regeneration.

Acute hepatitis

In western practice, acute hepatitis is almost exclusively viral hepatitis. It is currently classified into five types: virus A hepatitis (infectious hepatitis, short incubation hepatitis), virus B hepatitis (serum hepatitis, long incubation hepatitis), Epstein–Barr virus hepatitis, cytomegalovirus hepatitis and non-A, non-B hepatitis. Non-A, non-B hepatitis is probably caused by an as yet undetected virus or viruses; it is now the major cause of post transfusion hepatitis.

Patients rarely present for surgery during the acute phase but when they do, the presence of jaundice and hepatocellular failure should be managed as already described.

Hepatitis A

The causative organism is endemic in all parts of the world but the incidence of the disease is almost impossible to quantify because of subclinical and anicteric infections and the widely differing proportions of people presenting for treatment. Spread is usually by the faecal-oral route and small epidemics occur in schools or other institutions. Another vector is raw or undercooked shellfish. Hepatitis A most commonly affects young people (under 20 years) and it should be a guarded diagnosis in patients over 40 years, lest a more serious underlying pathology is missed.

After a variable incubation period of 2–6 weeks, there is a gradual onset of a non-specific viral illness with fever, malaise, anorexia, nausea and vomiting. If the disease progresses liver tenderness occurs followed by a dark urine, pale stools and jaundice. Liver enzymes are at very high levels but a strong cholestatic picture with very high bilirubin levels is rare. LFT's, jaundice and symptoms begin to improve after 1–2 weeks but return to normality may take up to 3 or 4 months.

The mortality is extremely low (0-0.2% of known cases). Corticosteroids may be given if there is marked cholestasis. There is no progression to chronic liver disease but there is a variable (0–10%)

185

spontaneous relapse rate which has been reported in association with exercise, stress and alcohol intake. It is this feature which bedevils the investigation of postoperative hepatic malfunction.

Immune serum globulin is effective in preventing the development of hepatitis A if there has been known contact.

Elective surgery in those suffering from hepatitis A should be postponed (probably for 4 months) as liver function has been shown to deteriorate after anaesthesia and surgery.

Hepatitis B

It used to be thought that this virus was only spread parenterally but recent evidence has established that, in certain circumstances, the virus can be transmitted in various body fluids such as saliva, vaginal discharges, seminal fluid, breast milk and weeping wounds. Those with a high risk of being carriers include male homosexuals, prostitutes, tattooed patients, drug addicts, those on immunosuppressives, renal dialysis patients, the mentally subnormal living in institutions, prison inmates, immigrants, travellers from an endemic region, those who have received multiple blood transfusions and those with disorders of the blood and reticulo-endothelial system.

Approximately 90% of patients with acute hepatitis B recover completely and do not persist as carriers. Fewer than 1% develop massive hepatic necrosis, but this complication is much more common than in hepatitis A. The carrier state of HB_5Ag (the antigen found on the surface of the antigen) is of great concern to the medical progression. It now seems probable that liver injury associated with hepatitis B is an immune cellular response mediated by 'T' cells. The carriers, who appear healthy, have apparently created a harmless symbiosis which, if disturbed, may result in an acute episode, chronic active hepatitis or a profound antibody response leading to hepatic necrosis. This can occur after cessation of immuno-suppressive therapy. The prevalence of carriers varies from 0.1% in northern Europe to 5% in Mediterranean countries and to 20% in parts of Africa and Asia. Despite the awareness of the modes of transmission, all health care workers have a high risk of infection, especially those frequently exposed to blood.

Presentation, in the acute illness, is essentially the same as for hepatitis A but the incubation period is longer (1–6 months) and the onset of symptoms is more gradual. In uncomplicated cases, treatment is symptomatic with an emphasis on isolation and barrier nursing. All blood samples should be taken in gloves (to protect the venesector) enclosed and transported in special bags and all laboratory staff must be warned of the diagnosis.

Gamma globulin containing high titres of anti HB$_s$ (hyperimmune globulin) has been used in the prophylaxis against hepatitis B. A vaccine is also now available and may be offered to those health workers in regular contact with hepatitis B carriers.

Occasionally one has to anaesthetize a known carrier of hepatitis B. All hospitals have a theatre procedure for dealing with this problem and it should be adhered to. Although there are local variations the overall principles are similar. All the relevant hospital staff, of whatever rank, should be aware of the danger. All clothing worn by the patient, his bedclothes, and the attendant's clothing should be disposable. Instruments should be disposable where possible. All nursing staff dealing with the case should be fully trained. People carrying out procedures on the patient must wear gloves and eye protection. The anaesthetic circuit needs to be autoclavable and the endotracheal tube disposable. There should be a surfeit of clearly labelled waste disposal bags.

Chronic hepatitis

The classification of chronic hepatitis is under frequent revision but it can be described under two main headings: chronic persistent hepatitis and chronic active hepatitis. Both are rare outside specialist units.

Chronic persistent hepatitis is a relatively benign condition. The majority of cases have no known aetiological factor but others have been known to follow hepatitis B, non-A, non-B hepatitis, alcoholic hepatitis or be associated with inflammatory bowel disease, cytotoxic drugs or chronic ingestion of paracetamol, aspirin and methyldopa. The clinical presentation varies widely. Jaundice is rare and the patients usually show little evidence of hepatocellular failure despite transaminase levels over five times normal. Diagnosis is by liver biopsy and the long term outlook is excellent with no progression to cirrhosis.

Chronic active hepatitis is an aggressive condition with fluctuating jaundice and hepatocellular failure. Progression to cirrhosis is the usual end point. Its aetiology is multifactorial. Some cases follow hepatitis B, non-A, non-B hepatitis, alcoholic hepatitis, Wilson's disease, alpha$_1$ antitrypsin deficiency, cytotoxic drugs, paracetamol and methyldopa. Many cases have no known cause. Some patients are treated with steroids.

When presenting for surgery, jaundice and hepatocellular failure should be managed as previously described.

Drugs and the liver

Metabolism

Most drugs undergo biotransformation in the liver which converts them into water soluble compounds. These can then be excreted in the urine or bile. Those with a molecular weight of over approximately 200 are excreted in the bile. The enzymes which carry out this function are located on the smooth endoplasmic reticulum of the hepatocytes and are referred to as 'the microsomal mixed function oxidase system'. The hepatic detoxification process is a two stage sequence, both or either stage being used by different drugs. Initially there is oxidation, reduction or hydrolysis of the parent drug, the resulting compound then being conjugated with glycine, sulphate or glucuronic acid. At either stage, if the product is sufficiently water soluble it can be excreted into bile or urine. For instance ethyl alcohol is only oxidized, bilirubin can be conjugated immediately and barbiturates require both stages. In some instances, the breakdown products are themselves active (e.g. those of diazepam, thiopentone) and in others they are hepatotoxic (chloroform).

Two drugs competing for the same enzyme may cause the drug with the lower affinity to have an increased half-life. Drugs interfering with bilirubin at any of its stages of metabolism may precipitate or intensify existing jaundice (see Table 4.3). This is a serious problem in cirrhotics presenting for anaesthesia.

Table 4.3. Some drugs affecting bilirubin metabolism

Salicylates Sulphonamides	} displace bilirubin from albumin
Rifampicin Filix mas extract Cholecystographic media	} affect uptake into hepatocyte
Novobiocin Progesterones	} inhibit conjugation with glucuronide
Phenobarbitone	potentiates action of glucuronyl transferase
Chlorpromazine PAS Thiouracil Chlorpropamide Nitrofurantoin Contraceptive pill Sulphadiazine Methyltestosterone Anabolic steroids	} produce cholestasis

Any drug producing haemolysis increases the bilirubin load.

Current thinking suggests that there are relatively large variations between individuals with respect to the activity of the enzyme systems, but that when a drug is given repeatedly to the same individual, metabolism proceeds at a fairly constant rate (provided enzyme inhibition or induction has not occurred). The conclusion is that the half-life of many drugs is genetically controlled in healthy subjects who are on no medication and that the ideal dose will vary from person to person. Fortunately, there is usually a sufficient margin of safety for drugs to be prescribed on a body weight basis. Where this is not so (e.g. hepatocellular failure) dosage must be adjusted to give the correct serum level. There is a high degree of correlation between the half-life of a drug, the degree of abnormality in the prothrombin time, the serum albumin concentration, hepatic encephalopathy and ascites.

A wide variety of substances are known to induce enzymes (see Table 4.4) and some drugs induce their own metabolism. Many patients present for surgery who are on enzyme inducing medication. In chronic liver disease with a reduced number of active hepatocytes, the drug load per cell is increased and this in itself may increase the intracellular enzymes.

A number of substances inhibit the activity of drug metabolizing enzymes but the only one of clinical significance is disulfiram (Antabuse).

Table 4.4. Drugs causing enzyme induction (drugs with most marked effect in brackets)

Alcohol
Barbiturates and other anticonvulsants (phenobarbitone and phenytoin)
Hypoglycaemic agents (chlorpropamide, glibenclamide, tolbutamide)
Anti inflammatory drugs (phenylbutazone)
Antibiotics (rifampicin)
Phenothiazines (chlorpromazine)
Steroids (cortisol, prednisolone, methyl testosterone)
General anaesthetic agents (possibly)

Toxicity

The classification of the hepatotoxicity of drugs has changed several times over the years. There are only two basic mechanisms: direct toxicity (almost always due to a metabolite) and an abnormal immunological reaction. Both have been credited with the ability to produce cholestasis and hepatocellular necrosis. Improved investigations and histology have shown that many drugs thought to act only by one of the two mechanisms do in fact exert their influence by using both. Chlorpromazine, for instance, is often quoted as a model for an immune based cholestasis but evidence is accumulating that it is also directly hepatotoxic. Drugs relevant to the anaesthetist which are known to have a potentially adverse effect on the liver are given in Table 4.5.

Table 4.5. Drugs known to have caused hepatotoxicity

Ethylalcohol	
Anaesthetic agents	Ethylchloride
	Chloroform
	Halothane
	Methoxyflurane
	Cremophor containing compounds
Sedatives	Thioridazine
	Chlorpromazine
	Chlordiazepoxide
	Promazine
	Prochlorperazine
Anticonvulsants	Phenytoin
	Carbamazepine
	Dantrolene
Anti inflammatory agents	Salicylates
	Phenylbutazone
	Allopurinol
	Indomethacin
Anti hypertensives	Methyldopa
Antimicrobials	Sulphonamides
	Erythromycin
	Nitrofurantoin
	Rifampicin
	Isoniazid
	Tetracyclines
	Penicillin
Hypoglycaemic agents	Chlorpropamide
	Tolbutamide
Cytotoxic agents	Methotrexate
	Azathioprine
	Cyclophosphamide
	6-mercaptopurine
Heavy metals	Arsenic
	Yellow phosphorus
Antidepressant drugs	Imipramine
	Amitriptyline
Hormones	Methyltestosterone
	Contraceptive pill

Direct Toxicity. This is caused by a metabolite of the drug binding covalently with a liver macromolecule essential to the cell. Cellular malfunction and ultimately necrosis result. The intensity of the

190

damage is increased by enzyme induction, the reaction is dose dependent and occurs early. Animal models exist, and other major organs, especially the kidney, are affected.

Immune mediated reactions. The drug or its metabolite is thought to bind to an intracellular or cell surface macromolecule so as to make the combination antigenic to the host and capable of sensitizing lymphocytes. Children (prepuberty) are usually unaffected, the response of the adult is unpredictable, and animal models have not been found. There appears to be a familial incidence and theoretically there is no damage on the first exposure. Classically, there is a latent period between the subsequent exposure and the onset of symptoms whilst the immune reaction occurs.

Halothane hepatitis

This is considered as a separate entity because of its importance in anaesthesia. Despite the difficulties in studying halothane related liver damage because of its extreme rarity, there seems an increasing willingness to accept that under some circumstances it may cause hepatitis. An argument frequently made is that there are many milder or sub-clinical cases not recorded because patients are not followed up.

The direct toxicity mechanism has received support from a rat model in which an increase in potentially toxic reductive metabolites (also found in man) occurred during hypoxaemia. This implies that halothane toxicity might be worsened by postoperative hypoxaemia. These metabolites are capable of being stored in fat for later release and there is an increased incidence of obesity in cases of halothane hepatitis. The obese are also most likely to be hypoxaemic post-operatively.

There is also considerable evidence for an immune based mechanism. There is a definite association with multiple exposures. The first signs of the disease (usually pyrexia) do not appear for over a week following the relevant anaesthetic. Challenge experiments have proved positive in known sufferers and a specific serological marker has been found in a number of the cases of fulminant hepatic failure following repeat halothane anaesthesia.

The conclusion must be that the exact mechanism is uncertain. However, based on factors thought to be possible causes, it is reasonable not to administer a second halothane anaesthetic to patients who are obese, elderly, likely to have enzymes induced, or who are having radiotherapy (produces free radicals). Other risk factors are the propensity to develop postoperative hypoxia, operations or anaesthetics which seriously reduce liver blood flow, a known case of halothane hepatitis in a relative and the suspicion of a mild reaction after the first exposure. There is no evidence of the normal period of hypersensitivity after the first exposure but a common practice, which has no logical basis, is to assume that a second exposure is safe after a period of six weeks has elapsed. The diagnosis of halothane hepatitis has however been made with exposure intervals of over a year.

Acute (fulminant) hepatic failure

Acute liver failure in a previously normal person is rare and results from a serious process, e.g. viral hepatitis, septicaemia, drugs or poisoning. Patients require intensive therapy and the mortality is very high (50–80%). Hepatic failure is described as fulminant if neurological signs appear within two months of the onset of the illness. In fulminant hepatic failure, the commonest sources of blood loss are oesophageal varices and gastric erosions, sometimes complicated by the diffuse intravascular coagulation syndrome. Ascites does not occur but there is salt and fluid retention evident as oedema. Encephalopathy develops rapidly, with an absence of classical signs (e.g. flapping tremor) and its severity can be judged on the depth of coma. Hypoglycaemia with raised plasma insulin levels is usually present and should always be excluded as a contributory factor to encephalopathy. Other endocrine disturbances associated with cirrhosis such as hypogonadism, gynaecomastia, bone disease and Cushing's syndrome do not have time to develop.

These patients have a poorly understood sensitivity to many drugs, especially when cerebral symptoms have become apparent. Several mechanisms have been proposed but an abnormal cerebral sensitivity at the cellular level is gaining in acceptance.

Other problems are early hyperventilation with a low $PaCO_2$ and respiratory alkalosis. Accompanying this is hypoxaemia, thought to be due to intrapulmonary shunting or pulmonary oedema. Coexisting pulmonary infections are frequent. Hypotension secondary to inappropriate vasodilation is frequent and usually requires an increase in circulating volume with blood or plasma. Arrhythmias often co-exist and they should be treated if they compromise the cardiac output. Cerebral oedema can underly much of the symptomatology of encephalopathy and a few centres, if a person is sufficiently ill to require ventilatory or circulatory support, monitor the intracranial pressure. Once consciousness is at all impaired, the risk of gastric aspiration is high and may be a make-weight consideration in whether or not to ventilate.

It is obvious that only life saving procedures should be undertaken on this group of patients, with all the precautions outlined above for jaundice and hepatocellular failure.

FURTHER READING

Bailey, M.E. (1976) Endotoxin, bile salts and renal function in obstructive jaundice. *Br. J. Surg.* **63**, 774–8.

Baum, M., Stirling, G.A. & Dawson, J.L. (1969) Further study into obstructive jaundice and ischaemic renal damage. *Br. Med. J.*, **2**, 229–31.

Browne, R.A. & Chernesky, M.A. (1984) Viral Hepatitis and the anaesthetist. *Can. Anaesth. Soc. J.*, **31**, 279–86.

Dawson, J.L. (1965) The incidence of postoperative renal failure in obstructive jaundice. *Br. J. Surg.*, **52**, 663–5.

Editorial (1977) The hepato-renal syndrome. *Lancet*, **1**, 940.

Fee, J.P.H., Black, G.W., Dundee, J.W. *et al.* (1979) A prospective study of liver enzyme and other changes following repeat administration of halothane and enflurane. *Br. J. Anaesth.*, **51**, 1133–40.

Neuberger, J., Gimson, A.E.S., Davis, M. *et al.* (1983) Specific serological markers in the diagnosis of fulminant hepatic failure associated with halothane anaesthesia. *Br. J. Anaesth.*, **55**, 15–19.

Neuberger, J., Vergani, D., Mieli-Vergani, G. *et al.* (1981) Hepatic damage after exposure to halothane in medical personnel. *Br. J. Anaesth.*, **53**, 1173–7.

Neuberger, J. & Williams, R. (1984) Halothane anaesthesia and liver damage. *Br. Med. J.*, **289**, 1136–39.

Oxman, M.N. (1984) Hepatitis B vaccination of high risk hospital personnel. *Anesthesiology*, **60**, 1–3.

Pohl, L.R. & Gillette, J.R. (1982) A perspective on halothane induced hepatotoxicity. *Anesth. Analg.*, **61**, 809–11.

Sear, J.W. (1984) Effect of renal and hepatic disease on pharmacokinetics of anaesthetic agents. *In:* Prys-Roberts, C. & Hug, C.C. Jnr. (eds), *Pharmacokinetics of Anaesthesia*. Blackwell Scientific Publications, Oxford. 64–88.

Sherlock, S. (1981) *Diseases of the Liver and Biliary System*. 6th Edn. Blackwell Scientific Publications, Oxford.

Strunin, L. (1977) *The Liver and Anaesthesia*. Saunders.

Zuckerman, A.J. (1984) Who should be immunised against Hepatitis B? *Br. Med. J.*, **289**, 1243–4

5/Nutritional disorders

Obesity

Malnutrition

Hypercatabolism

The essential nutrients required by the body to maintain the normal processes of life and to meet the demands of activity and growth comprise protein, carbohydrate, fat, trace elements and vitamins. The requirement in terms of calorific intake depends on the body size, the basal metabolic rate, the degree of activity, the environmental temperature and the age and sex of the individual. If these requirements are exceeded (as in obesity) or fail to be met (as in starvation), specific and quite different problems are presented to the anaesthetist. Although there can be a relative excess or deficiency of individual dietary components, these are either rare or of no particular consequence to the anaesthetic management, other than requiring modifications as outlined in the management of obesity or malnutrition. The specific excesses of iron (haemochromatosis) and alcohol are discussed in Chapters 9 and 10 respectively.

Obesity

Obesity, which results from an excessive intake of calories, is the commonest nutritional disorder in the infants, children and adults of western civilizations. Its incidence is increasing and it is defined as a body weight which exceeds the expected or ideal weight by more than 10%, taking into account height, age, body build and sex. An alternative definition is that state in which more than 25% of the body weight in males (30% in females) is attributable to fat. The majority of obese people have no other definable pathological condition apart from satisfying the desire to eat too much food for their needs. A minority become overweight as a side effect of endocrine dysfunction (Cushing's syndrome, hypothyroidism and hypopituitarism, q.v.).

The content of this section assumes that all efforts to reduce the patient's weight are either inappropriate or have been abandoned.

History

Ask about the effects of previous anaesthetics. Try and uncover the symptoms of those diseases commonly associated with obesity which may affect anaesthesia (heart disease, cerebrovascular disease, hypertension, hiatus hernia and diabetes mellitus, q.v.). Do not forget the possibility of an underlying anxiety neurosis as this may influence the choice of premedication. Suspect the rare but important coexistence of endocrine dysfunction.

Enquire about somnolence as a pointer to the uncommon Pickwickian syndrome. Try and get a measure of the person's normal level of activity, general mobility and exercise tolerance.

Discuss the possibilities of regional anaesthesia with both the patient and the surgeon prior to surgery. If an awake intubation is anticipated this should be fully explained in as sympathetic a manner as possible.

Examination

Ensure that the patient has been weighed; visual estimates are frequently inaccurate. Double scales or even the public weighbridge may be needed! Look at the patient and decide whether the standard operating table will be adequate or whether special arrangements will have to be made. Take the opportunity to look for venous access points and at the condition of the skin over pressure areas.

CVS. Look for signs of cardiac failure which can be difficult to detect in the obese. Sacral oedema is easily missed. Measurement of the blood pressure with a standard size cuff over-estimates the true values by as much as 20 mmHg in gross obesity.

RS. Examine the extent of rib movement on deep inspiration. If it is severely restricted, ventilation is almost totally diaphragmatic and very prone to postural deterioration. It is therefore wise to observe the breathing when supine and check that it is both adequate and comfortable in this position. Look for sternal fat pads which will make laryngoscopy difficult, and check the movement of the neck, the degree of mouth opening, the patency of the nostrils and the state of the teeth. If the jaws have been wired together for weight reduction liaise with the dentist to remove the wires.

LS. Arthritis is more common in the obese, so examine the knees and hips for mobility, especially if the lithotomy position is anticipated.

Skin. Intertrigo, boils or vaginal candidiasis could point to occult diabetes.

Investigations

FBC, LFT's and random blood sugar. These should all be normal in uncomplicated obesity. Polycythaemia may have developed secondary to chronic hypoxia.

CXR. This will assist in the detection of cardiomegaly, cardiac failure and aortic atherosclerosis. If the latter is present it will be general throughout the body. A radiograph is an important baseline for major operations. Its necessity for minor procedures can be left to clinical judgement.

ECG. Rhythm and conduction disturbances are adequately reproduced. A thick fat layer does, however, reduce the voltages recorded so that cardiac hypertrophy may remain unnoticed. There are often considerable differences in the ECG between inspiration and expiration because diaphragmatic breathing swings the cardiac vectors with respect to the electrode placements. A prolonged Q-T interval and a reduced QRS voltage are non-specific abnormalities which may be found and suggest an increased anaesthetic risk. Look for evidence of ischaemia.

Blood gases. These are indicated in all severely obese subjects regardless of the operation, and for major operations in the less severely obese. Although values may be normal, the commonest pattern is a normal $PaCO_2$ with a PaO_2 reduced by up to 20% from the expected value corrected for age, breathing air. Hypoventilation with a raised $PaCO_2$ is both rare and serious. If artificial ventilation is anticipated postoperatively a preoperative baseline is invaluable. When taking an arterial sample remember that the PaO_2 is dependent upon posture and is lowest when supine. Hence the position of the patient should be recorded with the results.

Lung function tests. These will reveal combinations of decreased total lung capacity, decreased inspiratory capacity and expiratory reserve volume, reduced vital capacity, reduced functional residual capacity and increased closing volume. Lung function tests usually have little influence on the anaesthetic technique, their main use in gross cases being the recording of baseline data. The most useful indicator of pulmonary function is arterial blood gases.

Preoperative preparation

Introduce the physiotherapists who will be important postoperatively, encouraging maximal chest expansion and general mobility. Consider the use of subcutaneous heparin prophylactically to prevent postoperative deep vein thrombosis.

Premedication. The choice is personal but avoid reducing the ventilatory drive in someone with borderline pulmonary mechanics. An anti-sialogogue is usually helpful and improves the performance of any topical local anaesthetic used subsequently.

PEROPERATIVE PHASE

Take all procedures, however trivial, very seriously. Many of the problems occur because of the sheer size of the patient. Adequate manpower must be available to transfer the patient from the ward to the theatre. In general it is a good idea to induce anaesthesia on the operating table (which can be tipped) rather than to have to lift the patient twice.

Always think carefully about the pros and cons of regional and general anaesthesia. Many people like to combine them for better overall control of both the airway and the patient and to provide analgesia and relaxation with little central depression. Peripheral nerve blocks, spinals and epidurals can be technically difficult to perform because of the problems in locating landmarks beneath the fat. However, the distribution of fat may be such that a local anaesthetic block may not be as difficult as at first envisaged. Obesity also has the reputation of making the dermatome level achieved in spinal and epidural anaesthesia unpredictable. Even if it is intended for the patient to remain fully awake during regional blockade, beware of the distress, both mental and ventilatory, which the supine or head down position may cause.

With either local or general anaesthesia, try hard to secure a really good drip. Superficial veins may not be obvious and it can be time consuming cannulating a vein which can neither be seen nor felt easily. Watch for extravascular or intra-arterial injection. If the patient is first on the list bring them to the anaesthetic room early to get a relaxed start. Always have adequate assistance and sufficient personnel to manhandle the patient in an emergency. Put on the ECG and BP cuff prior to induction.

Check that the sucker is working. There is a strong possibility of regurgitation because of a hiatus hernia. Ensure that all the equipment for difficult intubation is to hand, especially a long-bladed laryngoscope.

Induction. Opinion is divided over the advantages and disadvantages of gas and intravenous methods. Overall the object is to avoid producing an unconscious patient who cannot breathe, and who cannot be ventilated or intubated. This can be circumvented by an awake intubation followed by induction of anaesthesia, but this may be unpleasant for the patient. The authors' usual practice is slow intravenous induction in the left lateral position, conversion to spontaneous ventilation on inhalational agents and then if intubation is planned, laryngoscopy to assess the degree of difficulty and to spray the vocal cords with local anaesthetic. The patient is then intubated with or without the aid of suxamethonium. No matter how skilled the anaesthetist, the induction of obese people is often harrowing and inelegant. Facemask ventilation can be exceedingly difficult and may on occasions produce copious gastric contents, especially if there is a hiatus hernia. Cricoid pressure should, of course, be used to prevent aspiration.

Maintenance. Drug requirements can be difficult to estimate because of a reduction in the proportion of body water in relation to body weight. The dose of water soluble drugs therefore needs to be reduced on a mg/kg basis. Prolonged use of fat soluble drugs such as halothane can lead to delayed recovery.

Depending upon the anticipated length of the operation and position of the patient, decide between spontaneous or artificial ventilation. End tidal CO_2 monitoring gives a guide to the adequacy of ventilation. Be careful not to overdose with neuromuscular blocking drugs. A nerve stimulator can be very helpful. Do not forget that IPPV does not necessarily require paralysis. Check that your ventilator is sufficiently powerful to ventilate the patient.

Obesity undoubtedly creates operative difficulties for the surgeon and hence prolongs anaesthesia, even for relatively minor operations. Large abdominal surgical packs may seriously reduce venous return and cause precipitous falls in blood pressure. Indirect arterial pressure monitoring is inaccurate in the obese and for major operations we advise direct arterial monitoring. This may not be technically easy but the radial artery is usually palpable.

Intraoperative fluid balance is difficult to assess. Central venous pressure monitoring is helpful with large blood losses, but this can again be technically difficult to institute. Landmarks may be hard or impossible to find. There is an increased risk of puncturing the lung and causing a pneumothorax or haemothorax with subclavian and internal jugular routes. Urine output can be usefully monitored.

Take care of the arms; do not let them fall off the table and do not cause nerve injuries through bad placement of restraints.

POSTOPERATIVE PHASE

Beware of the theatre emptying of staff once the operation is completed. Ensure that there is adequate help to lift the patient into the bed and to tip or position him as necessary.

In gross obesity or following major surgery, careful monitoring either in an ICU, recovery area or high dependency unit is mandatory.

If the patient has been breathing spontaneously with an endotracheal tube it is probably best to allow him to extubate himself in the left lateral position. If a non-depolarizing muscle relaxant has been used it is essential to wait until good muscle power has returned before extubation. This may warrant a period of postoperative ventilation. The optimum time and the criteria for extubation are debatable. Some anaesthetists consider clinical observations give the best indication whereas others would wait until the peripheral nerve stimulator showed good recovery of neuromuscular function with a well sustained tetanus or train of four. Other tests of muscular power that can be used are grip strength, sustained head raising, the ability to produce a maximum inspiratory force of greater than 25–30 cm of water, a vital capacity of greater than 15 ml/kg, and a tidal volume equal to approximately the preoperative level. Whatever decision is made, the patient must be awake prior to extubation.

Be very careful with the use of postoperative opioids because of the danger of ventilatory depression. Regional blocks may be used to provide analgesia (local anaesthetic or opioid). Postoperative hypoxia is particularly marked in the obese so they must have oxygen enriched air. Often their ventilation is markedly improved by propping them up to 45°.

Do not forget that the stress of an operation can produce a temporary or permanent diabetic state in the obese. If serious postoperative surgical complications develop which prevent adequate spontaneous ventilation (e.g. septicaemia, pulmonary embolus etc.) it is sometimes better to cut ones losses earlier rather than later and perform a tracheostomy to aid management. When to do this will always remain a personal and variable decision.

Malnutrition

Ill health as a result of an inadequate diet may affect adults or children. The two commonest childhood conditions worldwide, kwashiorkor and marasmus, occur almost exclusively in underdeveloped countries. Kwashiorkor results from a deficiency of protein in the presence of an adequate or even excessive calorie intake. The extremely low calorie diets which are responsible for the syndrome of marasmus are also deficient in proteins and many other essential nutrients. In endemic areas there will be no difficulty diagnosing these conditions but more minor degrees of malnutrition are less easily recognized.

Marginal undernutrition (which is not infrequent in the western world) profoundly affects the patient's ability to recover from

199

surgery. It has been estimated that nearly half of the adult patients presenting for major abdominal surgery in Britain suffer from a degree of malnutrition. The causes are multifactorial: it may arise when there is not enough food to eat (e.g. poverty), when there is inability to swallow (e.g. carcinoma of the oesophagus, bulbar palsy), when there is chronic disease preventing normal metabolism of nutrients (e.g. tuberculosis, renal failure), when there is malabsorption (e.g. coeliac disease, Crohn's disease) and when there is a lack of desire to eat (e.g. anorexia of malignancy).

The anaesthetic consequences of undernutrition are similar whatever the cause. Specific deficiencies and their implications are only mentioned briefly as appropriate.

PREOPERATIVE CONSIDERATIONS

History

Have a high index of suspicion of malnutrition if the patient is a member of an 'at risk' group. In western society these are principally immigrant children, the impoverished elderly, the mentally ill, those suffering from malignant disease (especially of the GIT), those whose neurological disease makes swallowing difficult, expectant mothers (mainly of low social economic status), those who have had major gastrointestinal surgery (e.g. gut resections), those suffering from small intestinal disease (e.g. Crohn's disease, coeliac disease) and alcoholics.

The patient may be too depressed to give an adequate history. If not, there is a universal presence of the non-specific symptoms of weakness, lethargy and feeling 'run-down', which are not helpful in assessing the severity of undernutrition. If there is a reliable history of weight loss this is important. A weight loss in six months of over 10% of the body weight is significant. In the absence of an accurate weight record, an adult patient may complain of loose fitting trousers or skirts. Parents might say that their child is not growing out of his clothes.

Longstanding undernutrition is not associated with ketosis and the rate at which weight is lost decreases, as the body adapts to a decreased supply of food. The bulk of muscle and other tissues is reduced, basal metabolism falls and unnecessary voluntary movement is omitted. It is important to distinguish between the weakness and pain in limbs due to undernutrition and that due to degenerative arthritis.

Examination

General. A formal assessment of nutritional status must include the patient's weight. A weight (corrected for height and body build)

Background. Hypercatabolism is an acute state produced by a wide variety of events such as trauma, burns, sepsis, surgery and renal failure. Often several of these features exist in combination. In essence, the patient needs more energy than his ordinary or reduced nutritional supply can provide for the acute stress situation, and consequently endogenous energy stores of fat and protein are broken down to provide the substrates for intermediate metabolism.

The increase in the metabolic and nitrogen excretion rates and the higher blood glucose and insulin levels occurring during hypercatabolism contrast with the reduced energy expenditure, reduced nitrogen excretion and low blood glucose and insulin levels that are present in undernutrition when ketoadaptation and conservation of resources is the theme. The raised blood sugar levels of hypercatabolism are secondary to the release of stress hormones and the high insulin levels are produced to control the high blood sugar.

PREOPERATIVE CONSIDERATIONS

Firstly, get a full understanding of the background events which led to the hypercatabolic state. Take advantage of any previous anaesthetic experience to forewarn of possible difficulties. These patients are nearly always on an ICU and may present for repeated anaesthetics for procedures such as tracheostomy, orthopaedic operations or skin grafting. Take careful note of all the parameters that have been monitored, especially the pulse rate, blood pressure, temperature, ventilatory rate, fluid intake, urine output and the lability or stability of these factors. If the patient is being artificially ventilated, as they often are, find out what the inspired O_2 concentration is, what inflation pressures and minute volume are required, and whether any problems have been encountered. Note, if present, a parenteral feeding line (not to be used for anaesthetic drugs or replacement fluids) and the intravenous feeding prescription (so that this can be continued intraoperatively). Plan your venous access. If there is no drip available for your drugs, using strict asepsis cannulate a suitable vein on the ICU before going to theatre. If the patient is aware of his surroundings a sympathetic explanation of the anticipated procedure should be given even if he is not able to sign his own consent form. This is especially important for tracheostomy as the patient may think that this is to be permanent. Thoughtful and kindly handling outweighs drug premedication.

Investigations

Results should be available from the same day. Check FBC (any anaemia will hopefully have been corrected), urea and electrolytes, arterial blood gases and chest X-ray. The ECG needs continuous monitoring. Blood clotting studies may be indicated. Where possible, correct any acute biochemical changes before surgery. Mild non-specific changes in LFT's are common with all forms of hyperalimentation.

PEROPERATIVE PHASE

Ensure plenty of help with the transfer of the patient. Because of the high minute volume often required, underventilation is a real danger when 'bagging' him *en route* to the operating theatre. It is best to move the patient directly from the bed to the operating table because of the number of drips, tubes, catheters, drains etc. which have to accompany the patient. For a non blood-spilling operation (e.g. tracheostomy) the surgeon may be willing to perform the operation with the patient in his ICU bed. Before inducing anaesthesia ensure that all the monitoring used on the ICU (ECG, arterial and central venous pressures, pulmonary artery catheters etc.) is connected and operational. It is mandatory to monitor the patient at least as well as on the ICU. Movement often provokes unexpected haemodynamic perturbations.

At the time of the original insult, a far-sighted anaesthetist may have inserted an epidural catheter in which case, if appropriate, consider using it. Often though, once the hypercatabolic state is established there are coexistent clotting defects which preclude regional anaesthetic techniques.

If the patient is not already intubated preoxygenate fully. Aspirate the nasogastric tube. Induction of anaesthesia will be rapid because of the presence of a high cardiac output. Care is needed not to give an overdose of drugs. Suxamethonium can cause acute rises in serum potassium within days to weeks after trauma or, more particularly after burns. If rapid intubation is advisable because of stomach contents, ensure that the serum potassium is within normal limits preoperatively and keep a watchful eye on the ECG.

The high level of CO_2 production and the increased ventilatory activity required to 'blow it off' mitigates against spontaneous ventilation for even the shortest procedures. It is easy with the ventilatory depressant effect of opioids and volatile anaesthetic agents to very quickly develop a severe respiratory acidosis. Because the metabolic rate is very high, the normal nomograms for isocapnic ventilation are no longer applicable and higher minute volumes than normal will be needed, especially if there is also some underlying pulmonary pathology. The high CO_2 production with an increased deadspace can be disastrous for the patient if partial rebreathing circuits are used carelessly. End-tidal CO_2 monitoring is invaluable. Maintain the F_IO_2 at least as high as that required for adequate gas exchange before the operation. With the increased O_2 uptake of hypercatabolism and the frequent occurrence of pulmonary dysfunction there is a high risk of making the patient hypoxic. Repeat blood gas estimations peroperatively. With a high F_IO_2, the N_2O percentage may not be high enough to prevent awareness and intravenous supplements will be required.

The osmolarity of feeding solutions is always high. Increasing such a fluid to act as a maintenance solution during anaesthesia merely produces a prompt osmotic diuresis. A sudden withdrawal of hypertonic glucose often results in a rebound hypoglycaemia within twenty minutes.

There has been recent interest in the methods of reducing the catabolic response to surgery. In theory, there are great benefits to be derived by minimizing the metabolic and hormonal changes. As yet these have not been proven to be of practical benefit. The response can be attenuated by regional blockade or by high doses of intravenous opioid. It is only abolished by a very extensive local anaesthetic blockade which is maintained postoperatively, or by *massive* doses of intravenous opioid. Until definite advantages emerge, these techniques are not advised because of their inherent dangers.

Postoperative phase

Care should obviously be continued in the ICU. It is likely that the patient will require postoperative ventilation until the anaesthetic drugs have been metabolized and the underlying condition has improved. If extubation is anticipated the patient must be capable of very vigorous and sustained ventilatory efforts because of the high CO_2 production. Sufficiently high doses of opioid to ensure good postoperative analgesia can sometimes only be given if the patient is ventilated.

FURTHER READING

Cork, R.C., Vaughan, R.W. & Bentley, J.B. (1981) General anaesthesia for morbidly obese patients — an examination of postoperative outcomes. *Anesthesiology*, **54**, *310–3*.

Elliott, M.J. & Alberti, K.G.M.M. (1983) Carbohydrate metabolism — Effects of preoperative starvation and trauma. *Clinics in Anaesthesiology*, **1**, No. 3, 527–50. W.B. Saunders.

Fisher, A., Waterhouse, T.D. & Adams, A.P. (1975) Obesity: its relation to anaesthesia. *Anaesthesia*, **30**, 633–47.

Fox, G.S., Whalley, D.G. & Bevan, D.R. (1981) Anaesthesia for the morbidly obese: Experience with 110 patients. *Br. J. Anaesth.*, **53**, 811–16.

Goode, A.W. (1981) The scientific basis of nutritional assessment. *Br. J. Anaesth.*, **53**, 161–7.

Michel, L., Serrano, A. & Malt, R.A. (1981) Nutritional support of hospitalised patients. *N. Engl. J. Med.*, **304**, 1147–52.

Powell-Tuck, J. & Goode, A.W. (1981) Principles of enteral and parenteral nutrition. *Br. J. Anaesth.*, **53**, 169–81.

Schneider, A.J.L. & Biebuyck, J.F. (1983) Intraoperative management of patients receiving total parenteral nutrition. *Clinics in Anaesthesiology*, **1**, No. 3, 647–67. W.B. Saunders.

Traynor, C. & Hall, G.M. (1981) Endocrine and metabolic changes during surgery: anaesthetic implications. *Br. J. Anaesth.*, **53**, 153–60.

Vaughan, R.W. & Wise, L. (1975) Postoperative arterial blood gas measurement in obese patients: effect of position on gas exchange. *Ann. Surg.*, **182**, 705–9.

6/Endocrine and metabolic disease

The endocrine pancreas
Diabetes mellitus
Insulinoma

The pituitary gland
Panhypopituitarism
Diabetes insipidus
Acromegaly

The adrenal glands
The adrenal medulla
  Phaeochromocytoma
The adrenal cortex
  Cushing's syndrome
  Adrenocortical insufficiency
  Iatrogenic adrenocortical
    suppression
  Conn's syndrome

The thyroid gland
Hypothyroidism
Hyperthyroidism
Enlarged thyroid

Parathyroid glands
Hyperparathyroidism
Hypoparathyroidism
Hypercalcaemia
Hypocalcaemia

Carcinoid syndrome

THE ENDOCRINE PANCREAS

The two varieties of glandular tissue in the pancreas are the exocrine acini (which secrete digestive juices into the duodenum) and the endocrine islets of Langerhans. The cells in the islets are named alpha (secreting glucagon), beta (secreting insulin) and delta (secreting somatostatin). Although glucagon and somatostatin are involved in glucose homeostasis, their clinical importance is very much less than that of insulin.

Diabetes mellitus

The physiology and pathology of insulin deficiency

Normally, approximately 50 units (1/4 of the store) of insulin are released daily in response to carbohydrate foods. It enhances the entry of glucose into muscle and fat cells by facilitated diffusion across the cell membrane. It stimulates glycogen formation (in liver and muscle), inhibits glycogenolysis and gluconeogenesis, and encourages fat deposition, both by inhibiting lipase and by the transport of glucose into fat cells. Insulin also facilitates potassium transport into cells. Feedback mechanisms maintain the blood glucose in normals between 3.5 and 7.0 mmol/litre.

209

On the basis of aetiology two main divisions of insufficiency are recognized.

Primary (Idiopathic). The majority of patients fall into this group (approximately 2% of the adult population) and are further sub-divided:

1 Juvenile-onset type. This usually develops during the first 45 years of life in patients of normal, or less than normal weight. In most, the onset of symptoms is rapid and progressive over several weeks or months. They quickly develop ketoacidosis and their serum insulin is zero. They are therefore 'insulin-dependent'.

2 Adult or maturity onset type. This presents in late middle age or old age. The patients have some insulin secretion, but not enough. They are therefore described as 'insulin independent' and they are less prone to develop ketoacidosis. Often they present indirectly, with the complications of the disease. The situation is always made worse by obesity which requires a higher basal plasma insulin and an excessive insulin response to a glucose load to maintain serum glucose within normal limits. This group of patients may become insulin dependent when stressed by infection or surgery.

Secondary. A very small minority of cases of diabetes occur as a result of a recognizable pathological process, or secondary to some other condition:

- Pancreatic insufficiency from chronic pancreatitis, haemochroma-tosis, pancreatectomy or carcinoma of the pancreas.
- Secretion or ingestion of substances which antagonize insulin at the cellular level, e.g. steroids (Cushing's syndrome), growth hor-mone (acromegaly), adrenaline (phaeochromocytoma), thyro-toxicosis, glucagonoma.
- Pregnancy (increased insulin requirements).
- Liver disease.
- Drugs, especially steroids, including the contraceptive pill, and thiazides.
- Major injuries, especially burns.

ACUTE INSULIN INSUFFICIENCY

In contrast to hypoglycaemia (from an excess of insulin) when cere-bral function is affected early because the brain depends heavily upon glucose, the effects of insulin deficiency take hours or days (sometimes a week or two) to produce a life-threatening state. The condition can present in a continuous spectrum from near normality to terminal coma (if untreated). The major metabolic actions of

210

insulin are concentrated in skeletal and cardiac muscle, adipose tissue and the liver. Muscle and adipose tissue are dependent upon insulin to ensure cellular uptake of glucose by facilitated diffusion. In contrast the uptake of glucose by the brain (except possibly part of the hypothalamus), the kidney, the intestinal mucosa and erythrocytes is unaffected by insulin. Consequently, cerebral function is well preserved until the gross metabolic disturbances caused by diabetic hyperglycaemia affect it secondarily.

In insulin deficiency, glucose uptake from the intestine continues normally and glucose production is stimulated in the liver. There is no, or very little, uptake of glucose into muscle or adipose tissues and the serum glucose rises. Once the serum level exceeds the individual's renal threshold (average 10 mmol/litre), the glucose acts as an osmotic diuretic, carrying with it sodium and potassium ions. The result is polyuria, polydipsia, and electrolyte deficiency. In addition, the gradual elevation of serum, but not intracellular, glucose produces effective intracellular dehydration.

Initially, energy supplies are maintained by the catabolism of proteins and fats. For total conversion, fat requires the products of intermediate carbohydrate metabolism (principally oxaloacetate) to allow acetyl Coenzyme A (acetyl CoA), which is produced by the breakdown of triglyceride, to enter the Kreb's cycle. Without insulin these intermediate substances are absent, or at best in very low supply, and free fatty acids enter the blood stream and travel to the liver. Here, free acetoacetic acid is liberated (from condensed acetyl CoA units) and broken down to beta hydroxybutyric acid and acetone. These three compounds are known as ketone bodies. The two acids can produce a severe metabolic acidosis and acetone can be detected by its sweet smell both in urine and on the breath.

The final picture is therefore, that of an acidotic, dehydrated, hypovolaemic, hypotensive, electrolyte-depleted patient who eventually becomes comatose because of the effects of these disturbances on neural function.

LONG TERM COMPLICATIONS

Vascular. Vascular complications are responsible for 75% of all diabetic deaths. Both large and small vessels are affected. Ischaemic heart disease is five times more common than in normals. Atheroma of major arteries of the lower limbs is fifty times commoner than in normals. Cerebrovascular disease is frequent.

In small vessel disease, diabetic microangiopathy specifically affects the vascular basement membrane. It can cause retinopathy, renal failure and superficial gangrene of the skin of the foot (in the presence of palpable arterial foot pulses).

211

Neurological. Peripheral neuropathy (up to 30% of cases) is the commonest problem. It is a mainly sensory neuropathy with numbness, night cramps and paraesthesia in both feet, loss of proprioception and absent ankle jerks. Severe cases result in chronic painless ulcers which frequently become infected and may progress to gangrene. Charcot's joints occur but are now rare.

Autonomic neuropathy is less frequent, but of great importance. It causes postural hypotension and the autonomic effects of hypoglycaemia (pallor, sweating, tachycardia) may be absent. Less important (for anaesthesia) are the associated symptoms of impotence, diarrhoea and urinary retention with overflow.

Occlusion of vasa nervorum can produce isolated, frequently transient, nerve palsies (mononeuritis). These are usually of the 3rd cranial, ulnar or lateral popliteal nerves.

Renal. Intrinsic parenchymal disease is seen as both diffuse and nodular glomerular sclerosis. Small vessel disease causes reduced blood flow and infarction. Infarction of the papillae results in haematuria. Both acute and chronic pyelonephritis are more common, especially if there is frequent glycosuria. Renal failure is responsible for up to a third of diabetic deaths occurring in the under 40 year age group. Diabetics are now considered as candidates for renal transplantation.

Eye. Retinal changes occur in up to 20% of diabetic patients. Nonproliferative changes (haemorrhages, exudates, microaneurysms) do not affect vision. Proliferative changes (new vessel formation near the disc followed by fibrosis) can cause blindness. Subhyaloid and vitreous haemorrhages are more common than in normals.

Diabetics occur frequently on ophthalmic lists and may be totally or partially blind (q.v.).

Skin. Lipodystrophy, insulin sensitivity and chlorpropamide photosensitivity are unimportant in anaesthesia. Pressure points and existing broken skin require special care.

Infection. Intercurrent infection is common in diabetics (urinary tract, vulva, skin and chest), and can precipitate loss of control. Tuberculosis is not unusual, especially in the elderly.

EFFECT OF TREATMENT

The object of control, by whatever method, is to prevent hyper and hypoglycaemic states. Good control definitely reduces intercurrent infection and *may* reduce the incidence and progression of neurological defects. Vascular defects appear to be independent of control. Hypoglycaemia is the major serious complication of insulin therapy.

Modes of presentation and their anaesthetic management

General points applying to all diabetics are considered now and features of the different modes of presentation are discussed subsequently.

PREOPERATIVE CONSIDERATIONS

History and examination

Ask about the common presenting features (polyuria, fatigue, pruritus vulvae, thirst), whether there is a family history, if female whether she has had babies over 4.5kg, and about drugs (corticosteroids, thiazides). Pass rapidly over the systems which may be involved (see above), following up a positive finding appropriately. In a known diabetic, assess the degree of control.

CVS. Evidence of angina, myocardial infarction, intermittent claudication, gangrene and postural hypotension (systolic fall of > 30 mmHg on standing) should be sought.

NS. Involvement may show as numbness, pain, paraesthesia, leg ulcers, strokes, transient ischaemic attacks, impotence or gustatory sweating. Postural hypotension is a late sign of autonomic neuropathy: loss of heart rate variability during deep breathing is the most reliable early sign.

Renal. Symptoms may include polyuria (glycosuria or renal failure), frequency, dysuria, pruritus, or the secondary symptoms of anaemia or hypertension.

Skin. Look for boils and at the pressure areas.

Investigations

FBC, U & E's. These should be normal.

Blood glucose. This is an essential investigation in all diabetics. The desired value is between 5 and 10 mmol/litre. Glycosylated haemoglobin is useful to assess whether there have been prolonged periods of hyperglycaemia but this investigation is more relevant to the physician who is dealing with long-term control.

Urine analysis. Look for glucose (hyperglycaemia), ketones (poor control), protein (renal complications) and at the bacteriology (infection).

ECG. This should be normal. Look for evidence of ischaemic heart disease.

213

CXR. This should be normal. It is a useful screen for pulmonary infection, including tuberculosis.

Local or general?

There is no evidence that, with appropriate management, one is better than the other. For some operations, general anaesthesia (GA) is the only possibility. Where there is a choice, surgery is usually quicker under a GA, but postoperative nausea may make a rapid return to good diabetic control more difficult.

Local. The advantages of regional anaesthesia are reduction of the stress response, hypoglycaemia is noted early in the awake patient, there is a low incidence of postoperative nausea, and postoperative diabetic control is easy. The disadvantages of regional block are those problems normally associated with cardiovascular disease (q.v.), neurological conditions (q.v.), and patchy or unsuccessful anaesthesia. Some anaesthetists permit patients to maintain their normal diet if they are planning a regional block. Although a good system if it is totally successful it has several disadvantages. Because of stomach contents, conversion to a general anaesthetic is more risky, there is likely to be vomiting instead of nausea in response to a transient period of hypotension, and any convulsion secondary to intravascular injection of local anaesthetic risks producing aspiration.

General. Almost all general anaesthetic techniques have been used successfully. Ether is contraindicated because it produces hyperglycaemia. Co-existing cardiac or renal disease needs appropriate treatment.

With either technique, one of the most important things is to prevent intraoperative hypoglycaemia. During anaesthesia the clinical signs (sweating, tachycardia, hypotension) can result from many unrelated causes. Hypoglycaemia should, however, always be eliminated as a precipitant because of its potential for brain damage.

The presence of autonomic neuropathy has two important corollaries. Firstly, it prevents the symptoms and signs of hypoglycaemia occurring, and secondly, it confers a tendency to transient ventilatory arrest which is intensified in the presence of opioids and anaesthetic agents. The cause of this is not known. Beta-adrenoceptor blockade also prevents the sympathetic signs of hypoglycaemia. Patients with autonomic neuropathy are also at risk during changes of intraoperative posture and may develop hypotension on institution of IPPV.

All diabetics are at increased risk of spinal cord infarction and cerebrovascular insufficiency during hypotension. Induced hypotension should therefore only be undertaken in the fittest, youngest patients.

Intraoperative fluid replacement can be as normal except that lactate (NB Hartmann's solution) and fructose containing solutions should be avoided. Pressure areas need careful protection. Intraoperative details of insulin regimens are given later.

POSTOPERATIVE PHASE

Aim to get the patient back to a normal diet and insulin (or oral hypoglycaemics) as soon as possible. There is some evidence that better control is attained if an insulin infusion is maintained for 72 hours after surgery. This is relevant to the more major operations and is important because better diabetic control improves wound healing. Insulin requirements are increased postoperatively because of the stress response and if infection is present.

Write clear instructions for the nursing staff about how frequently to check the blood glucose (e.g. 2 hourly) and who to call if it falls outside prescribed limits (e.g. 5–10 mmol/litre).

Remember that diabetics are prone to infection (examine the chest regularly) and arrange physiotherapy and antibiotics as necessary. Always suspect an occult infection if diabetic control worsens unexpectedly. Increased insulin requirements usually precede the symptoms of infection.

FEATURES OF SPECIFIC CONDITIONS

Diabetics can present to the anaesthetist in six ways:
- Previously undiagnosed.
- Controlled by diet.
- Controlled by oral drugs.
- Controlled by insulin.
- In ketoacidosis.
- With rare complications.

The condition requiring surgery, especially if associated with infection (e.g. cholecystitis, abscess) may induce a diabetic state or worsen the control of a known diabetic. Good control is usually impossible until the underlying cause is dealt with and surgery should *not* be postponed. Others lose control because of the surgery, especially if it is on the bowel. Methods of dealing with the modes of presentation are described below.

The previously undiagnosed

Approximately one quarter of all diabetic patients undergoing surgery are undiagnosed on admission to hospital. Almost all of these fall into the 'adult onset type' who have a definite but insufficient insulin production. It is therefore necessary to have a high index of suspicion that diabetes may be present in any patient, especially if obese and over 60 years old.

The diagnosis is confirmed by blood glucose measurements. The criteria for diagnosis suggested by the World Health Organization and the National Diabetes Data Group of the National Institutes of Health are:
- A fasting blood glucose over 7.8 mmol/litre on two separate occasions.
- A blood glucose over 11.1 mmol/litre at 2 hours and on one other occasion during a 2 hour test after ingestion of 75 g of glucose.

In hospital practice, if a blood glucose sample taken between 9 and 10 am is in the normal range, it is very unlikely that the patient will be diabetic because this is the time of the peak serum glucose following breakfast.

If the patient is found to be diabetic, elective surgery should be postponed until good control has been achieved by whatever means are appropriate. Urgent surgery can proceed (unless the patient has ketoacidosis, see later) but the patient may need to be treated as insulin dependent and put on an infusion regimen in the perioperative period.

Controlled by diet

These patients can effectively be treated as normals. They occasionally become insulin dependent in the early postoperative period when they are best managed by an insulin infusion (see later).

Controlled by oral drugs

Sulphonyl ureas. These drugs act by stimulating endogenous insulin release. It is important to be aware of the duration of their action, e.g. tolbutamide 8 hours, glibenclamide 12 hours and chlorpropamide 36 hours. Because of its long duration of action, chlorpropamide should ideally be changed to tolbutamide or glibenclamide one week before operation. For minor operations, if the blood glucose is well controlled and usually below 7 mmol/litre, it is sufficient to omit the drugs (except chlorpropamide, see above) on the morning of surgery and recommence them postoperatively.

Those with poor control or having a major operation are best converted to an insulin, dextrose and potassium regimen on the day of surgery as outlined below.

The hypoglycaemic effect of sulphonyl ureas is enhanced by aspirin, phenylbutazone, the sulphonamides (which displace it from its binding sites), chloramphenicol and anticoagulants (which inhibit its metabolism). The prescribing of these in the perioperative period needs caution.

Biguanides. These drugs increase the peripheral uptake of glucose but their exact mode of action is uncertain. They also inhibit lactate metabolism and give rise to lactic acidosis. Because of this, it is recommended that all patients on these drugs are converted to an insulin, dextrose and potassium regimen as outlined below. Examples of the biguanides are metformin and phenformin whose duration of action is 6–8 hours.

For patients on oral drugs there are no special perioperative requirements and all general anaesthetic techniques have been used with success. Dextrostix are adequate as an indicator of blood glucose to reassure the anaesthetist. In the postoperative period the patient may need insulin temporarily.

Controlled by insulin

Elective surgery. There are over thirty commercially available preparations of insulin. Their most important feature is the duration of action. Most patients are maintained on a mixture of insulins to optimize the convenience of administration and the correct time of insulin release. Short acting insulins (e.g. soluble, actrapid), have a peak effect at 2–4 hours and last 8–12 hours. Medium acting insulins (e.g. isophane, semilente, monotard) have a peak effect at 6–10 hours and last up to 24 hours. Long acting insulins (e.g. lente, protamine zinc, ultratard) have a peak effect at 12–15 hours and last for at least 36 hours.

The general principle is, in the few days prior to surgery, to switch the patient to purely short acting insulins, usually on a twice daily basis. By doing this, there is effectively no active long acting insulin preparation left on the day of surgery. If possible put the patient first on the morning list.

The immediate pre and peroperative management of diabetics has been the subject of many recommended regimens, all of which presumably work well for their protagonists. Any successful regimen must accomplish two things:
• Prevent intraoperative hypoglycaemia.

217

● If it is a prolonged procedure have sufficient insulin and glucose in the serum to prevent the onset of ketosis.

Only two regimens which we have found to work well and which do not cause confusion on a general ward are outlined here. This is not meant to imply that other methods are necessarily inferior.

● For minor procedures early on morning lists (after which one can expect a rapid return to normal eating), the 'no insulin and no food' on the morning of operation works well. The serum potassium and blood glucose should be measured prior to surgery. Lunch can be taken with an appropriately reduced dose of soluble insulin based on previous requirements.

● All other patients are best treated with an insulin, dextrose and potassium infusion as recommended by Alberti and Thomas. One advantage of this scheme over some others is that because the dextrose and insulin are given together, any accidental change in the drip rate does not alter the proportions of dextrose and insulin given. Thus, there is less chance of consequent hyper or hypoglycaemia. The potassium supplement is required because insulin drives potassium into the cells and serum hypokalaemia results. If there is likely to be a long delay in returning to normal eating, the infusion needs to be given through a central line (separate to fluid balance solutions) to prevent thrombophlebitis.

On the day of surgery, whatever the time of surgery, omit the subcutaneous insulin and at 8–9 am set up an IV infusion composed of:

$$\underline{10\% \text{ dextrose } 500 \text{ mls} + 10 \text{ units soluble insulin}}$$
$$+ 10 \text{ mmol KCl}$$

to run over 5 hours.

Check the blood glucose and serum potassium before starting the infusion and after 2–3 hours. Monitor the glucose peroperatively every 30 minutes. Continue this scheme as long as the glucose is between 5 and 10 mmol/litre. If the blood glucose falls to less than 5 mmol/litre reduce the insulin to 5 units, and if it rises to between 10 and 20 mmol/litre increase it to 15 units. Blood glucose can be measured by dextrostix or a glucocheck machine but confirm the level by a laboratory test if there is doubt. Postoperatively, monitor the glucose 2 hourly and continue the IV scheme until the patient is eating normally. Greater concentrations than 10% dextrose can be given if fluid overload is a problem.

The effect of insulin is antagonized by corticosteroids, oral contraceptives and thiazide and loop diuretics. Beta-adrenoceptor blockers may prolong hypoglycaemia.

Emergency surgery. If the patient has been previously well controlled (e.g. requires wound debridement after an accident) the only additional problem is that of hypoglycaemia because of the long acting insulins which have already been given. This can be countered by the appropriate infusion of dextrose (using a central line if $> 10\%$ is needed). Otherwise, treat as an elective case unless they are ketoacidotic (q.v.).

In ketoacidosis

Only infrequently is it necessary to operate urgently on a patient in ketoacidosis, and when it is, it is usually an intra-abdominal problem (e.g. perforated diverticular abscess). There are two diagnostic difficulties: firstly, severe abdominal pain may be caused purely by ketoacidosis and disappear with treatment and secondly, severe peritonitis may present with minimal pain because of neuropathy.

Once surgery has been decided upon, although each case must be managed individually, the general principles described below are a useful basis from which to start. It is a serious undertaking. The object of management is not to try and correct everything as quickly as possible, achieving in an hour or so what normally takes 1–2 days. Doing this produces dangerous swings in serum osmolarity (which can result in cerebral oedema) and imbalances the serum and CSF pH (which disturbs the ventilatory compensation of acidosis). It is sufficient, prior to urgent surgery, to correct acute hypovolaemia and produce a falling blood glucose.

Presentation. The likely abnormalities are:
- fluid losses of approximately 100 ml/kg
- electrolyte losses, sodium of 8 mmol/kg, potassium of 4 mmol/kg
- hyperglycaemia and hyperosmotic plasma
(osmolarity = glucose + urea + $2(Na^+ + K^+)$)
- a metabolic acidosis, compensated by hyperventilation and a low $PaCO_2$
- hypotension if severely hypovolaemic and acidotic.

Management.
- Take the patient to an intensive care area where facilities for resuscitation and ventilation are available.
- Take blood for glucose, electrolytes, urea, Hb and blood gases. Catheterize, get urine for microscopy and culture and sensitivity. Do a CXR.
- Monitor the ECG.
- Give IV fluids (0.9% saline) quickly, until the patient has a high normal CVP and is well perfused.
- Give 20 units of soluble insulin IV stat and start an infusion at 10 units/hour.

219

● Add potassium to the infusion fluids to prevent hypokalaemia. Monitor the T wave on the ECG (see Fig. 7.1). Once acute hypovolaemia has been corrected and the urine output is adequate, 10–20 mmol of KCl is usually needed with each litre of fluid.
● The use of bicarbonate is controversial and discussed later, but if the pH is below 7.1 the acidosis itself is potentially life-threatening and it is reasonable to give 1 mmol/kg of bicarbonate over the first one or two hours. More potassium will be necessary.
● Acute gastric dilation is common so pass a nasogastric tube for the aspiration of stomach contents.
● Give a broad spectrum antibiotic.
Monitor the blood glucose every 30 minutes. Once it has started to fall, it indicates that insulin is acting successfully, sugar is entering muscle and adipose tissue, and surgery can commence.

Anaesthetic considerations. All patients with ketoacidosis need to have their $PaCO_2$ controlled. This implies the use of IPPV. N_2O, O_2, opioid and relaxant is the method of choice. Gastric dilation requires crash induction with cricoid pressure to prevent aspiration of stomach contents.

It is essential to do blood gases immediately prior to induction. This $PaCO_2$ can be regarded as the physiological optimum for correction of that individual's metabolic acidosis. There are then two approaches.

Firstly, the patient can be ventilated to this $PaCO_2$ during surgery (for which an end-tidal CO_2 meter is useful). Ventilation to normocapnia may produce an acute and dangerous fall in the pH. However, if the $PaCO_2$ is very low, there can be a serious fall in cardiac output during anaesthesia. Under these conditions an alternative which may be preferable is to infuse bicarbonate and allow the $PaCO_2$ to rise by reducing the ventilation. It must be stressed that great care is needed to prevent dangerous swings in pH and serum potassium (which can be sufficient to produce cardiac arrest).

Throughout the operation do blood gases every 15 minutes and glucose every 30 minutes. As the ketoacidosis is corrected at the cellular level, ventilatory requirements will change continuously.

Reversal of relaxants may be impaired in the presence of acidosis. In serious cases, a period of postoperative ventilation is appropriate until the diabetes is under better control.

Continued postoperative treatment is as for the insulin dependent patient.

Rare conditions

Hyperosmolar non-ketotic diabetic coma. This is rare, and even more so to present with a surgical condition. The principles of management are similar to ketoacidosis but there is no acid base imbalance. The pathogenesis of the illness is not understood. Normally, there is only a very mild underlying diabetic state.

Blood glucose should only be reduced very gradually, because of the risk of inducing cerebral oedema. The likelihood of venous and arterial thrombosis is very high and patients may need to be heparinized.

Lactic acidosis. This condition should be suspected in a diabetic patient who is acidotic but who has no ketosis. It can be due to the action of biguanides (usually on alcohol) but it also occurs in uraemia, liver failure, septicaemia and pancreatitis.

Diagnosis is made on an anion gap $(Na^+ + K^+) - (Cl^- + HCO_3^-)$ of over 15–20 mmol. Treatment is that of the underlying condition and by correction of the acidosis with bicarbonate.

Insulinoma

This rare tumour, of which 10% are malignant, causes hypoglycaemia especially during fasting. It is usually a single benign adenoma found in the pancreas but it can be multiple or ectopic. There is a family history of diabetes mellitus in 25% cases. Other endocrine adenomas, e.g. pituitary, parathyroid and adrenal, may co-exist.

The diagnosis of inappropriate insulin secretion in a fasting hypoglycaemic patient can be difficult to make. Treatment is surgical removal.

The main anaesthetic problem is that of maintaining normoglycaemia. Watch for hypoglycaemia during the preoperative starve and put up a 10% dextrose drip. Handling of the tumour often causes hypoglycaemia which may go undetected during general anaesthesia.

It is vital to be able to monitor the blood glucose every five minutes during surgery and to have some 50% dextrose solution drawn up ready to give for acute hypoglycaemia. Hence, a central venous line is needed. Some workers consider that if, after removal of the tumour there is not a sustained rise in blood sugar after 30 minutes, there are other tumours remaining. There may be a temporary postoperative diabetic state.

PITUITARY GLAND

This small gland (0.5–1.0 g, 1 cm in diameter) is located in the sella turcica at the base of the brain. Together the hypothalamus and the pituitary form a control unit that regulates growth (growth hormone), lactation (prolactin), thyroid (thyrotropin releasing hormone (TRH), and thyroid stimulating hormone (TSH)), adrenal (corticotrophin releasing factor (CRF), and adrenocorticotropin hormone (ACTH)), and gonadal (follicle stimulating hormone (FSH), and luteinizing hormone, (LH)) function from the anterior pituitary and the state of hydration (antidiuretic hormone (ADH)) from the posterior pituitary.

The three commonest pituitary tumours releasing excess hormones cause acromegaly (growth hormone), Cushing's syndrome (ACTH) and lactation (prolactin). Tumours releasing gonadotrophins and thyrotropins are exceedingly rare. All tumours may cause neurological symptoms or signs, particularly visual field defects because of pressure on the optic chiasma. Prolactin secreting tumours, apart from their space-occupying effect, should not pose much problem to the anaesthetist. Acromegaly is discussed under pituitary gland disorders and Cushing's syndrome under adrenal gland disorders.

Abnormally low release of hormones may be due to tumours, surgical hypophysectomy or radiation. This results in a hypopituitary state which may affect all hormones (panhypopituitarism), ADH (diabetes insipidus), ACTH (Addison's disease), TSH (hypothyroidism) or growth hormone.

Panhypopituitarism

The clinical condition resulting from destruction of the anterior pituitary is accompanied by secondary atrophy of the gonads, the thyroid gland and the adrenal cortex. The commonest cause is a pituitary tumour. When it results from postpartum necrosis of the pituitary gland it is called Sheehan's disease.

Adults have absent axillary and pubic hair, genital and breast atrophy, pale skin and nipples and poor muscle development. If it occurs before puberty, growth is stunted. The important anaesthetic implications, however, are those of undersecretion of thyroid hormone and ACTH which are discussed later in this chapter.

Diabetes insipidus

Diabetes insipidus is a disorder due to impaired renal conservation of water because of inappropriately low levels of ADH. In the majority of cases the cause is unknown (idiopathic) but it can follow trauma or pituitary or hypothalamic surgery. Surgically-induced diabetes insipidus usually manifests itself during the first postoperative week and may then either resolve or become chronic.

The patient notices polyuria and polydipsia. The urine has a low specific gravity (under 1.010) and the volume can be up to 24 litres daily in extreme cases. Plasma osmolality rises. Normal function of the thirst centre ensures that polydipsia closely matches polyuria so that unless fluid is withheld (e.g. preoperative starvation), dehydration does not normally occur.

If the patient has some residual ADH function this can be enhanced by chlorpropamide, clofibrate or carbamazepine. The condition is, however, usually treated with desmopressin (a synthetic analogue of vasopressin) 10–20 µg applied nasally once daily. It can also be given IM or IV. Symptomatic relief should be evident and the desmopressin taken normally in the perioperative period. Alternatively, vasopressin can be used (by infusion) but it is more likely to cause hypertension.

In practice, intraoperative fluid management is not difficult. Monitor urine output and serum osmolality. The serum osmolality can be estimated from the sum of the concentrations of the serum glucose and urea and twice those of sodium and potassium (normal range 283–285 milliosmole/litre). If the osmolality reaches over 290 milliosmole/litre, hypotonic fluids should be given and desmopressin given IM or IV.

Acromegaly

Acromegaly is a chronic disease of middle life characterized by overgrowth of bone, connective tissue and viscera due to prolonged excessive release of growth hormone. If this defect occurs before puberty the long bones continue to grow and gigantism results.

Acromegaly affects both sexes equally. Once diagnosed it is treated by pituitary ablation with radiotherapy, or by surgical removal if there is a major visual impairment. There is enlargement of the heart, liver and thyroid. Although it is a rare disorder, it is important to the anaesthetist because of airway management and the high incidence of hypertension and diabetes mellitus. These patients have large lips, jaw, tongue and epiglottis. Face mask ventilation may be impossible. Hypertrophy of pharyngeal and laryngeal structures may make the anatomy difficult to interpret, the cords may not be seen, and the larynx may be resistant to external manipulation, all resulting in a difficult intubation.

PREOPERATIVE CONSIDERATIONS

History

The onset of symptoms is insidious but the advanced acromegalic is easily recognized. Common complaints are needing larger hats, gloves, rings and shoes, and headaches, visual disturbances, amenorrhoea, loss of libido and arthralgia. A third of patients originally seek medical advice for an unrelated illness. Ask about the symptoms of diabetes mellitus (q.v.) and hypertension (q.v.). When diabetes is present it is usually easily controlled. Drug therapy frequently includes a diuretic and antihypertensive agents.

In the treated patient, gauge the arrest of the disease by the progress of symptoms since treatment. Look for signs of hypopituitarism. Any previous anaesthetic record may indicate the degree of difficulty with airway management.

Examination

General. Note the characteristic enlarged hands, feet, nose and jaw and the coarseness of facial features. Examine the mobility of any joints affected by osteoarthritis. Look for kyphoscoliosis and degenerative signs in the back if an epidural or spinal block is envisaged.

RS. Examine the airway, note the size of the jaw and check neck movements carefully. Ask to see the patient's tongue which is often enlarged. Listen for a hoarse voice indicating thickening of the vocal cords or soft tissue obstruction of the pharynx. The patency of the nasal airway is prone to obstruction by polypoid growth. Carefully consider in the light of these findings the options for endotracheal intubation.

CVS. Hypertension occurs in 25%. Check that cardiac failure is not present. If anticipating arterial cannulation, test the ulnar collateral supply to the hand because it is frequently compromised. If this is the case, brachial or dorsalis pedis arterial cannulation may be preferable to radial.

NS. Look for peripheral neuropathy, due to nerve trapping, especially if anticipating local anaesthetic blocks.

Investigations

FBC and U & E's. These should be normal.
CXR. Look at the heart size, for the presence of cardiac failure or kyphoscoliosis and at the position of the trachea.

Skull X-ray. The sella turcica will be enlarged. These films may also predict the difficult intubation already anticipated clinically.
ECG. Look for left ventricular hypertrophy.
Urinalysis. Check for glucose.
Blood glucose. Do a random blood sugar to uncover occult diabetes.

ANAESTHETIC MANAGEMENT

First consider whether local or regional anaesthesia is possible or advisable. Whether a local or a general anaesthetic is chosen, always be prepared for a difficult intubation. Have available a long-bladed laryngoscope, long endotracheal tubes of varying sizes (a smaller diameter tube than predicted may be needed if there is supra or subglottic stenosis) and any other aids or introducers likely to help.

Management of the airway on a facemask is likely to be difficult and only suitable for short operations. Use a large facemask and make sure the large tongue does not cause obstruction. A size four oral airway is usually necessary. A nasopharyngeal airway can be successful but often there is considerable haemorrhage and difficulty in passing one because of hypertrophied nasal mucosa.

If intubating, the best technique depends upon the individual patient and anaesthetist. Although theoretically correct, deepening anaesthesia by spontaneous ventilation with volatile agents (and assessing the problem at laryngoscopy before attempting intubation or giving a muscle relaxant) is often very difficult to do smoothly. If the intubation on preoperative assessment, or from a previous anaesthetic record, appears relatively straight forward, preoxygenation, IV induction and suxamethonium is probably the sequence of choice. Handle all tissues gently: blood in the larynx can make things much worse. The most difficult cases need appropriately skilled management, possibly with awake intubation. Facilities for performing tracheostomy must be readily available.

Manage hypertension, diabetes and kyphoscoliosis as outlined in other chapters.

Postoperatively, do not extubate until there is good muscle power and the patient is awake. There is a tendency to postoperative hyperglycaemia.

THE ADRENAL GLANDS

These are located at the superior pole of each kidney and are composed of two distinct parts, the medulla and the cortex which are of different embryological origin.

The adrenal medulla

This is functionally part of the sympathetic nervous system and is derived from neural crest tissue. Under normal conditions it secretes adrenaline (80%) and noradrenaline (20%) into the circulation. Here they have a similar effect to direct sympathetic stimulation. The half-life of adrenaline and noradrenaline in the circulation is only a few minutes. The adrenal medulla is not essential for life, and its ablation has little apparent effect.

In the doses secreted by the medulla, adrenaline has alpha and beta-adrenoceptor stimulating activity with the beta effects predominating. The net result is an increase in heart rate, cardiac contractility, cardiac output and systolic blood pressure. The vessels to skeletal muscle are dilated and those to skin, mucosae and the kidneys are constricted. Overall, this results in a lowering of peripheral vascular resistance and diastolic blood pressure.

Noradrenaline is predominantly an alpha stimulant and the peripheral resistance rises in almost all vascular beds. There is an increase in both systolic and diastolic pressures with a reflex reduction in heart rate.

Phaeochromocytoma

This is a rare tumour of adrenal medullary tissue which literally means 'dusky coloured'. Most cases are diagnosed preoperatively but the condition should be suspected during operation for any posterior mass between the kidney and diaphragm. Approximately one fifth of cases present *de novo* during pregnancy.

Phaeochromocytoma can arise from other chromaffin tissues of the sympathetic nervous system (e.g. para-aortic ganglia) but less than 2% are outside the abdomen. 10% are bilateral. Only very rarely are they malignant, but they can occur as part of a multiple endocrine adenoma syndrome (type II) with parathyroid adenoma, neurofibromatosis and medullary thyroid carcinoma.

60% of tumours secrete noradrenaline, 35% secrete noradrenaline and adrenaline and 5% secrete adrenaline alone. They represent less than 0.1% of hypertensives.

The following account of the preoperative preparation represents the most usual approach followed. However, there are some specialist centres which permit an incomplete state of adrenoceptor blockade preoperatively and use a sustained fall in BP intraoperatively as evidence of complete tumour removal. There are several potential complications and success requires excellent rapport between the anaesthetist and surgeon. Details of this can be found in 'Further reading'.

PREOPERATIVE CONSIDERATIONS

The condition mainly presents with hypertension in young adults. This may be sustained (usual) or paroxysmal (unusual). Symptoms include 'attacks' of pallor, palpitation, anxiety, headache, sweating and nausea. Angina and dysrhythmias of all types can occur. The systolic BP goes very high and cerebrovascular accidents and myocardial infarcts may cause premature death. Adrenaline secreting tumours produce hyperglycaemia and there may be a compensatory bradycardia with noradrenaline producing tumours.

The diagnosis is confirmed by elevated catecholamine levels in the blood or urine or by elevation of the urinary metabolite, vanillyl mandelic acid (VMA). Aortograms or an intravenous pyelogram may be used for localization of the tumour.

The elective case should be prepared well before surgery. The aim is to produce the appropriate amount of adrenergic receptor blockade preoperatively, so that there is no fall in blood pressure from systemic vasodilatation or reduction of sympathomimetic stimulation of the heart after removal of the tumour. Short acting drugs can then be used intraoperatively to deal with surges of catecholamine release as the tumour is handled. These can be minimized by the surgeon clamping the tumour's venous drainage early.

Initially, hypertension should be treated by an alpha-adrenoceptor blocker (phentolamine in an emergency, otherwise phenoxybenzamine). Beta-adrenoceptor blockers should only be added later to control tachycardia and dysrhythmias. If they are given before alpha-adrenoceptor blockade is achieved, they can reduce the skeletal muscle vasodilatation (if adrenaline is being secreted) and increase the peripheral vascular resistance and with it the blood pressure. Blood pressure stabilization usually takes several days to be effected.

The following criteria have been recommended as signs of adequate treatment:
• BP not greater than 165/90 mmHg for 48 hours before surgery.
• Orthostatic hypotension should be expected, but the BP on standing should not fall to below 80/45 mmHg.
• No S-T segment or T wave changes on ECG for at least 2 weeks.
• No more than one premature ventricular contraction present in 5 minutes.

PEROPERATIVE PHASE

Many techniques have been used with success; only the principles are outlined here (see Further reading).

Reduce endogenous catecholamine release by generous premedication. Have a selection of emergency drugs drawn up (e.g.

propranolol, practolol, phentolamine, lignocaine, sodium nitro-prusside (SNP)). On arrival in the anaesthetic room connect the ECG and insert a CVP line, peripheral drip and arterial line. Consider using a pulmonary artery catheter.

After preoxygenation and slow IV induction, laryngoscope and intubate gently so as to minimize a hypertensive response. Enflurane or isoflurane are preferable volatile agents to halothane for deepening anaesthesia because of their higher threshold for catecholamine-induced dysrhythmias. Agents which release histamine may aggravate catecholamine secretion and hence, muscle relaxants such as curare and alcuronium should be avoided. Pancuronium can, on occasions, produce hypertension. Vecuronium or atracurium may emerge as the relaxant of choice.

During maintenance, ensure an adequate depth of anaesthesia and aim to produce a systolic blood pressure of approximately 100 mmHg systolic, with the aid of, for example, enflurane, isoflurane or SNP. Set arbitrary limits (e.g. systolic BP of >150 mmHg, pulse rate of >90/minute) above which you will treat with the appropriate drugs.

Treat any dysrhythmias as outlined in Chapter 1 but do not forget that they can occur for other reasons than handling of the tumour (e.g. underventilation, awareness). Do not hesitate to ask the surgeon to stop in a crisis. Pay meticulous attention to fluid balance as considerable quantities of blood are sometimes lost.

After removal of the tumour hypotension should be treated with fluid replacement rather than by the use of catecholamines. This is one of the important factors in reducing operative mortality.

The unsuspected case

Suspicions may be aroused by an excessive hypertensive response to laryngoscopy and intubation or during surgery. *Always* get the surgeon to stop while you check for other simple, disastrous causes (e.g. underventilation, light anaesthesia, blocked endotracheal tube, pneumothorax, lack of oxygen).

If you are convinced of the likelihood of the diagnosis, establish alpha-adrenoceptor blockade with phentolamine (up to 10 mg diluted in 10 mls saline given slowly IV) to reduce the BP. Phentolamine lasts only minutes and needs repeated dosage. Continue management as in the elective case.

The adrenal cortex

The adrenal cortex is a true endocrine gland derived from embryonic mesothelium. It is essential for life. All its products are based on the cholesterol skeleton and daily it produces on average 20 mg of hydrocortisone (glucocorticoid), 0.15 mg of aldosterone (mineralocorticoid), and 20 mg of androgenic hormones.

The release of hydrocortisone is directly controlled by ACTH (from the anterior pituitary) which in turn is controlled by CRF (from the hypothalamus). The serum level of hydrocortisone produces negative feedback inhibition at both anterior pituitary and hypothalamic levels. There is a diurnal variation with a 'low' at midnight and a 'high' just after breakfast. Its role is principally in the control of intermediary metabolism with an overall catabolic effect. Protein breakdown, nitrogen excretion and gluconeogenesis are all increased and the peripheral utilization of glucose is decreased. It has an anti-insulin action.

The secretion of glucocorticoids is increased during periods of stress (serum levels rise only minutes after the start of surgery) and is essential for survival. The exact reason for this is as yet undefined, but is thought to be due to the fact that circulating glucocorticoids may be necessary for the maintenance of vascular reactivity to catecholamines. In addition, glucocorticoids are necessary for catecholamines to exert their full free fatty acid mobilizing action.

Aldosterone has its most important effect on the renal tubules conserving sodium and excreting potassium, hydrogen and magnesium ions. The control of its secretion is complex. It is secreted in response to stress (via ACTH), a high extracellular potassium, and as the final end point in the renin-angiotensin system.

Only four clinical syndromes resulting from malfuntion of the adrenal cortex are of importance in anaesthesia: over and under production of glucocorticoids, iatrogenic suppression of the adrenal cortex, and over production of aldosterone.

Cushing's syndrome

This results from a chronic excess of glucocorticoids due either to excess pituitary ACTH, ACTH from an ectopic site (e.g. carcinoma of lung, kidney or pancreas) or adrenal hyperplasia with loss of feedback control. It affects three times as many females as males and usually presents between the ages of 30 and 50 years. The diagnosis is made by demonstrating increased plasma and urine concentrations of cortisol. Treatment is by surgical removal of the source of excess ACTH or glucocorticoid.

The glucocorticoids are present in such large amounts that they exert a significant mineralocorticoid action, and there may be potassium depletion and weakness. Protein catabolism reduces the muscle bulk, the skin becomes thin and striae form, wounds heal poorly, minor injuries cause ecchymoses, and there is a reduction in bone matrix causing osteoporosis. The decreased peripheral utilization of glucose may produce diabetes (in up to 20% of cases) and the immune response and fibroblastic activity are inhibited.

PREOPERATIVE CONSIDERATIONS

History

Ask about the symptoms associated with the complications of the disease: diabetes mellitus (q.v.), hypertension (q.v.), chronic infections (chest and urinary tract), muscular weakness, obesity (q.v.), bone pain and vertebral collapse. Indigestion may be due to peptic ulceration. Aggressive behaviour or euphoria can result from 'steroid psychosis'.

Examination

General. Note the typical appearance of central obesity (may cause difficult surgical access), rounding of the face, the 'buffalo hump' (can make positioning difficult for intubation) and cutaneous striae.
CVS. Check the BP. Hypertension is common. Look for peripheral oedema due to salt and water retention and for left ventricular failure.
RS. Look for kyphoscoliosis (q.v.) and signs of pulmonary infection. Assess the ability to cough and breathe deeply.

Investigations

FBC. This should be normal but there may be iron deficiency anaemia if there is bleeding from peptic ulceration. Erythrocytosis, granulocytosis and lymphopenia have all been found secondary to a raised serum cortisol.
U & E's. Hypokalaemia with hypochloraemic alkalosis occurs in 10–20%.
Urinalysis. Glycosuria may be present. Check the blood glucose.
CXR. Look for kyphoscoliosis, osteoporosis, cardiac enlargement and the presence of left ventricular failure. The thoracic cavity may be small and lower lobe basal collapse present.
ECG. This may reveal left ventricular hypertrophy or hypokalaemia (see Fig. 7.1).
FEV_1, FVC and arterial blood gases. These tests of lung function are indicated in severe disease with vertebral collapse and kyphoscoliosis.

PREOPERATIVE PREPARATION

Few patients with untreated Cushing's syndrome present for incidental surgery. In preparation for curative hypophysectomy or

230

adrenalectomy optimize pulmonary and cardiac function but do not delay surgery unnecessarily for a long period as there is a high risk of myocardial infarction. Correct hypokalaemia. Prophylaxis against deep vein thrombosis may be advisable because of hyper-coagulability.

PEROPERATIVE PHASE

Manage the complications of kyphoscoliosis (q.v.), hypertension (q.v.) and diabetes mellitus (q.v.) as indicated elsewhere. Always take extreme care moving or positioning the patient because of the danger of causing fractures and skin damage.

Look for a good venous access site away from bruises. The veins may be buried, thin-walled and fragile and cannulation therefore requires skill and patience. Fix the cannula carefully with adhesive tape. It is easy to denude the skin when removing the tape. After removing a cannula the site bruises easily and bleeding is prolonged, so apply pressure gently and firmly.

The presence of hyperadrenocorticism does not influence the choice of drug or technique. Nevertheless, respiratory muscle weakness necessitates IPPV for all but the shortest procedures. Reduce the dose of muscle relaxants both because of muscle weakness and hypokalaemia. Avoid infection by using a sterile endotracheal tube.

Take care not to overload with sodium containing IV fluids because of the mineralocorticoid effect of excess cortisol.

If surgery is on the adrenal glands have drugs ready to block the peripheral actions of catecholamines (e.g. phentolamine, practolol, lignocaine) released during inevitable handling of the medulla.

The patient secretes large amounts of glucocorticoids (up to 500 mg/day in extreme cases) and this should only be reduced gradually. The exact replacement for each patient is best decided by discussion with the endocrinologist, who usually supervises the reduction in dose over the first two postoperative weeks. A typical regimen would give 200 mg hydrocortisone the night before the operation and 300 mg hydrocortisone by infusion on the day of the operation. Intra-operatively, after the tumour is removed, or the vein clamped, tachycardia and hypotension may result from insufficient circulating cortisol and 100 mg hydrocortisone can be given IV. However, always rule out other, simple causes of the same signs (e.g. blood loss).

POSTOPERATIVE PHASE

Postoperative ventilatory function is often poor because of muscular weakness. The first postoperative day should be spent in a high dependency area with oxygen enriched air to breathe and regular physiotherapy. Treat infections early with antibiotics.

Glucocorticoid insufficiency (vomiting, weakness, tachycardia, low grade fever, hypotension) and electrolyte abnormalities can occur. This requires treatment with hydrocortisone and electrolyte replacement and a change in the weaning regimen. This frequently involves an adjustment in the ratio of hydrocortisone and fludrocortisone given.

Adrenocortical insufficiency

The incidence of primary adrenocortical insufficiency (Addison's disease) is about 1 per 100 000. It affects both sexes and all ages. When it is caused by destruction of the cortex by granulomatous disease (most commonly tuberculosis), meningococcal septicaemia, fungal infections, cancer, haemorrhage, infiltrations (amyloid, haemochromatosis, leukaemia) and autoimmune processes, both cortisol and aldosterone are lacking. When the deficiency is secondary to a lack of pituitary ACTH, aldosterone secretion remains normal.

These states tend to be chronic and may have superimposed (Addisonian) 'crises' when the adrenal gland is unable to meet the demands of stress for increased glucocorticoids.

PREOPERATIVE CONSIDERATIONS

History and examination

The onset of chronic disease is insidious. The patient feels generally unwell, weak and has anorexia, nausea, vomiting or abdominal pain with weight loss. Pigmentation (due to melanocyte stimulating hormone, MSH, secretion) occurs particularly in exposed portions of the body (resembling a suntan), at points of pressure and friction and in the palmar creases. The most notable finding is *hypotension* (usually with a postural drop) and tachycardia. If the cause is autoimmune, there may be coexistent diabetes mellitus, hypothyroidism or hypoparathyroidism.

The diagnosis is made by a reduced plasma cortisol response to ACTH. Maintenance therapy is cortisone acetate and fludrocortisone.

Investigations

FBC. This may show mild normochromic anaemia.

U & E's. These are normal in mild disease but when severe or in a

crisis, hyponatraemia and hyperkalaemia (due to aldosterone defi-
ciency) are evident. The urea may then be raised due to dehydration.
ECG. This may show evidence of hyperkalaemia.
Blood glucose. This may be low.
Blood gases. These show mild metabolic acidosis.

ANAESTHETIC CONSIDERATIONS

The known chronic case presents few operative problems and should
be treated similarly to patients on steroid therapy (q.v.). Problems
arise when the patient presents for the first time because of the stress
of an acute illness requiring surgical correction. This is *very* rare.
The picture is indistinguishable from oligaemic shock. The patient is
usually apathetic and may be suffering from hypoglycaemia. Diagnosis is made by thinking of the possibility of hypoadrenalism and as
a result of investigations, especially those of the serum electrolytes.

If suspicions have been raised, it is best to asume that the diagnosis is that of adrenal insufficiency. Full investigations can be
carried out later. In emergency cases a rapid preparation for surgery
is as follows:
• Give hydrocortisone 100 mg IV stat followed by infusion of 100
mg over 24 hours.
• Rehydrate with sodium containing fluids.
• Give IV dextrose, 50 mls of 50% immediately, then by infusion.
• If there is a high serum potassium with associated ECG changes,
give calcium gluconate (10 mmol) and if necessary add insulin to the
dextrose infusion.
Unexplained hypotension may be corrected empirically by hydrocortisone after other simple reasons have been eliminated (e.g.
hypovolaemia, hypoxia). Monitor the serum glucose and the T wave
on the ECG. These patients are weak and debilitated and need
reduced doses of all drugs, especially neuromuscular blockers.

Postoperatively they are weak with poor ventilatory power.
Manage steroid cover as for those maintained on steroids with iatrogenic suppression of the cortex (q.v.).

Iatrogenic adrenocortical suppression

Patients present on steroid therapy for a variety of reasons (asthma,
rheumatoid arthritis, SLE, etc). Their adrenal suppression and tendency to a cushingoid state depends on the maintenance dose. In
addition to their adrenal suppression the anaesthetic considerations
are those of the basic disease and Cushing's syndrome.

In normal healthy patients, there is a prompt secretion of cortisol
immediately after the commencement of surgery which, after major

operations does not return to normal for up to 3 days. The rise in the plasma cortisol parallels the severity of surgery. The maximum output possible from normal adrenals is approximately 300 mg/day, but the amount secreted in response to major surgery does not usually exceed 150 mg/day.

Patients who have been on long-term steroid therapy may be unable to increase their cortisol output in response to surgery because of suppression of the pituitary-adrenal axis. This failure of cortisol secretion has been blamed for reports of 'collapse' and intra-operative hypotension in patients on long-term steroid therapy. The integrity of the pituitary-adrenal axis is not routinely tested and the traditional advice has been to increase steroid dosage in proportion to the surgical stimulus. Typical recommendations are, starting immediately before surgery, to give

- 100 mg hydrocortisone IM 6 hourly for 3 days for major surgery
- 100 mg hydrocortisone 6 hourly for one day for minor surgery
- for very short, non-stimulating procedures 100 mg hydrocortisone only.

These guidelines would include patients who have been on steroids within the last year although adrenal function is now thought usually to be normal within a week of stopping steroid therapy.

Recently there has been a swing in opinion suggesting that these dosages are excessive and may have deleterious effects (delay wound healing, increased likelihood of infection and GI haemorrhage). Consequently current recommendations have suggested reducing steroid cover to 25 mg hydrocortisone IV at induction of anaesthesia followed by 100 mg hydrocortisone infused IV over 24 hours for major surgery. 25 mg hydrocortisone IV at induction should be sufficient for minor surgery. Obvious causes of hypotension (e.g. hypovolaemia, vasodilation) should be corrected before empirically increasing steroid administration at any point in the postoperative period.

Conn's syndrome

This is due to an adrenal adenoma secreting aldosterone. It is rare, accounting for less than 1% of hypertensives. It is twice as common in women as in men.

The clinical features reflect the physiological effect of aldosterone:

Sodium conservation. The patient becomes hypertensive and the blood volume is expanded.

Potassium depletion. Muscle weakness, areflexia, tetany and paraesthesiae occur. The ECG abnormalities of hypokalaemia (S-T depression, flattened T waves and the appearance of U waves, see Fig. 7.1) and idioventricular arrhythmias may be present. Metabolic alkalosis follows *pari passu* with hypokalaemia because of the excess excretion of hydrogen ions.

The diagnosis should always be suspected when hypertension and unprovoked hypokalaemia coexist. Treatment is surgical removal of the adrenal gland containing the adenoma. If they are bilateral, medical therapy with the mineralocorticoid antagonist, spironolactone is preferred.

The main anaesthetic implications are those of hypokalaemia which should be corrected before surgery (with spironolactone and potassium supplements) and those of hypertensive cardiovascular disease (see Chapter 1).

THE THYROID GLAND

Physiology. The thyroid gland, located immediately below the larynx, secretes the hormones thyroxine (T4) and triiodothyronine (T3) whose function is the regulation of tissue metabolism. 90% of the hormonal release is T4 of which some is subsequently deiodinated to T3. Both hormones have qualitatively similar effects but T3 is more potent and is shorter acting. Iodine (about 1 mg weekly) is essential for the formation of thyroid hormones. Iodine deficiency in the first two years of life results in irreversible mental retardation (cretinism).

To maintain a normal basal metabolic rate, thyroid hormone secretion is regulated by a specific feedback mechanism. TRH, from the hypothalamus, directly increases the anterior pituitary gland output of TSH which, in turn, increases both the secretion and formation of T3 and T4. These are both stored bound to thyroglobulin in thyroid follicles but are released from the gland in the free form. They are then bound to thyroxine-binding globulin, thyroxine-binding prealbumin and a small proportion to albumin. The unbound fraction, which can now be measured, increases the overall metabolic rate and, in children, stimulates growth.

The clinical problems associated with the thyroid gland arise because of excessive or deficient hormone secretion (hyperthyroidism or hypothyroidism) or, alternatively, because of physical enlargement of the gland which may, or may not, be associated with hormonal dysfunction.

Hypothyroidism

Hypothyroidism affects 1.4% of adult females and 0.1% of adult males. It is also referred to as myxoedema which, strictly, is the non-pitting oedema caused by mucopolysaccharide accumulation in subcutaneous tissues.

235

Reduced thyroid function may be secondary to hypothalamic or anterior pituitary dysfunction, but surgical resection (after which hypothyroidism takes at least one month to develop) and auto-immune destruction of the thyroid gland are the commonest causes in adults.

The symptoms and signs can be attributed to either deceleration of cellular metabolic processes or the accumulation of hygroscopic mucopolysaccharide. The prognosis is excellent provided thyroid replacement is maintained.

PREOPERATIVE CONSIDERATIONS

History

Always have a high index of suspicion because this disease is one of the 'great imitators'. Common symptoms are weakness, fatigue, lethargy, dry coarse skin, voice change, intolerance of cold, moderate weight gain despite anorexia, poor memory and hearing, arthralgia, constipation and swelling of the hands, face and extremities. Be careful not to confuse the poor memory of hypothyroidism ('myxoedema madness') with that of cerebrovascular insufficiency or senile dementia. Check that those patients already treated with thyroxine are no longer clinically hypothyroid. See later if there are symptoms or signs of an enlarged gland.

Examination

General. Body and scalp hair are reduced and the skin is coarse, cool and sallow.
CVS. Bradycardia is common, with a low systolic but raised diastolic blood pressure. The heart sounds may be distant and the heart enlarged. A pericardial effusion is common but rarely leads to clinical problems.
NS. Cerebellar ataxia may be present. Delayed relaxation of deep tendon reflexes, peripheral neuropathy and carpal tunnel syndrome all resolve with hormone replacement.

Investigations

Serum thyroxine. A reduced free T4 index is diagnostic of hypothyroidism unless the patient is on large doses of salicylates or phenytoin. Measurement of the active hormone has superseded the use of protein bound iodine as an estimate of total serum T4 concentration. The total T4 gives a false normal result in 15% of patients with hypothyroidism.

236

TSH measurement establishes whether the disease is primary or secondary. If the TSH is high, the gland is failing to produce thyroxine. When the TSH is normal or low the hypothyroidism is likely to be secondary to a hypothalamic or pituitary disorder, in which case there may be deficiencies of other pituitary hormones, the most important being ACTH. If this is not recognized thyroid hormone replacement may result in an Addisonian crisis. Note that a dopamine infusion can cause suppression of an elevated TSH into the normal range.

Serum cortisol. This may be low if pituitary insufficiency is the cause of hypothyroidism.

FBC. This should be normal.

U & E's. The GFR is reduced and the ability to excrete free water is reduced. Inappropriate ADH secretion may lead to a low serum sodium.

ECG. This may indicate bradycardia and cardiomegaly.

CXR. This may reveal cardiomegaly or a pericardial effusion. Check that there is no retrosternal extension of the thyroid gland.

Preoperative preparation

The patient who is on replacement hormone treatment and who is clinically euthyroid does not present any particular anaesthetic problem and can be treated as normal.

Because of the high mortality associated with surgery and untreated hypothyroidism, postpone elective surgery until oral replacement (50 μg/day of thyroxine, which may need to be increased) is effective. This probably takes 10 days. In emergencies, T3 can be given by dilute intravenous infusion (0.1 mg per litre 5% dextrose at 60 mls/hour) but great care is needed, especially in the elderly, if angina and cardiac failure are not to be precipitated. Monitor the ECG for signs of myocardial ischaemia.

If there is any suspicion of an impaired stress response, hydrocortisone can be given empirically.

ANAESTHETIC CONSIDERATIONS

The ventilatory sensitivity to both hypoxia and hypercarbia is greatly decreased whilst hypothyroid. In premedication, therefore, be cautious in the use of ventilatory depressant drugs which may even precipitate myxoedema coma.

During anaesthesia, use reduced dosages of all sedatives, induction agents, analgesics and volatile agents. CO_2 production is decreased, so it is easy to produce hypocarbia when ventilating.

Watch for hypotension and if it is unexplained, consider adrenocortical insufficiency and give hydrocortisone empirically. Monitor the core temperature to detect hypothermia which occurs easily and take positive measures to avoid it.

Postoperatively, similar care is required with sedatives and analgesics.

Hyperthyroidism

Like hypothyroidism, hyperthyroidism is commoner in females. 1.9% of the female and 0.2% of the male population are affected, the peak incidence being between 20 and 40 years. The major symptoms reflect the hypermetabolic state (the basal metabolic rate is increased 30–60%) which is produced by excess circulating thyroid hormone. The basic cause of the disease is not understood but an immunoglobulin G (either long acting thyroid stimulator (LATS), or other immunoglobulin) can often be isolated as the mediator of thyroid stimulation. The disorder can be inherited.

Graves' disease (diffuse thyroid enlargement with hypermetabolism and exophthalmos) is the commonest disorder, but hyperthyroidism may be caused by autonomous nodular goitres and subacute thyroiditis.

PREOPERATIVE CONSIDERATIONS

History

Agitated fatigue, palpitations, muscle weakness and heat intolerance are frequent complaints. Weight loss is common, despite an increased appetite. Bowel habit may be increased in frequency and, rarely, there is diarrhoea. In premenopausal women amenorrhoea may occur and in older patients, angina or heart failure may be worsened. Hyperthyroidism is often asymptomatic in the elderly.

Examination

General. Thyroid enlargement is common. Refer to later section for assessment and management. Thyroid bruits are sometimes heard because of the increased blood flow. The ocular signs of hyperthyroidism include stare, lid lag, lid retraction and proptosis. Look for raised, thickened skin on the legs or feet (pretibial myxoedema, rare). The hair is usually fine and silky.

CVS. Tachycardia, atrial dysrhythmias, widened pulse pressure, systolic flow murmurs and increased intensity of the first heart sound are classical signs. Check that the thyrotoxic state has not precipitated heart failure, which along with atrial dysrhythmias, may be the only presenting symptoms and findings (especially AF in the elderly).

NS. A fine tremor of the fingers and tongue, together with hyper-reflexia, is characteristic.

Investigations

FBC. Leukopenia may occur as a side effect of antithyroid drugs.
ECG and CXR. These may show evidence of the cardiac effects.

Treatment

In younger patients, the usual practice is medical treatment with antithyroid drugs (e.g. carbimazole, propylthiouracil or potassium perchlorate). If there is not a remission within 2 years, subtotal thyroidectomy is often then recommended. Elderly patients do not often present for surgery because radioactive iodine is used to ablate thyroid tissue and render them euthyroid. Both for thyroidectomy and for coincidental surgery the patient's thyroid state should be assessed clinically, and the euthyroid state confirmed by a free T4 index. Beta-adrenoceptor blockade is frequently used to suppress a tachycardia but as yet the adequacy of this method of treatment as a preparation for surgery is in question. It seems wise to add potassium iodide preoperatively which inhibits hormonal release from the thyroid gland.

Preoperative preparation

If surgery is being performed on the thyroid gland the antithyroid drugs are often changed to oral iodine (e.g. potassium iodide 60 mg three times daily) for the week preceding surgery, in order to reduce the vascularity of the gland. Check that the drugs have been taken.

When premedicating, sedate the patient well, especially if nervous. Continue beta-adrenoceptor blockade on the day of surgery.

PEROPERATIVE PHASE

There is no contraindication to the usual anaesthetic agents or techniques though it is wise to avoid drugs which stimulate the sympathetic nervous system (e.g. ketamine, ether, cyclopropane and possibly pancuronium). This is because exaggerated adrenergic effects may result. For the same reason, avoid hypercarbia. Similarly, use a direct acting sympathomimetic amine (e.g. methoxamine or phenylephrine) in reduced dosage if vasoconstriction is required.

If surgery is on the gland itself, take the usual precautions for head and neck surgery as outlined later.

POSTOPERATIVE PHASE

The considerations relating to the operation of thyroidectomy are referred to later. The important complication of hyperthyroidism *per se* is thyroid crisis. With adequate preoperative preparation it should not occur. However, if there is an excessive release of thyroid hormones, they cause exaggerated symptoms of thyrotoxicosis, either during the operation or, more commonly in the early postoperative period.

It is characterized by a rapidly rising pulse rate, abdominal pain, pyrexia, sweating, diarrhoea, restlessness and ultimately dysrhythmias and cardiac failure. It has a mortality of 20–40%. A thyroid crisis must be distinguished from the postoperative complications of sepsis, septicaemia, haemorrhage and transfusion or drug reactions. Treatment is aimed at reducing tachycardia by beta-adrenoceptor blockade, inhibiting further release of thyroid hormone by intravenous iodine (e.g. sodium iodide 250 mg 6 hourly) and cooling the patient externally (but do not use salicylates which increase the release of thyroid hormones). Hydrocortisone may also be needed to treat acute adrenal insufficiency due to the increased biotransformation and utilization of corticosteroids. Propylthiouracil 400 mg 6 hourly by mouth inhibits further thyroid hormone synthesis.

The enlarged thyroid

The enlarged gland may, or may not, have an associated abnormal hormone secretion and the possibility of hypo or hyperthyroidism should always be considered. Refer to earlier sections for the relevant clinical findings.

Thyroid swelling can be benign or malignant; it may be diffuse, a single nodule or multinodular, and can extend retrosternally into the thorax. Surgery is indicated when there are pressure symptoms, if there is a suspicion of malignancy and for selected thyrotoxic cases.

PREOPERATIVE CONSIDERATIONS

History

Probably the commonest complaint is that of the adverse effect on one's appearance. Pressure symptoms may cause difficulty in swallowing or difficulty in breathing. Rarely, a bleed into the gland can cause acute enlargement and severe ventilatory obstruction which needs relieving urgently. Stridor may be noticed, particularly on the alteration of neck posture. A change of voice requires indirect laryngoscopy before surgery to evaluate recurrent laryngeal nerve function, and may be indicative of malignancy.

Examination

Thyroid swelling is best demonstrated by inspecting the anterior neck and asking the patient to swallow with the neck moderately extended. Feel for the position of the trachea, remembering that it can be grossly deviated. This, and tracheal compression are important factors in anticipating a difficult intubation. Retrosternal extension can be demonstrated by jugular venous distension and suffusion of the face on extending the patient's arms over his head (Pemberton's sign). Note the position (often sitting up) in which the patient has least difficulty breathing and plan the conduct of anaesthesia accordingly.

Investigations

Thyroid function tests. These should always be performed in order to confirm that the patient is euthyroid.
CXR. This is helpful in revealing a retrosternal extension and will also demonstrate any tracheal deviation.
Lateral neck X-rays. A view of the thoracic inlet is particularly helpful to see tracheal narrowing and to anticipate the size of endotracheal tube required.

PEROPERATIVE PHASE

Do not oversedate the patient if the gland is large enough to cause severe ventilatory embarrassment. Otherwise, there are no contraindications to usual premedicants.

The major problem is difficult intubation. If the gland is only moderately large, and the trachea is undeviated, there is unlikely to be any problem in intubation. Where possible, an armoured tube is preferred in order to reduce the likelihood of kinking of the tube with movement of the head. When a difficult intubation is anticipated the pros and cons of awake intubation should be considered and a range of endotracheal tube sizes and types, as well as introducers, be available. With a co-operative patient, a good compromise is gas induction. If the patient is only able to breathe satisfactorily while sitting, retain this position until intubation is achieved. Skilled efforts to intubate are essential as tracheostomy is not an attractive alternative. Only paralyse the patient if the airway can be managed safely.

Take all the usual precautions of head and neck surgery (i.e. check that all connections are secure, protect the eyes, secure the endotracheal tube with sticky tape rather than bandage, and provide moderate head up-tilt). There are protagonists for both spontaneous ventilation and IPPV; if the operation is likely to be long and difficult, IPPV is certainly preferred. Because of head-up tilt, remember the possibility of air embolism in the spontaneously breathing patient.

With thyroid carcinoma especially, be aware of the possiblity of tracheal damage and have tracheostomy tubes available. At the end of surgery, on extubation, look at the cords to ensure that both sides are moving fully, in case of recurrent laryngeal nerve damage. Suck out the pharynx carefully to remove any blood or mucus, but try not to cause too much coughing which increases the likelihood of reactionary haemorrhage.

POSTOPERATIVE PHASE

On the return of spontaneous ventilation tracheal collapse can occur. This is a particular problem after the removal of large goitres which have eroded tracheal cartilages or, after thyroidectomy for malignancy, when tracheal cartilage may have been removed inadvertently during a difficult dissection. Reintubate the patient immediately and consider tracheostomy.

Always take the patient to a well-staffed recovery area because of the danger of postoperative ventilatory obstruction. The cause of any obstruction needs identification and the appropriate action to be taken promptly.

Reactionary haemorrhage causes pressure on the trachea and, if it is severe, requires immediate evacuation of the haematoma.

Recurrent laryngeal nerve injury should have been apparent on laryngoscopy at extubation. It will probably not cause obstruction unless bilateral or if there is concomitant oedema. If the nerve injury does not resolve, tracheostomy may have to be done.

Stridor due to laryngeal oedema does not usually present until 2 or 3 days after operation and may require reintubation.

If the parathyroid glands have also been inadvertently removed, tetany may occur (8 hrs–8 days after operation). This needs treatment with up to 20 mls 10% calcium gluconate, given slowly IV and repeated as necessary.

242

THE PARATHYROID GLANDS

Normally, four parathyroid glands are located immediately behind the thyroid gland. They are small ($6 \times 3 \times 2$ mm) and look like brown fat. They are, therefore, difficult to locate, either when removing intentionally, or in avoiding, during thyroidectomy.

The glands release a polypeptide hormone, parathormone (PTH), whose function is to maintain the ionized calcium concentration of cellular and extracellular fluids. Its secretion in response to hypocalcaemia, via Vitamin D, increases the small intestinal absorption of calcium, reduces renal excretion of calcium and increases that of phosphorus, and stimulates the release of calcium from bone. By contrast, hypercalcaemia depresses the synthesis and release of PTH. Another hormone, calcitonin, which is of thyroid origin, opposes the action of PTH on bone. Its release is stimulated by a high ionized calcium level but its clinical importance is doubtful, and there is little effect if it is absent altogether.

Hyperparathyroidism

There are four types, the only common factor being a raised blood parathormone level.

Primary hyperparathyroidism is the commonest. Oversecretion of PTH occurs from an autonomous adenoma which is usually benign. It can be part of the multiple endocrine adenoma type II syndrome.

Secondary hyperparathyroidism is a normal physiological response to a low serum calcium. The usual causes are Vitamin D deficiency, malabsorption or chronic renal failure.

In tertiary hyperparathyroidism the parathyroid glands are made autonomous by development of an adenoma after secondary disease.

In pseudohyperparathyroidism a malignant tumour secretes PTH. It can be from lung, breast, pancreas or kidney.

Hypoparathyroidism

This is characterized by hypocalcaemia and consequent neuromuscular symptoms. The commonest cause is surgical, but rarely it is an autoimmune process. Although the symptoms usually develop within days of operation, there can be a delay of months to years after neck surgery before the diagnosis is made.

Pseudohypoparathyroidism is a rare, hereditary disorder characterized by signs and symptoms of hypoparathyroidism (in fact it is a failure of end-organ response to the hormone) in conjunction with distinctive skeletal and developmental defects (short stature, round face, short neck and multiple discrete bony abnormalities).

The anaesthetic implications of hypo and hyperparathyroidism are only those of disordered serum calcium, which has other causes apart from alterations in parathyroid function.

Hypercalcaemia

The physiologically relevant measurement is ionized calcium but the total calcium is measured in the laboratory, almost half of which is bound to albumin.

Hypercalcaemia has many causes (Table 6.1) and a diagnosis and full work up is imperative. The anaesthetic problems then also become those of the background disease. The features of hypercalcaemia *per se* are psychiatric disturbances, dehydration, nausea, vomiting, thirst, polyuria, constipation, muscle fatigue and hypotonicity. The ECG has prolonged P-R and shortened Q-T intervals. The most serious complications are renal calculi and nephrocalcinosis with progression to chronic renal failure (q.v.) and hypertension (q.v.).

Hypercalcaemia is treated by depositing calcium out of solution with one of several schemes involving sodium phosphate, steroids and calcitonin. The action of these agents is not rapid and if the serum Ca^{++} is above 3.5 mmol/litre there is imminent danger of cardiac arrest. The best emergency method of lowering a high serum Ca^{++} is to increase its excretion by infusing isotonic saline accompanied by frusemide. Renal dialysis is another effective method.

In the uncomplicated case, there are no special anaesthetic considerations. A high serum calcium enhances the release of acetyl choline, but has not been reported to have any measurable effect on the clinical use of muscle relaxants.

Table 6.1. Differential diagnosis of hypercalcaemia

Malignancy, with or without metastasis	breast, lung, kidney, cervix, multiple myeloma, lymphoma, leukaemias
Sarcoidosis	
Hyperparathyroidism (1°, 3°, or pseudo)	
Hyperthyroidism	
Vitamin D toxicity	
Immobilization, especially Paget's disease and paraplegia	
Acute renal failure	
Adrenal insufficiency (iatrogenic or Addisonian crisis)	
Milk alkali syndrome	

Hypocalcaemia

This has several causes (Table 6.2) and presents with paraesthesia, muscle cramps, circumoral pallor, tetany, laryngeal spasms and convulsions. Latent tetany can be detected by Chvostek's and Trousseau's signs, the former being very useful after thyroidectomy. The ECG shows a prolonged Q-T interval.

After parathyroidectomy (or thyroidectomy), if all the functioning parathyroid tissue has been removed, there is a precipitous fall in the serum calcium (peak effect seen variously from 8 hours to 8 days) resulting in tetany. Treatment is by slow injection of IV calcium gluconate 10% (10–20 mls).

Anaesthetic considerations are as for the underlying disorder. Prior to surgery always correct the serum Ca^{++}. Although there are no large series, patients with previous longstanding hypocalcaemia have the reputation of being 'sensitive' to anaesthetics and muscle relaxants.

Table 6.2. Causes of hypocalcaemia

Hypoparathyroidism (usually post surgery)
Vitamin D deficiency
Chronic renal failure
False low in hypoalbuminaemia
Acute pancreatitis
Sudden correction of chronic acidosis (fall in ionized fraction)

Carcinoid syndrome

Carcinoid tumours are slowly growing neoplasms of enterochromaffin cells. They are rare but when present usually arise in the small intestine and also in organs derived from the embryonic foregut (bronchus, stomach, pancreas or thyroid). The carcinoid *syndrome* occurs in less than 25% of patients with carcinoid tumours. It usually implies metastases in the liver. The mediators in the syndrome are principally serotonin and bradykinin, although other substances (e.g. histamine, substance P) can be secreted.

The commonest clinical feature is episodic cutaneous flushing (probably bradykinin mediated) which may be accompanied by a tachycardia but no change in BP. Intestinal hypermotility (serotonin mediated) with borborygmi, cramps and explosive diarrhoea can accompany the episodic flushes. Chronic diarrhoea is more common. Bronchoconstriction is less common but may be severe.

Rarely, fibrous tissue deposits occur, particularly on the right side of the heart, producing tricuspid incompetence and pulmonary stenosis (see Chapter 1). The serum proteins may be low because of tryptophan (serotonin precursor) uptake by the tumour and may need correcting before surgery.

The humoral effects can be controlled by medical treatment but the response is variable and long-term therapy may be limited by side effects. The treatment of choice is surgical removal of the primary growth. They very rarely also present for heart valve replacement. The incidental finding of a carcinoid tumour at laparotomy (often in the appendix) in an asymptomatic patient is most unlikely to cause problems.

The rarity of the syndrome means that no one has a large series of patients on which to base perioperative management. The general principles are outlined below and the patient needs to be managed in conjunction with an endocrinologist.

Direct preoperative assessment towards the cardiovascular system and decide whether symptoms are due predominantly to serotonin or bradykinin (or possibly histamine). Bradykinin symptoms should be treated with aprotinin by IV infusion (200 000 units 4 hourly) starting 1 hour before surgery. Serotonin symptoms should be treated with antiserotonin drugs (e.g. methysergide 2–4 mg, 3–4 times daily or 4–12 mg 6 hourly). Some authorities recommend both treatments for all patients with the carcinoid syndrome. Although theoretically sound, the value of the serotonin antagonist, ketanserin, has yet to be fully evaluated.

The anaesthetic technique should avoid any agents likely to release histamine (morphine, curare etc.). The complications liable to occur are hypotension, bronchospasm and flushing and hyperkinetic states with hypertension and tachycardia, particularly on tumour handling. Thus invasive monitoring is strongly advised with CVP and arterial lines. Epidural and spinal block are contraindicated because hypotension may precipitate a bradykinergic crisis. This may also be provoked by catecholamines and vasopressors. Consequently, if hypotension occurs, it is better treated with volume replacement.

Continue close observation into the postoperative period since deaths have been reported then.

FURTHER READING

Alberti, K.G.M.M. & Thomas, B.J.B. (1979) The management of diabetes during surgery. *Br. J. Anaesth.*, **51**, 693–710.

Campkin, T.V. (1980) Radial artery cannulation: potential hazard in patients with acromegaly. *Anaesthesia*, **35**, 1008–9.

Desmonts, J.M. & Marty, J. (1984) Anaesthetic management of patients with phaeochromocytoma. *Br. J. Anaesth.*, **56**, 781–9.

Edis, A.J. (1979) Prevention and management of complications associated with thyroid and parathyroid surgery. *Surgical Clinics of N. America*, **59**, 83–92.

Ewing, D.J., Campbell, I.W. & Clarke, B.F. (1980) Assessment of cardiovascular effects in diabetic autonomic neuropathy and prognostic implications. *Ann. Int. Med.*, **92**, (part 2), 308–11.

Feek, C.M., Stewart, J., Sawers, A. *et al.* (1980) Combination of potassium iodide and propranolol in preparation of patients with Grave's disease for thyroid surgery. *N. Engl. J. Med.*, **302**, 883–5.

Gangat, Y., Triner, L., Baer, L. *et al.* (1976) Primary aldosteronism with uncommon complications. *Anesthesiology*, **45**, 542–4.

Hale, P.J., Crase, J. & Nattrass, M. (1984) Metabolic effects of bicarbonate in the treatment of diabetic ketoacidosis. *Br. Med. J.*, **289**, 1035–8.

Hamilton, W.F.D., Forrest, A.L., Gunn, A. *et al.* (1984) Beta adrenoceptor blockade and anaesthesia for thyroidectomy. *Anaesthesia*, **39**, 335–42.

Heath, D.A. (1980) The emergency management of disorders of calcium and magnesium. *Clinics in Endocrinology and Metabolism*, **3**, 487–502.

Hoffenberg, R. (1980) Thyroid emergencies. *Clinics in Endocrinology and Metabolism*, **3**, 503–12.

Kehlet, H. (1975) A rational approach to dosage and preparation of parenteral glucocorticoid substitution therapy during surgical procedures. *Acta Anaesthesiol. Scand.*, **19**, 260.

Kitahata, L.M. (1971) Airway difficulties associated with anesthesia in acromegaly. *Br. J. Anaesth.*, **43**, 1187–90.

Knudsen, L., Christiansen, L.A. & Lorentzen, J.E. (1981) Hypotension during and after operation in glucocorticoid-treated patients. *Br. J. Anaesth.*, **53**, 295–301.

Manger W.H. & Gifford, R.W. (1977) *Pheochromocytoma*. Springer-Verlag, New York.

Mason, R.A. & Steane, P.A. (1976) Carcinoid syndrome: its relevance to the anaesthetist. *Anaesthesia*, **31**, 228–42.

Murkin, J.M. (1982) Anesthesia and hypothyroidism. A review of thyroxine physiology, pharmacology and anesthetic implications. *Anesth. Analg.*, **61**, 371–83.

Page, M.Mc.B. & Watkins, P.J. (1978) Cardiorespiratory arrest and diabetic autonomic neuropathy. *Lancet*, **1**, 14–16.

Plumpton, F.S., Besser, G.M. & Cole, P.V. (1969) Corticosteroid treatment and surgery (parts 1 and 2). *Anaesthesia*, **24**, 3–18.

Robinson, A.G. (1976) DDAVP in the treatment of central diabetes insipidus. *N. Engl. J. Med.*, **294**, 507–11.

Southwick, J.P. & Katz, J. (1979) Unusual airway difficulty in the acromegalic patient: Indications for tracheostomy. *Anesthesiology*, **51**, 72–3.

Symreng, T., Karlberg, B.E., Kagedal, B. *et al.* (1981) Physiological cortisol substitution of longterm steroid-treated patients undergoing major surgery. *Br. J. Anaesth.*, **53**, 949–54.

Van Heerdan, J.A., Edis, A.J. & Service, F.J. (1979) The surgical aspects of insulinomas. *Ann. Surg.*, **189**, 677–82.

Wade, J.S. (1980) Respiratory obstruction in thyroid surgery. *Ann. R. Coll. Surg. Eng.*, **39**, 15–24.

Weatherill, D. & Spence, A.A. (1984) Anaesthesia and disorders of the adrenal cortex. *Br. J. Anaesth.*, **56**, 741–9.

7/Renal disease

Acute renal failure
Description and definition
Aetiology
Prevention and detection in the
  perioperative period
Management of oliguria
Management of acute renal failure

**Anaesthetic management of patients
with acute renal failure**
Preoperative considerations
Peroperative phase
Postoperative phase

Chronic renal failure
The features relevant to the
  anaesthetist
Prescribing drugs

**Anaesthetic management of non-
dialysed patients with chronic
renal failure**
Preoperative considerations
Peroperative phase
Postoperative phase

Patients on long-term dialysis
Haemodialysis
Peritoneal dialysis

**Patients with a functioning renal
transplant**

ACUTE RENAL FAILURE

The anaesthetist meets acute renal failure in two ways. Firstly, he becomes involved with the avoidance, recognition and treatment of acute renal failure in the 'at risk' patient both during surgery and on the ICU. Secondly, he has to anaesthetize patients who are already in established acute renal failure. The latter present either for the investigation of renal outflow obstruction or for surgical treatment of the precipitating cause (e.g. major trauma, burns, drainage of infections, vascular repair).

Established acute renal failure in the perioperative period is a serious condition associated with an overall mortality of approximately 50%. A high incidence is found after open heart, major vascular and trauma surgery.

DESCRIPTION AND DEFINITION

Acute renal failure occurs when there is a rapid deterioration in the ability of the kidney to perform its task of excretion, metabolism and acid-base homeostasis. Irrespective of the exact aetiology, waste products of protein metabolism such as urea and creatinine accumulate in the blood and there is inadequate excretion of hydrogen ions. Sodium and water balance is disturbed and hyperkalaemia may occur. Traditionally, acute renal failure is defined as a sudden reduction of urine output to below 400 mls/day. Although this is its commonest presentation, it is an imperfect definition because up to 30% of cases (especially those resulting from loop diuretic or antibiotic toxicity) are polyuric and acute renal failure develops with the production of normal or increased volumes of isotonic urine.

AETIOLOGY

Classically, acute renal failure is divided into pre-renal, renal and post-renal causes (see Table 7.1), their order of occurrence being pre-renal > renal > post-renal. A division of this nature is necessarily arbitrary, and there are obvious areas of overlap between the groups. Some texts, for example, would classify toxins as pre-renal, based on

Table 7.1. Causes of acute renal failure

Pre-renal	1. Hypovolaemia—	haemorrhage
		dehydration
		burns
		septicaemia
		obstetric disasters
		under-replacement
	2. Hypotension—	loss of circulating volume
		myocardial infarction
		pulmonary embolism
	3. Hypoxia	
	4. Incompatible blood transfusion	
	5. Jaundice and cirrhosis	
	6. Septicaemia or endotoxaemia especially Gram negative organisms	
	7. Tissue damage (myoglobin)	
	8. Tetracycline	
	9. Pancreatitis	
	10. Severe hypertension	
Renal	1. Acute glomerulonephritis	
	2. Severe acute pyelonephritis	
	3. Systemic disease involving kidneys, e.g. connective tissue disorders, diabetes mellitus	
	4. Nephrotoxic drugs and chemicals	
Post-renal	Tubular blockage—	myeloma protein
		uric acid
		sulphadiazine
	Outflow blockage—	stones
		tumours (NB prostate)
		retroperitoneal fibrosis

where they are administered, whilst others would classify them as renal, based on where they exert their effect. Acute renal failure may have a diverse aetiology and often complicates a serious medical or surgical condition of systems other than the kidney and urinary tract.

Pre-renal causes possess a common theme of low circulating blood volume, low cardiac output, hypotension, hypoxia and serious infection. Frequently more than one of these features are present in combination. Directly nephrotoxic drugs to be avoided include the aminoglycosides (amikacin, gentamicin, kanamycin, neomycin, tobramycin), tetracycline, amphoteracin, cephaloridine, colistin, vancomycin, troxidone (used for petit mal epilepsy), gold, penicillamine, methoxyflurane and enflurane. Gentamicin produces a thickening of the glomerular basement membrane.

Tetracycline is the only antibiotic which produces a true pre-renal uraemia. Whilst depending upon renal function for excretion, it has a general catabolic effect throughout the body. Patients with renal impairment, who excrete the drug more slowly than normal, therefore have a disproportionate increase in the quantity of nitrogenous waste products. Consequently, there is an abrupt rise in the serum urea.

Several of the newer antibiotics, which when they were introduced were said to be free of nephrotoxicity, have since been shown not to be. Information on this subject is changing so rapidly that it is unrealistic to state rigid guidelines on prescribing. The best solution is to contact a renal physician who will be able to give the current local recommendations. There is some evidence that netilmicin may emerge as the drug of choice but this has yet to be confirmed by large-scale studies.

PREVENTION AND DETECTION IN THE PERIOPERATIVE PERIOD

Post-renal causes. The anaesthetist has no control over the development or prevention of post-renal uraemia. He does, however, become involved when the obstruction is relieved surgically. The two commonest procedures are the passing of retrograde ureteric catheters and the transcutaneous drainage of the renal pelvis. This allows renal function to recover prior to definitive surgery.

Post-renal obstruction causes progressive and inexorable renal impairment. If it is due to bilateral ureteric stones (NB some patients have only one ureter) or urethral obstruction (prostate), there is a gross reduction in urine output which in severe cases results in total anuria. When it is secondary to malignant obstruction (e.g. carcinoma of the cervix or bladder) or retroperitoneal fibrosis, the urine volume is well maintained. In contrast to pre-renal and renal causes there may be accompanying pain from the ureters or bladder.

Renal function usually recovers well even after prolonged outflow obstruction. Although relief of the obstruction is a matter of some urgency there is no reason to take a patient to theatre in a life-threatening condition. The day, or few days, necessary to improve his condition has little effect on the ultimate prognosis but greatly reduces the risks of anaesthesia.

Pre-renal and renal causes. In contrast to post-renal uraemia, the development of certain types of pre-renal or renal failure (Table 7.1) can be avoided by the appropriate perioperative management. It is one of the anaesthetist's responsibilities to ensure that this occurs.

The first requirement is to identify an 'at risk' group and the predisposing factors are listed in Table 7.2. The second is to monitor those 'at risk' carefully, and search positively for the first signs of renal failure. This is important because with correct and vigorous treatment the progression to established renal failure may, at times, be averted.

Table 7.2. Factors predisposing to perioperative renal failure

Jaundice
Sepsis
Diabetes mellitus
Existing chronic renal failure
Pregnancy
Undernourishment
The use of nephrotoxic drugs
Old age

The cornerstone of prophylaxis is to keep the patient well hydrated with a satisfactory blood pressure. He should never be allowed to become hypovolaemic, hypotensive or hypoxic. Aim for a moderately high CVP (>6 mmHg) and if necessary use inotropic agents at *low* dosage levels to maintain renal perfusion. Pushing these to moderate or high levels is counterproductive because of the resultant vasoconstriction. Measure the U & E's and serum creatinine at least daily in the perioperative period and chart the urine volume every two hours. Usually the latter is no problem because the patient has a urethral catheter to aid the management of other pathologies. Take great care to ensure accurate collections.

The concentrating power of the kidney may be assessed by the urinary specific gravity or osmolality. The colour of the urine, which

251

is due to urochromes, is totally unrelated to its quality in terms of excretion and acid-base homeostasis.

When a person is managed as described above, any sustained fall in the urine output (always check for a blocked catheter) in the presence of a constant fluid load, must be investigated. It is incorrect to wait until some arbitrary figure of daily urine output has been reached (e.g. 400 mls/day) before taking the situation seriously.

A reduction in urine flow can precede the rapid rise in blood urea and creatinine levels by 24 to 72 hours. Once renal failure has occurred, in the untreated patient the serum potassium rises at 0.5 to 3.0 mmol/day (this may be intensified by excessive tissue damage) and acidosis occurs from the production of approximately 1 mmol hydrogen ion/kg/day. All these changes are intensified by catabolism. Later, hypertension, anaemia and clotting abnormalities may occur.

MANAGEMENT OF OLIGURIA

Some patients are not brought to the attention of the anaesthetist until the blood urea is already elevated. In those who have not had effective circulatory support, pre-renal uraemia may still be reversible, provided that restoration of circuating fluid volume and improvement of renal blood flow occur at a stage when renal excretory, concentrating and re-absorptive mechanisms are still adequate. Established acute renal failure will inevitably supervene if the factors causing the low urine output are not corrected promptly.

When first encountering a patient with a low (approximately 0.5 ml/minute) or deteriorating urine flow, it is important to differentiate between true renal failure and an exaggerated physiological response to hypovolaemia. This differentiation is important because, depending upon the cause of the oliguria, the correct treatment is either to increase fluids or to restrict them. The renal response of a healthy kidney to poor perfusion is the excretion of small volumes of highly concentrated urine ($>$500 mosmol/litre) which is low in sodium content ($<$10–20 mmol/litre) because of maximum tubular reabsorption. In addition, the urine to plasma urea concentration is greater than 8 to 1. Once acute renal failure is established, the urine excreted (usually of small volume) is iso-osmotic with plasma (approximately 290 mosmol/litre) with a high concentration of sodium ($>$40 mmol/litre). The urine to plasma urea ratio is less than 3.

All oliguric patients require catheterization so that the urine output can be measured accurately. Initial management should be directed to the primary cause and to the correction of any *hypoxia and haemodynamic abnormalities* that may be present.

If oliguria persists, despite adequate resuscitation and there is a satisfactory blood pressure and a moderately high CVP (>6 mmHg) it is appropriate to give an IV diuretic challenge. A suitable regimen is mannitol (up to 0.7 g/kg) followed by frusemide in increasing doses of 40 mg, 80 mg, 160 mg and 250 mg. Between each prescription allow at least 1–2 hours to assess the response. Note that giving frusemide to patients who are hypovolaemic can itself produce acute renal failure. There are two possible responses to the diuretic challenge:

• No effect. This confirms renal failure with the possible need for dialysis and fluid restriction.

• An increased output of hypotonic or isotonic urine. This means that acute renal failure has been aborted or that oliguric failure has been converted to polyuric failure. If the latter has occurred the patient's biochemistry will still deteriorate quickly. Careful monitoring of the U & E's and acid-base status must continue in order to differentiate these two conditions.

Once acute renal failure has been diagnosed it should be managed as outlined below.

MANAGEMENT OF ACUTE RENAL FAILURE

The overall philosophy of management is to keep the patient alive by whatever means are required, until spontaneous recovery of renal function occurs. Simultaneously, the basic cause of the renal failure should be treated aggressively. The ease of management depends greatly upon the precipitating cause. Patients with extensive soft tissue trauma, septicaemia, multiple fractures and burns are the most difficult. They readily become catabolic and thus have increased metabolic activity and protein breakdown superimposed upon grossly inadequate or temporarily non-existent renal function. Once renal failure is established, measure all daily fluid losses from vomit, urine, faeces etc.

Hyperkalaemia develops early in the course of acute renal failure and is completely asymptomatic. The ECG (See Fig. 7.1) and serum potassium must be monitored for changes and wide QRS complexes and peaked T waves treated urgently. These are usually evident with a serum potassium of approximately 6 mmol/litre but if the development of hyperkalaemia is very gradual, the ECG can remain unaffected until the serum potassium is much higher. The terminal cardiac event is ventricular tachycardia progressing to ventricular fibrillation. The first line emergency treatment is calcium chloride (to stabilize the myocardium) and sodium bicarbonate (to reduce the acidosis). Never give these together in the same intravenous line or

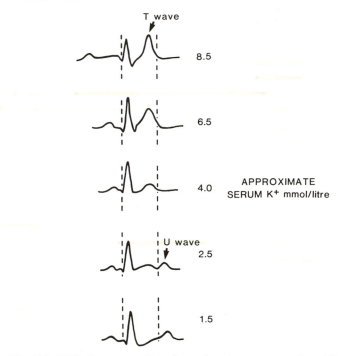

Fig. 7.1. ECG changes resulting from altered serum potassium. Note the high voltage, peaked T wave with hyperkalaemia and the low voltage T wave and U wave with hypokalaemia.

calcium bicarbonate will precipitate out. These measures can be followed by glucose and insulin but this serves only to transfer potassium ions to the intracellular space. To remove excess potassium from the body, which is ultimately required, needs the use of ion exchange resins, dialysis or haemofiltration.

The optimum management for an individual patient is often difficult to decide upon and is usually undertaken by specialist renal physicians. The choices are conservative management, peritoneal dialysis, haemodialysis or haemofiltration.

The problem with conservative management is that, whilst awaiting spontaneous recovery, the biochemistry of the body continues to deteriorate and this does not provide the optimum setting for renal function to improve. Consequently, many centres limit their trial of conservative therapy to only 24 to 48 hours before active steps are taken. This has the important effect of allowing adequate nutrition, which is now thought to be crucial in early recovery. Whenever possible, use the enteral route, otherwise commence intravenous feeding. Parenteral nutrition presents considerable problems because of the inevitable fluid load, the use of hypertonic glucose and the potassium content of some amino acid solutions. Skillful dialysis and adjustment of the regimen are required to minimize disturbances.

Peritoneal dialysis is better for the safe removal of excess fluid, is technically simpler and is better tolerated in children and the elderly. Its disadvantages are that it can splint the diaphragm, thus encouraging pulmonary infection, it only corrects uraemia slowly and it may be contraindicated after abdominal surgery or trauma.

Haemodialysis is far more efficient in removing the waste products of metabolism but can potentiate cardiac irregularities and requires the patient to be heparinized. Emergency dialysis used to be done with arteriovenous (A-V) shunts but now single cannula dialysis via the subclavian vein is increasing in popularity.

Haemofiltration is a recent development. It employs the use of an extracorporeal circulation which is usually perfused from an A-V shunt. A semipermeable membrane allows an ultrafiltrate of plasma to be produced and the losses are replaced from new solutions via a separate intravenous line. It has been shown to have great advantages in very sick patients with unstable haemodynamics and has also been used to remove excess fluid following cardiopulmonary bypass.

The use of haemodialysis or haemofiltration is essential in hypercatabolic patients, peritoneal dialysis being too inefficient for controlling the uraemia, acidosis and hyperkalaemia which occur.

The ventilatory response to metabolic acidosis reduces the $PaCO_2$ and thus minimizes the pH change. If the patient has insufficient ventilatory reserve to make this compensation, there will be a rapid rise in the serum hydrogen ion concentration. Consequently, ventilatory support with IPPV is not infrequently required, especially if there is co-existing pulmonary trauma, chest infection, pulmonary oedema or septicaemia. Haemodialysis itself increases the pulmonary shunt by the sequestration of white blood cells in the lung and the activation of complement. A problem associated with ventilation, and especially the use of PEEP, is the inappropriate secretion of ADH which further suppresses urine formation.

Infection is a major risk and can occur in any body system or organ. If it is unchecked it rapidly progresses to septicaemia. Routine cultures of blood, sputum, urine and drainage fluids are required.

Stress ulcers in the stomach and duodenum occur in up to 25% of patients with acute renal failure. Combined with the bleeding tendency these patients have, intestinal blood loss may be brisk and massive. Many units now give prophylactic cimetidine but it only reduces ulcer bleeding if it is combined with a two hourly antacid. In acute renal failure magnesium salts should be avoided. Anaemia and hypertension tend to be later complications. It is important to remember that any drugs prescribed must have their doses adjusted if their excretion depends upon good renal function.

Anaesthetic management of patients with acute renal failure

The background presentation, physiology and management of acute renal failure has already been described. Many patients presenting for surgery have other major surgical or medical problems around which any anaesthetic must be tailored. For the management of these individual problems *per se* the reader should refer to the appropriate sections.

The philosophy of any anaesthetic procedure must be first to optimize the patient's condition within the time available (this is usually undertaken by a renal physician), and secondly to give an anaesthetic which least jeopardizes existing renal function.

PREOPERATIVE CONSIDERATIONS

History

Establish the cause of acute renal failure, the time of onset, progress of symptoms, prognosis and mode of treatment. Ask the staff about the patient's morale and record the patient's mental state. Be suspicious that any bloody nasogastric aspirate or melaena might be from a stress ulcer or due to a blood dyscrasia. In patients with multiple problems, consider whether or not a tracheostomy could usefully be fashioned during the same anaesthetic. If the patient is ventilated or sedated, see how long drug dosages have lasted because the duration is often markedly altered by renal function. Note especially if on the one hand inotropes and a high CVP are necessary to maintain cardiac output, or, if on the other hand antihypertensives are needed for reducing the BP.

If the patient has had haemodialysis, record any problems encountered, especially post-dialysis hypotension or pulmonary oedema, both of which occur most easily in patients who are very sensitive to changes in circulating fluid volume. Check the daily allowance of IV fluids. Prior to surgery contact the renal physicians and ask their advice on intra-operative fluids and whether or not transfused blood needs special treatment (e.g. washed cells).

If the patient is fit enough discuss the possibility of regional or local techniques.

256

Examination

Examine the significance of the precipitating factors in relation to the proposed procedure (e.g. fractured spine, crush injuries etc.). Look at the condition of the skin and check the quality of the drip sites. If a new or additional one is required, it can often best be established in a relaxed atmosphere on the ICU before moving to theatre. If a shunt is present make a mental note to protect it peroperatively.

RS. If breathing spontaneously look for cyanosis (may be masked by anaemia) and assess the ventilatory rate, the chest expansion and the use of the accessory muscles of respiration. Note the presence of air hunger and any anxious facial expression. The patient will probably be hyperventilating to maintain his pH.

Borderline ventilation when sitting may become inadequate when supine. If the patient is able to co-operate, the preoperative vital capacity and tidal volume are sensible measurements. The comparison between them gives an indication of the ventilatory reserve. Auscultate carefully for equal air entry and crepitations. Ventilation may deteriorate with both haemodialysis and peritoneal dialysis. Check the ability to breathe deeply and cough and examine a specimen of sputum for macroscopic evidence of infection or blood.

If the patient is on a ventilator note the settings required to maintain adequate blood gases. This will affect the anaesthetic technique and great care may be necessary to prevent hypoxia and/or hypercarbia whilst transporting the patient to theatre.

CVS. Check the stability of the BP under the treatment regimen. Examine for signs of anaemia (pale, tachycardia, bounding pulse). Auscultate for murmurs (usually flow murmurs in the aortic region and at the left sternal edge, but rarely can be endocarditis), or added sounds (LVF). Check the postural fall in blood pressure. Examine the neck veins or measure the CVP. Look for sacral and ankle oedema and listen for the crepitations of pulmonary oedema. Note any petechiae or ecchymoses secondary to a blood dyscrasia (often best seen under the BP cuff).

GIT. Examine the nasogastric aspirate and faeces for the presence of blood. Regular nasogastric tube aspiration or vomiting can reduce the rate of rise of serum potassium. In patients on peritoneal dialysis an opalescence in the dialysis fluid often indicates infection.

NS. From a conversation (if this is possible) make a crude estimate of the mental state. Record any preoperative neurological symptoms, signs or injuries. The muscular twitchings of uraemia usually occur late with a very high blood urea, and do not occur in dialysed patients. Therefore, if odd neuromuscular movements are present, or there is blunted consciousness always suspect an occult cause (e.g. cerebral oedema).

Investigations

U & E's These are obviously very important, particularly the serum potassium shortly before surgery.

FBC. Anaemia in acute renal failure is measurable after one week and maximal by one month. If the Hb is unexpectedly low, taking into account all the features of the case, look for other occult sites of blood loss, especially from the GIT. The presence of a raised white cell count should suggest infection.

Clotting studies. Acute renal failure often produces clotting abnormalities which might require the use of FFP or platelet concentrate. Remember that patients are heparinized during haemodialysis.

CXR. Look at the heart size, and for the presence of pulmonary oedema or pleural effusions.

ECG. Look for signs of K^+ toxicity (see Fig. 7.1) and for dysrhythmias. A sinus tachycardia is common.

Sputum. Do regular cultures.

Blood gases. These are useful as a baseline and to give a guide to the extent of the ventilatory compensation necessary to counter the metabolic acidosis. Avoid causing any unnecessary trauma to an artery which may be needed subsequently for an A-V shunt or fistula.

Preoperative preparation

The basic preparation is as in 'management of acute renal failure'. For urgent operations with a normal ECG and a serum potassium of 6.0 mmol/litre or less, the operation can probably proceed immediately.

If on haemodialysis, it is usual to dialyse until 4 to 6 hours preoperatively and to give a calcium resonium enema. Peritoneal dialysis can continue until the time of operation but during both the transport to theatre and the operation itself it is more convenient to spigot the cannula.

Premedication. This may not be required. If it is, try to avoid intramuscular injections which cause bruising. Beware of ventilatory depressant drugs in a patient who is hyperventilating to compensate for acidosis.

PEROPERATIVE PHASE

Always remember that a patient with acute renal failure may require haemodialysis in the future. Therefore, it is vital to avoid potential shunt and fistula sites with intravenous and arterial cannulae.

The effect of anaesthesia. The only two anaesthetic agents that have not been implicated in reducing urine production are nitrous oxide and droperidol. Volatile anaesthetics, narcotics, sympathomimetic drugs, endogenous catecholamines and surgery itself all reduce urine flow by a variety of mechanisms including hypotension, vasoconstriction and the release of ADH. Free flouride ions from the breakdown of methoxyflurane and enflurane are directly nephrotoxic.

The most important factors of all in protecting the kidney are unrelated to the choice of anaesthetic drugs. *The features which must be avoided at all costs are hypoxia, hypovolaemia and hypotension*. There are obviously several ways of achieving this.

Monitoring. It is essential to monitor the BP and ECG from before the induction of anaesthesia through to the postoperative period. The need for an invasive measurement of blood pressure obviously differs from case to case, but an arterial cannula should only be used if it is going to play a vital role. Whenever possible, avoid the radial and brachial arteries. The dorsalis pedis is probably the artery of choice.

A central venous catheter also has the potential for damaging potential fistula sites. Although it is useful for assessing fluid balance and for testing the response of a compromised cardiovascular system to a fluid load (see Chapter 1) do not use one without good reason. The best sites are the internal jugular or subclavian veins. The subclavian route is less preferable after recent haemodialysis because there is no facility for applying pressure if the patient bleeds.

The acid-base status can be followed either by repeated arterial blood sampling or from measurement of the end-tidal CO_2. The latter is preferable from the non-invasive viewpoint, but the former also confirms the adequacy of oxygenation. Because of the increased pulmonary shunt present in many of these patients, a good case can be made for the placement of an arterial line during major surgical procedures. It is likely to be needed afterwards anyway since the majority require postoperative ventilation on the ICU.

A nerve stimulator can be used to follow the progress of neuromuscular blockade. It is most useful in confirming the presence of a significant residual block at a time when 'top-up' doses would normally be given.

Any prolonged procedure is an indication for the use of a warming blanket and body temperature measurement.

Fluid balance. Optimal fluid balance is difficult to achieve. The major problem is that of fluid overload resulting in postoperative pulmonary oedema. Those patients on conservative management are at the greatest risk and often it is necessary to accept that postoperative dialysis will be necessary. It is almost invariable after major surgery.

Many anaesthetic agents produce arteriolar and venous dilatation. This results in a fall in blood pressure which responds to an infusion of fluid. Fluid has to be given since hypotension and hypovolaemia might further jeopardize the kidneys. Use normal saline because dextrose solutions produce acute hyponatraemia.

5% Dextrose is satisfactory for 'keeping a line open' when it is required for injecting drugs. It can be given up to the daily allowance plus estimated evaporative losses.

Frank blood losses obviously need replacement by normal saline, blood, blood products or a plasma expander (but not dextran which is nephrotoxic). When giving blood always watch the T wave closely on the ECG. The high serum potassium of stored blood (see Chapter 9) is not always rapidly reabsorbed by the red cells as it is in the 'normal' patient and hyperkalaemia can occur. Do not overtransfuse. A high haematocrit reduces renal plasma flow. A postoperative haemoglobin of over 11 g% is almost certainly contraindicated unless required for other purposes (e.g. to maintain oxygen flux in severe adult respiratory distress syndrome). If the haemoglobin had already fallen preoperatively because of renal disease alone, treat as a case of chronic renal failure.

Regional anaesthesia

The normal indications and contraindications to this type of anaesthesia apply. Problems can arise during spinal or epidural anaesthesia if a large fluid load is given to maintain the blood pressure. As vascular tone returns, pulmonary oedema may occur.

General anaesthesia

Induction. Always preoxygenate. If the patient is starved give the drugs slowly to minimize haemodynamic disturbances. Even doing this, the blood pressure can still fall dramatically. If a crash induction is necessary be ready to infuse normal saline to restore the blood pressure (see 'fluid balance').

When intubation is indicated, use a sterile endotracheal tube with a low pressure cuff because of the susceptibility to infection and the potential need for a period of postoperative ventilation.

Potassium release following suxamethonium is not exaggerated in people who are only moderately uraemic with a normal serum potassium. There are, however, many patients in acute renal failure who have a serum potassium which is high initially and/or associated tissue or neurological damage. In them the succeeding rise is more likely to reach dangerous levels.

Maintenance. Spontaneous ventilation is usually only suitable for short procedures such as diagnostic radiology, the reason being that the majority of patients in acute renal failure have some degree of ventilatory compensation for their metabolic acidosis. This compensation is suppressed by volatile agents which cause the $PaCO_2$ to rise and the alveolar ventilation to fall (see Chapter 2). There are consequent rapid changes in the pH and, if there is a large pulmonary shunt, unexpected falls in the PaO_2. Therefore, meticulous airway control is essential and the F_IO_2 should be set to 50%. If there is any doubt about the adequacy of the airway always intubate. End-tidal CO_2 measurement is very helpful and if it rises appreciably ($>1\%$), manual assistance of the ventilation is often sufficient to return it to the preoperative value.

Measure the blood pressure at least every five minutes. Hypotension secondary to a volatile agent may necessitate a change in technique.

Controlled ventilation is preferred for any long procedure and especially for those where blood and/or insensible fluid losses will be appreciable. The necessity for maintaining the $PaCO_2$ and the possibility of unexpected hypoxia have already been discussed. Many patients with acute renal failure are already being ventilated on the ICU prior to surgery. If so, and they have been stable, their F_IO_2, and minute ventilation can be maintained intraoperatively. Otherwise they should be ventilated with a large tidal volume, a minute volume sufficient to achieve their preoperative $PaCO_2$ and an F_IO_2 which prevents hypoxia.

Patients with renal failure often need only small doses of non-depolarizing relaxant, if any at all, to maintain IPPV. When they are required, atracurium and vecuronium have the advantage of non-renal excretion. The other non-depolarizing agents are all, at least in part, excreted via the kidney. Gallamine is contraindicated because this is its sole route of excretion. If pancuronium, alcuronium or curare is used, an extended duration of action can be expected and less frequent increments should therefore be given. It is often possible after intubation to ventilate the patient without the need for further muscle relaxant. Supplementation with 0.5% halothane can usually augment the neuromuscular block sufficiently to prevent any troublesome movement without causing hypotension.

Despite careful anaesthesia and meticulous attention to fluid balance, the blood pressure may start to fall gradually after approximately 2 hours surgery. Provided it is certain that the patient is not hypovolaemic, this is best treated by *low* dose inotropes (dopamine or dobutamine) to increase cardiac contractility and cardiac output. Moderate or high dosages of these agents are contraindicated because of possible vasoconstrictor actions. It is difficult to give exact figures for when to treat hypotension, but it is not unreasonable in patients with renal failure to aim never to allow the systolic blood pressure to fall below 100 mmHg.

POSTOPERATIVE PHASE

Reversal of neuromuscular block should only be attempted if there is evidence that recovery has commenced spontaneously (e.g. nerve stimulator, ventilatory efforts). If not, have no hesitation in deciding to continue ventilation. Recurarization is a real danger. A low body temperature combined with a prolonged action of non-depolarizing muscle relaxants can produce an extended paralysis. If the body temperature is low ($< 35°C$) at the end of the operation, reversal may be impossible until the body is rewarmed.

Return the patient to a high dependency area and maintain a high F_IO_2. If he is breathing spontaneously, instruct the staff to be alert to the possibilities of pulmonary oedema and recurarization. On rare occasions, pulmonary oedema needs acute treatment by IPPV. Dialysis or haemofiltration is then required for the bulk removal of excess fluid.

The BP, ECG and breathing need to be monitored closely for several hours and any irregularities must be treated early. The most frequent causes of abnormalities following careful anaesthesia are those common to any operation, such as hypoxia, a high $PaCO_2$, pain and the excessive use of analgesics.

Postoperative chest infections are common. Early physiotherapy is very important and if antibiotics are required, thought must be given to their potential nephrotoxicity.

CHRONIC RENAL FAILURE

In contrast to patients with acute renal failure, the majority of cases of chronic renal failure (CRF) are totally unavoidable. The several forms of glomerulonephritis continue to provide the largest group treated in renal units. Other causes are pyelonephritis, polycystic disease, diabetic nephropathy, hypertensive nephropathy, gout, analgesic abuse (phenacetin), the collagen diseases, hypercalcaemia, obstruction from an enlarged prostate gland, retroperitoneal fibrosis, and very rarely, incompletely resolved acute renal failure. Patients with diabetic nephrosclerosis account for a steadily increasing number of those receiving treatment.

The choice of treatment depends upon the patient's age, intelligence, social resources, employment, associated diseases, geographical situation and motivation. In the United Kingdom at the present time there are approximately 2500 patients on chronic haemodialysis, and 2000 patients with functioning renal transplants.

The features relevant to the anaesthetist

PRESENTATION

Chronic renal failure has a variable presentation because it can, indirectly, cause any organ system to be affected. Most commonly there is a non-specific history of lethargy, anorexia, polyuria, nocturia and general ill health. Nausea, vomiting, bruising, pruritus and weight loss follow. There are few physical findings except the signs of anaemia, hyperventilation, hypertension, and a pallid complexion. Mental confusion, pericarditis and neuropathy are late features.

Sometimes renal failure is discovered because significant albuminuria or hypertension is found at a routine medical examination. Renal impairment may progress to a relatively advanced stage without any symptoms but, as yet, most renal disease can neither be prevented nor treated. Its detection is aided by routine screening of urine samples from every patient admitted for surgery. Significant proteinuria (over 150 mg in 24 hours) should make one think not only of renal disease but of the consequences of the resultant hypoalbuminaemia. Proteinuria in patients with healthy kidneys may disappear on lying supine or be associated with congestive cardiac failure, fever or exercise. A specific gravity of 1.023 or more in a random urine sample implies normal renal concentrating power. A more accurate, but less readily available, measurement is urine osmolality. Maximal dilution and concentration produce urine osmolalities from 50 mosm/litre to 1400 mosm/litre.

Never test the concentrating power of the kidneys by fluid restriction if you suspect chronic renal failure. It may precipitate an irreversible deterioration in function.

PHYSIOLOGY AND MANAGEMENT

Once chronic renal failure has been discovered, the first line of attack is to search for any treatable cause (e.g. post-renal obstruction) and to treat complicating factors which may accelerate the deterioration in renal function.

The advanced stage of all types of CRF is characterized by uraemia and the production of urine with a fixed specific gravity of 1010. Under these conditions, because of the failure of the kidney to handle variations in water and salt intake, the patient on the one hand faces possible dehydration, hypoperfusion and volume contraction and, on the other hand, crystalloid overload may precipitate peripheral oedema, pulmonary oedema and hypertension.

Reduction of dietary protein to 40 g/day is usually adequate to keep the urea below 25 mmol/litre. A high calorie intake is nevertheless necessary to suppress breakdown of endogenous protein.

Fortunately, various compensatory mechanisms enable the patient in CRF to still have some regulating ability, the most important being an increase in the excretory power of the surviving nephrons (intact nephron hypothesis). A large intake of water (3 litres/day) results in an increased urine flow and, hence, increases the daily losses of urea, potassium and other toxins. Large doses of frusemide are sometimes prescribed to assist diuresis (rarely up to 1.5 g/day).

When the patient is producing large volumes of dilute urine, serum potassium is not a problem, but the inability to excrete hydrogen ions and other fixed acids leads to a metabolic acidosis. This is partly alleviated by oral bicarbonate. However, if arterial blood gases are done they always show a metabolic acidosis with ventilatory compensation. The level of the $PaCO_2$ is very important because it indicates the degree of hyperventilation. Mild to moderate hyperventilation is difficult to detect from clinical observation. Its presence is important because of the effects of anaesthetic agents and opioids on ventilatory drive. By increasing the $PaCO_2$ they may produce dangerous swings in pH and serum potassium. Another effect of the acidosis is to shift the oxygen dissociation curve of haemoglobin to the right, thus increasing oxygen delivery to the tissues. This mechanism is further enhanced by the increased levels of 2,3 DPG in chronic anaemia (see Chapter 9).

Anaemia in CRF results from marrow suppression secondary to a failure of production of erythropoietin. Red cell survival is also reduced. In addition, there is a qualitative platelet defect and frequently occult blood loss from the gut which exacerbates the condition. Adequate oxygen flux is maintained by a compensatory tachycardia and increased cardiac output. This can produce premature symptoms of angina and left ventricular failure.

Hypertension is almost invariable but the exact role of renin and aldosterone is uncertain. It should be treated vigorously and commonly needs several drugs for good control. A reduction in dietary sodium, which is sometimes useful in essential hypertension, is inappropriate because of the inevitable reduction in renal blood flow which follows. In very severe and terminal renal failure, salt and water retention worsen the hypertension but it may respond to a reduction in the extracellular fluid volume. This can be accomplished either by high dose diuretic therapy (if the kidney will respond) or by dialysis.

Thyroid function tests are often abnormal with low serum T_4 and T_3 levels. These figures reflect abnormal binding characteristics and the free T_4, T_3 and TSH assays are normal.

Chronic renal failure affects calcium metabolism in two ways; phosphate is retained and patients can no longer hydroxylate 25-hydroxy cholecalciferol to 1,25-dihydroxycholecalciferol (1,25-DHCC). Phosphate retention produces a reciprocal fall in serum calcium which can nevertheless create conditions that precipitate ionic calcium because of chemical instability. There may thus be paradoxical ectopic calcium deposition in the presence of a low serum calcium.

Overall the ionic hypocalcaemia produces a state of chronic, but appropriate, hypersecretion in the parathyroid glands. This secondary hyperparathyroidism results in a permanently high level of parathormone (PTH) which acts directly on bone osteoclasts. The response of the osteoclasts is modified when there is a deficiency of 1,25-DHCC to synergize with PTH at bone level. Consequently, the clinical picture is one of bone pains, generalized decalcification and pseudofractures, but bony swellings, subperiosteal erosions and bone cysts are rare.

There is evidence that the early control of rising phosphate levels may delay the onset of renal osteodystrophy. Restriction of dietary phosphorus and calcium supplements help. Aluminium hydroxide is used to bind phosphorus in the gut, but there is increasing concern that ingestion of aluminium hydroxide may lead to its accumulation in the brain causing 'dialysis dementia'. 1,25-DHCC is now available commercially and can be successful in preventing demineralization.

Tetany from the hypocalcaemia is most unusual, but the maintenance of the unbound calcium fraction depends heavily upon hypoproteinaemia and metabolic acidosis and corrective changes in these two variables can precipitate tetany.

Diabetics who develop renal failure often have a change in their insulin requirements. On the one hand, they can decrease because poor renal function reduces insulin degradation in the kidney; on the other, they can increase because of the effect of acidosis and uraemia at the cellular level where insulin acts.

Renal and other intercurrent infections need prompt antibiotic therapy. This in itself may cause problems from drug nephrotoxicity and ideally, though this is not always possible, antibiotics should only be administered after the results of culture and sensitivity are available. In general, ampicillin is safe, gentamicin needs dose reduction and measurement of serum levels, the cephalosporins should only be used with great care as a reserve and nitrofurantoin and the tetracyclines are contraindicated (see 'aetiology of acute renal failure').

The patient is followed up for life by the renal physicians who take an overall view and decide upon a long-term plan. Dialysis or transplantation are usually considered when the renal function is approximately 10% of the norm.

Prescribing drugs

Patients with chronic renal failure often react unpredictably to a normal drug dosage, implying that the initial dose of any drug should err on the low side. There are many reasons for this erratic response.

Although gastrointestinal absorption of drugs *per se* is essentially normal, antacids hinder the absorption of antibiotics, warfarin and fat soluble vitamins. Poor renal function reduces the protein binding of drugs for reasons which are unclear. If the patient also has hypoalbuminaemia, the free drug fraction can be greatly in excess of normal. This is a problem with sulphonylureas, warfarin, frusemide and sulphonamides. For many drugs the distribution volume is markedly altered. The most frequently quoted example is digoxin whose distribution volume is halved as compared with the normal.

As yet there is little hard data available to demonstrate the effects of chronic renal failure on drug metabolism. It is, however, well established that the reduction of hydrocortisone and the hydrolysis of procaine and suxamethonium are slowed.

The total clearance of an active drug and its active metabolites is the sum of the renal and non-renal clearances. The renal clearance of any drug, irrespective of the exact mechanism, is broadly proportional to the creatinine clearance. Consequently, those drugs relying heavily upon renal clearance have a greatly prolonged and exaggerated action. The two classic examples are non-depolarizing neuromuscular blockers (especially gallamine) and digoxin. The beta-adrenoceptor blockers, atenolol, nadolol, pindolol and sotalol are all excreted unchanged through the kidney.

In addition to these problems, CRF patients appear to be more sensitive than normals to a given serum level of a drug. This is particularly so with narcotics, barbiturates, phenothiazines and sedatives. It has been suggested that the chronically high serum urea in some way affects the uptake across cell walls and the blood brain barrier.

Anaesthetic management of non-dialysed patients with chronic renal failure

The background presentation, physiology and management is as described above. *Any anaesthetic given should jeopardize existing renal function as little as possible.* This revolves around maintaining the normal flow of oxygenated blood to the kidney by *avoiding hypoxia, hypovolaemia* and *hypotension*.

PREOPERATIVE CONSIDERATIONS

History

Establish the original cause of the renal failure, the duration of treatment and the limitations and quality of everyday life. Be clear what the outlook and long-term plans for therapy are, particularly with regard to possible future haemodialysis or transplantation. Discuss the patient's morale with the nursing staff; it is important to establish good rapport. Once these patients are accepted for haemodialysis they tend to be regular customers. Note the usual fluid allowance and the daily urine output.

If the renal failure was caused by a generalized systemic disease, enquire about the associated anaesthetic problems of the background condition (e.g. connective tissue disorders, diabetes mellitus). Polycystic disease of the kidneys may be associated with pulmonary cysts and 14% have intracerebral aneurysms.

Ask about exercise tolerance and the symptoms of anaemia, myocardial ischaemia, LVF, pericarditis and cerebrovascular insufficiency. Check what drugs (and what dosage) the patient is taking, especially antihypertensives, diuretics, immunosuppressives, resonium and sodium bicarbonate. Assess the patient's personality and mental state.

If the operation is suitable for it, and the patient and surgeon are co-operative, discuss the possibilities of regional or local techniques.

Examination

General. The patients tend to be underweight, so record their weight. Look at the quality of the skin, the state of the pressure areas and for signs of bruising or purpura. Take the opportunity to evaluate the ease of establishing an intravenous line. Note the signs of obvious anaemia. Look for pyrexia because of the susceptibility to infection.

CVS. Measure the BP with the patient supine and standing, looking for both absolute levels and any postural drop. A tachycardia is usual and is necessary to maintain the oxygen flux in anaemia. Auscultate for murmurs (a high cardiac output may cause flow murmurs in the aortic region and down the left sternal edge), added sounds (LVF) or rubs (pericarditis occurs late in uraemia). Quiet heart sounds in a person of normal build might suggest a pericardial effusion if there is severe uraemia. Listen for pulmonary crepitations and look for sacral and ankle oedema. Peripheral oedema can result both from RVF and from a low serum albumin. The important differentiator is the JVP.

RS. Mild hyperventilation can often best be noticed by the inability to perfectly co-ordinate speech and breathing, extra breaths being taken from time to time. Small pleural effusions present on a CXR are rarely detectable clinically. Basal crepitations are always significant and indicate a degree of LVF. Examine any sputum for possible infection and send it for culture.

Investigations

FBC. If the anaemia is not normochromic and normocytic with an Hb of 7–8 g% suspect an additional occult blood loss.
Clotting studies. These are normal unless the uraemia is severe.
U & E's. These are mandatory within a few hours of surgery. Treat a high serum potassium as outlined in acute renal failure.
ECG. A sinus tachycardia is almost invariable. Check for dysrhythmias and the signs of potassium toxicity (see Fig. 7.1).
CXR. Look for the signs of pulmonary oedema, cardiomegaly and pleural effusions. The latter are commonest in the nephrotic syndrome.

Preoperative preparation

Optimize the person's BP, serum potassium and metabolic state within the limits of the time available and in conjunction with their physician. Treat infections vigorously with antibiotics and physiotherapy.

Never transfuse blood preoperatively, even if blood loss is anticipated at operation, without first consulting a renal physician. The majority of CRF patients depend upon a low haematocrit to provide a high renal plasma flow and hence maximize the glomerular filtration rate (GFR). If the haematocrit is artificially raised to a normal level, renal function may suddenly deteriorate and may never recover. There is also a risk of precipitating pulmonary oedema. If it is anticipated that blood *will* be required, check with the renal physician whether washed cells are advisable (to avoid sensitizing the patient because of future transplantation).

PEROPERATIVE PHASE

The important considerations are almost identical to those of patients in acute renal failure and to those who are anaemic. Please refer. Only extra points specific to chronic renal failure are given here.

Continue antihypertensive therapy up to the time of surgery. Intraoperatively these drugs react synergistically with volatile agents and there may be unexpected falls in blood pressure. This is most easily corrected by switching off the offending agent or avoided altogether by using a total intravenous technique.

For all but the shortest procedures, a urethral catheter should be passed to monitor intraoperative urine production. With good hydration, an adequate CVP and blood pressure, urine flow should be maintained at 1 ml/kg/hour. If it is not, despite good hydration etc., mannitol (25 gm over 10–15 minutes) is the first line of treatment. A small dose of frusemide may then be tried.

Intraoperative fluid and blood replacement requires considerable skill in judgment. The object of blood replacement should be to maintain the final Hb to within 1 gm/100 mls of the initial level. Overtransfusion not only reduces the renal plasma flow (see above) but also creates a higher load of products which are toxic to the kidney.

If a patient has been maintained for a long period on conservative management, it is reasonable to assume that his $PaCO_2$, pH, oxygen dissociation curve characteristics and cardiac output have compensated to give maximum oxygen delivery to the tissues. To maintain this state his peroperative end-tidal CO_2 or $PaCO_2$ should be monitored and the ventilation adjusted to achieve the preoperative level.

POSTOPERATIVE PHASE

The postoperative course obviously depends on the nature and extent of surgery. After minor surgery, the patient should return as soon as possible to his preoperative regimen. After major surgery, it may be necessary to temporarily dialyse or haemofiltrate the patient (for the first week or so). Depending on the site and extent of the operation, peritoneal or haemodialysis can be used. The best modern technique is probably haemodialysis via a two-way subclavian cannula inserted at the time of operation.

Patients on long-term dialysis

This section assumes that the patient has *no* effective renal function and that recovery is impossible. It is therefore *unnecessary* to take extreme and complex measures to maintain intraoperative renal blood flow to prevent further damage.

Haemodialysis

Chronic renal failure patients being followed up by a renal physician are, if considered suitable, prepared for haemodialysis when their creatinine clearance is approximately 10 ml/minute. Under local anaesthesia, an A–V fistula is created, usually at the wrist of the non-dominant hand. This takes 4–8 weeks to fully develop and to dilate the veins of the forearm sufficiently to allow easy access.

Most patients are started on dialysis when uraemic symptoms develop which are not corrected by a protein restricted diet. The commonest regimen is to dialyse for 5 hours three times per week. After starting dialysis, urine flow falls off and patients are limited to a fluid intake of 600 mls/day plus the urine loss. Not adhering to this results in hypertension and pulmonary oedema. Dialysis does nothing to correct the anaemia and many patients require trans-fusions to keep the Hb above 6 g%. The anaemia can intensify when on dialysis; firstly, because the necessary heparinization aggravates any occult blood loss (e.g. from a duodenal ulcer) and secondly, because red cells are sequestered in the extra-corporeal system.

Renal osteodystrophy is a frequent finding and patients may be treated by 1,25–DHCC or present for a parathyroidectomy.

Tiredness, breathlessness, malaise, emotional instability, de-pression, angina and claudication occur all too frequently. It is tempting to think that haemodialysis restores the internal environ-ment to normal: it is vital to remember that this is not so. These patients are severely abnormal and for instance, commence dialysis with a serum creatinine of anything from 700 to 2000 mmol/litre.

The two major problems of fistulae are aneurysmal dilatation and left ventricular failure. The latter can occur when the fistula flow is above approximately 1 litre/minute. The commonest causes of death in people on haemodialysis are premature myocardial infarction, left ventricular failure and strokes. Following these is infection which is often from opportunist organisms.

ANAESTHETIC CONSIDERATIONS

Essentially the preparation and management is as for CRF. There are a few additional details.

Before operation discuss intraoperative fluids with the renal physi-cians. Overtransfusion of red cells is less important than in people who are not on dialysis because the GFR no longer needs to be maximized. However, which pack of cells is transfused is important because of future transplantation. Rapid transfusion in haemodialysis patients carries a high risk of producing hyperkalaemia because the red cells do not act as 'potassium sponges' as they do in normal patients.

It is important to co-ordinate the times of dialysis and surgery. Ideally, dialysis should finish 3–6 hours preoperatively, and after coming off the machine, FBC, U & E's and a clotting screen *must* be done. The patient should also be weighed. Many units give a calcium resonium enema routinely. Shortly after dialysis the patient is relatively hypovolaemic and his blood pressure is very sensitive to most intravenous and volatile anaesthetic agents. Hypotension should be corrected promptly by normal saline. Dextrose solutions produce a dilutional hyponatraemia and are to be avoided.

If the patient receives excess fluid intraoperatively, postoperative pulmonary oedema is a very real risk and it requires further dialysis.

The site of the A–V fistula should be noted and that limb must be carefully protected, It should never have a BP cuff applied to it, every effort must be made to establish the intravenous drip site in another arm or leg, and intraoperatively it should be wrapped in warm Gamgee. Some units use a stellate ganglion block or brachial block to dilate the blood vessels of the relevant arm. There is a theoretical objection, in that the major effect of the dilatation is on the small vessels and this may produce a 'steal' from the fistula. Probably, the major factor in ensuring fistula patency is the maintenance of cardiac output and blood pressure. Some centres measure fistula flow intraoperatively with an ultrasonic flowmeter.

Patients with fistulae can be very difficult to handle psychologically. They know their outlook and many are young with family responsibilities. Often a brash exterior hides chronic anxiety. A sedative oral premedication is probably the best choice and since they usually present for surgery on several occasions for a variety of procedures, there is frequently a previous anaesthetic record to guide prescription.

There is no contraindication to local or regional techniques provided that the clotting screen is normal and a high level of sterility is observed. Care must be taken not to allow the BP to fall and vasoconstrictors should be used at an earlier stage than in normal people to avoid an excessive fluid load. A block may wear off more quickly than expected, especially if it is in the arm with a fistula where there is a tremendous 'washout' potential.

Peritoneal dialysis

Until recently, peritoneal dialysis was only used as a semi-emergency technique to cover a period of acute renal failure. Now, many centres in the UK have up to 30% of patients on chronic ambulatory peritoneal dialysis. The commonest complication is infection (usually in the peritoneum) which can be detected by eye because the dialysate on return to the bag is opalescent. Failure to empty the peritoneum properly can result in congestive cardiac failure, basal atelectasis, and chest infection from a splinted diaphragm.

The advantage of the technique to the patient is that it is good at removing excess fluid and allows much greater dietary freedom.

ANAESTHETIC CONSIDERATIONS

Patients present for a variety of operations (genitourinary surgery, for congenital urinary tract abnormalities, blocked cannulae, renal transplantation). Their management is essentially the same as for patients with chronic renal failure. It is best to spigot the peritoneal cannula during surgery because the dialysis bags are a nuisance. Always check that the patient can breathe adequately when lying flat, that he is not in cardiac failure and does not have an underlying chest infection.

Patients with a functioning renal transplant

The preparation and management of these patients is as for chronic renal failure. They present for a wide variety of procedures, either related to their renal disease (e.g. nephrectomy, blockage of transplanted ureter, stenosis of transplanted artery) or for other reasons (e.g. vagotomy, caesarean section). Their serum creatinine can be normal, elevated and stable, or gradually rising.

Paradoxically, the person with a successfully functioning transplant is, from the anaesthetic viewpoint, probably the most predictable 'renal' patient. If their serum creatinine is within the normal range, they can effectively be treated as a normal person, with the proviso that great care should be taken to maintain their renal blood flow (by the methods described earlier in 'management of acute renal failure').

Rejection, although usually heralded by pain in the graft, malaise, oedema, hypertension, and arthropathy, may be completely asymptomatic so knowledge of the preoperative electrolytes is important.

Immunosuppressive drugs, usually prednisolone and azathioprine, are taken for life. Perioperatively the steroids should be increased (see Chapter 6) and if the GIT is going to be compromised because of the surgery, azathioprine can be given IV. Infection secondary to immunosupression is an important complication in transplanted patients. The infections can be bacterial, protozoal, viral or fungal and are often difficult to identify or treat. Because of this infection risk all procedures, no matter how trivial, must be performed with the utmost sterility.

Other problems which may result from immunosuppressive therapy are bone marrow depression, hepatotoxicity and neoplasia from azathioprine and the features of Cushing's syndrome (q.v.) from steroids.

Many patients with healthy transplants still have a functioning fistula and this should be treated carefully as already detailed (see haemodialysis). It may well be needed in the future if rejection occurs.

The majority of patients are maintained on antihypertensives which can interact with anaesthetic agents as described in the management of CRF.

FURTHER READING

Anonymous (1980) Acute renal failure after major surgery. *Br. Med. J.*, **280**, 2–3.

Barry, K.G. & Berman, A.R. (1961) Mannitol infusion III. The acute effect of the intravenous infusion of mannitol on blood and plasma volume. *N. Engl. J. Med.*, **264**, 1085–8.

Bastron, R.D. & Deutsch, S. (1976) Renal effects of anesthesia. In: *Anesthesia and the Kidney*. Grune & Stratton. 29–39.

Bastron, R.D. & Deutsch, S. (1976) Perioperative events and renal function. In: *Anesthesia and the Kidney*. Grune & Stratton. 45–51.

Berry, A.J. (1981) Respiratory support and renal function. *Anesthesiology*, **55**, 655–67.

Jarnberg, P.O. (1978) Acute effects of furosemide and mannitol on central hemodynamics in the early postoperative period. *Acta. Anaesthesiol. Scand.*, **22**, 184–93.

Weir, P.H.C. & Chung, F.F. (1984) Anaesthesia for patients with chronic renal disease. *Can. Anaesth. Soc. J.*, **31**, 468–80.

Wilson, R.F. (1977) Oliguria and acute renal failure. In: *Critical Care Manual*, **1**, Section J. Upjohn.

For the effect of jaundice on the kidney see Further Reading in Chapter 4.

8/Diseases of the connective tissue, bones and joints

Connective tissue disorders	Congenital skeletal deformities
Rheumatoid arthritis	The dwarfing syndromes
Systemic lupus erythematosus	Craniofacial malformations
Ankylosing spondylitis	
Marfan's syndrome	Gout and hypercuricaemia
Polyarteritis nodosa	
Scleroderma	Paget's disease
Temporal arteritis	
Wegener's granulomatosis	Osteoporosis and osteomalacia
Dermatomyositis	
Sjogren's syndrome	Osteoarthrosis
Still's disease	
	Unusual arthropathies

The disorders of this chapter are grouped together because of the similar way in which they affect anaesthesia. Common conditions are dealt with fully: the rarer ones have briefer notes related to their individual characteristics.

CONNECTIVE TISSUE DISORDERS

Rheumatoid arthritis

Rheumatoid arthritis is a disease with a world wide distribution which has a reduced incidence in primitive countries and tropical climates. It can occur at any age (with a peak incidence at 40 years) but its onset is less common under 20 and over 55 years. The prevalence in English adults is approximately 3% in women and 1% in men. Although there is a familial predisposition and an increased frequency of certain HLA types in those affected, there is no definite evidence of genetic transmission.

The cause is unknown, but it is thought that a trigger stimulates the formation of antibodies against the patient's own immunoglobulins, a process which in time can become self-generating.

The disease is usually insidious in onset and follows a chronic course with exacerbations and remissions. The overall picture is that of a connective tissue disorder, the dominant clinical feature of which is a chronic synovitis, most commonly affecting the small joints of the hands and feet.

PREOPERATIVE CONSIDERATIONS

History

Common general complaints are morning stiffness, weight loss, tiredness (often from anaemia), depression and social problems. Try to assess the level of mobility and exercise tolerance. Many are so immobile that they cannot generate the angina of effort or breathlessness on exertion which would indicate myocardial disease. Ask about neck, thoracic and other joint deformities. Symptoms of cervical spine instability can include aching over the occiput, the nape of the neck and the shoulders, and dizzy spells or loss of consciousness related to head movement (vertebrobasilar insufficiency).

Enquire of any other neurological symptoms. These usually have mechanical causes (carpal tunnel, ulnar nerve entrapment, spinal root compression (usually cervical)), but rarely there is a neuropathy secondary to vasculitis of the vasa nervorum. The latter commonly causes leg ulcers and more rarely digital ischaemia (there may be Raynaud's phenomenon) and ischaemic arteritis of the viscera with widely varying symptoms.

Throughout the interview listen for hoarseness or stridor and ask about dysphagia. These features may indicate laryngeal involvement in the rheumatoid process. A few patients are deaf due to arthritis of the auditory ossicles.

A drug history is vital since many drugs used in this disease cause GIT blood loss, affect platelet function, can depress the bone marrow, can cause proteinuria, and can affect the carriage of other drugs. A proportion of patients are on steroids and antidepressants (q.v.).

Take the opportunity to discuss the possibility and acceptability of a regional block if it is thought appropriate.

Examination

Make sure the patient is weighed; they are often deceptively light. *Musculoskeletal.* The small joints of the hands and feet are the ones most commonly affected but other larger joints (knees, elbows, hips) may also be involved. The position of maximum comfort for an inflamed joint is with the joint flexed, thus making the joint capsule as slack as possible. Fixed flexion deformities with muscle and tendon contractures result. Look also for the subluxation of joints (especially wrist and metacarpophalangeal joints) and ulnar deviation of the fingers. All these factors will affect the optimum intraoperative positioning of the patient and the best choice of drip site. Assess the hip and knee joints, especially if the lithotomy position is anticipated. Check the movement of the neck and the ability to adopt the intubating position. Temporomandibular involvement may reduce mouth opening. In severe cases indirect laryngoscopy may be indicated to assess the larynx.

RS. Watch the movements of the chest carefully during a deep inspiration and look for restricted rib movement. Clinical evidence of lung involvement is uncommon although pleurisy and small pleural effusions may be present in up to 20% of cases. These are more frequent in males.

CVS. Pericarditis although relatively common, only very rarely becomes constrictive or leads to tamponade. Postural hypotension occurs often in bed-ridden patients. Left-sided valvular incompetence caused by rheumatoid granulomas is recorded but rare. Vasculitis is evidenced by a purpuric-like rash, chronic leg ulcers, poor peripheral circulation, and renal, coronary and cerebral artery insufficiency. The stigmata of anaemia (q.v.) should be pursued. Anaemia may prevent cyanosis occurring.

GIT. A large spleen indicates possible thrombocytopaenia (Felty's syndrome) and rectal examination can reveal GIT bleeding.

Skin. Examine the state of the pressure areas, look for the presence of skin fragility and feel for subcutaneous nodules with a view to intraoperative positioning.

NS. Paraesthesia and weakness in the hands and arms can be secondary to cervical nerve root compression. Peripheral neuropathies secondary to vasculitis of vasa nervorum are usually sensory. The most frequent peripheral nerve entrapment is median nerve compression in the carpal tunnel.

Investigations

FBC. Normochromic, normocytic anaemia is common. However, if the Hb is below 10 g% then suspect a superimposed cause such as drug-induced GIT bleeding (common) or more rarely a co-existing pernicious or haemolytic anaemia. Impaired release of folate from erythrocytes can result in a macrocytosis. The anaemia is refractory to iron and, if acute treatment perioperatively is thought necessary, it needs blood transfusion. A clotting screen is wise prior to major surgery or regional anaesthesia since thrombocytopaenia is not always obvious clinically. In the absence of infection, the ESR is a sensitive index of the degree of activity of the rheumatoid process.

U & E's, LFT's. Many patients are on diuretics and steroids so check the serum potassium. A raised urea may indicate renal involvement with poor clearance of drugs. A low serum albumin, which is not infrequent, affects the binding and carriage of drugs.

Mild inflammatory changes in the portal tracts can elevate the alkaline phosphatase and 5-nucleotidase.

ECG. The rheumatoid process can involve all tissues of the heart leading to dysrhythmias and ischaemic changes.

X-rays. CXR—Small pleural effusions are found occasionally but are usually of little significance. Less often there are rheumatoid nodules which can occur throughout the lung fields and resemble neoplasms. They can be accompanied by a massive fibrotic reaction (Caplan's syndrome). Rarely, there is a true diffuse pulmonary fibrosis. Look for vertebral flexion deformities and evidence of rib cage joint fixation. Check the heart size.

Joints—In all but the most trivial cases it is mandatory to X-ray the cervical spine. X-rays should be taken in flexion and extension and on flexion may show posterior displacement of the odontoid peg beyond the normal limit of 3 mm.

Lung function tests. These are only indicated if there is severe chest involvement combined with an upper abdominal incison. A low FEV_1 and a high tidal volume to vital capacity ratio may predict the need for a period of postoperative assisted ventilation when diaphragmatic activity is impaired by pain and residual neuromuscular blocking drugs, or when ventilatory drive is depressed by analgesics. In these circumstances arterial blood gases on air are useful baseline data.

Preoperative preparation

With the help of physiotherapy encourage maximum mobility. Consider the use of splints to minimize deformities. Discuss the advantages of regional blockade with both the patient and surgeon. Imagine the position the person with rheumatoid disease will have to adopt to enable the block to be done and decide whether or not it is feasible. Immobility can make many blocks difficult.

PEROPERATIVE PHASE

Premedication. There is a wide range of possibilities but beware of ventilatory depression and remember steroid cover (q.v.) where appropriate.

Regional techniques. If using a regional technique with a conscious patient make great efforts to ensure the patient is comfortable before starting surgery. Joint contractures can make it necessary to adopt odd postures. Immobile joints can become very painful during a medium or long operation and pressure areas are at great risk.

Induction. Site the drip, if required, carefully so that the patient is at a minimum disadvantage postoperatively. Be meticulous in securing the cannula, or indwelling needle, because of the risk of cutting through fragile veins.

Position the patient carefully prior to induction. Always give good support to the head and neck and be very gentle with cervical manipulation. Consider the use of a vacuum head mould or judiciously placed sandbags. If the patient normally wears a cervical collar it may be better to keep it on. Let the patient position his own head to his limit whilst awake. It is often best to do this on the operating table to minimize movement. When moves have to be made with an unconscious patient ensure sufficient helpers to protect the rheumatoid joints, especially those of the neck.

If a facemask is to be used, a nasopharyngeal airway can be superior to an oral airway in terms of neck position. Topical local anaesthetic (cocaine) can usefully shrink the nasal mucosa to minimize bleeding. Holes cut in the side of the tube wall close to the end may prevent obstruction when the bevel lies on the pharyngeal wall.

Always have the equipment available for a difficult intubation. In severe cases, awake bronchoscopic or blind nasal intubation or even preoperative tracheostomy are possibilities. Although perhaps unpleasant they are superior to tetraplegia.

Use a sterile tube with a low pressure cuff.

Maintenance. The patient can be allowed to breathe spontaneously with an endotracheal tube or on a mask or given IPPV. For the latter smaller doses than normal of non-depolarizing muscle relaxants are required and in many cases they can be omitted altogether, the patient requiring only mild hyperventilation in the presence of opioids to permit mechanical ventilation.

POSTOPERATIVE PHASE

One serious problem is postoperative ventilatory insufficiency. Thus it may be advisable in chosen cases to continue IPPV until there is a well maintained tetanus or train of four on nerve stimulation, a satisfactory tidal volume, or a good inspiratory effort. Neuromuscular tests can be difficult to interpret in severe rheumatoid disease of the wrist and hands where there is both deformity and disease atrophy of the muscles. Assess spontaneous ventilation carefully (see Chapter 2) before extubation as re-intubation may not be easy.

Consider the use of regional blockade for postoperative analgesia. This may reduce the need for drugs which depress ventilation. Postoperative pulmonary infection is common so chest physiotherapy should be started immediately and all joints exercised passively to prevent the formation or worsening of contractures.

Always think about alternative routes of administration for rheumatoid drugs if the GIT is temporarily out of action. Continue steroid cover where appropriate.

Systemic lupus erythematosus (SLE)

This is chronic inflammatory disease of unknown cause which may affect the skin, joints, kidneys, nervous system, serous membranes and many other organs of the body. Women outnumber men in the ratio 9:1 and most of those affected are in the 20–50 year age group. Increasingly common, milder forms of the disease are being recognized and it has been estimated to have an incidence of up to 0.4% in American negresses.

The onset, or exacerbations of the disorder can be precipitated by sunlight, infection, surgery, emotional stress and drugs such as hydralazine, sulphonamides, anticonvulsants, methyldopa, procainamide, PAS and oral contraceptives.

The disease normally runs a chronic course with exacerbations and remissions, renal involvement being a bad prognostic feature.

PREOPERATIVE CONSIDERATIONS

History

Because of the ubiquitous nature of the disease, symptoms and signs occur in all organ systems. There is general debility, ill health, weight loss and tiredness which is often secondary to anaemia. When taking the history beware of CNS involvement causing psychiatric problems, which can be anything from mild anxiety to frank psychosis. CNS lesions can also present as epilepsy, focal lesions or migraine. Most patients have a history of polyarthritis or arthralgia but relatively few have joint deformities or tendon contractures. Ask about physical activity and note symptoms of breathlessness, angina, PND and orthopnoea. Oedema may be due to either cardiac or renal involvement. Cardiac failure from cardiomyopathy is rare, as is non-bacterial endocarditis of the aortic and mitral valves. Do not forget that chest pain can result from pleurisy and pericarditis.

The drug history is vital. Many patients are on steroids, diuretics, anti-hypertensives, and anti-inflammatory agents.

Examination

The reported involvement of the various body systems varies considerably from series to series.

Musculoskeletal. Check on joint deformities and tendon contractures. *Skin.* Look for areas of vasculitis and examine the state of the skin in general. Note gangrene (fingertips) if present. Purpura and ecchymoses may reflect underlying blood platelet and clotting problems, renal insufficiency, the side effects of corticosteroids, or vasculitis. Find the best drip sites. Note the presence of a wig from alopecia and allow the patient to wear it to theatre to save embarrassment.

CVS. This is involved in nearly 50%. Suspect myocarditis when there is a tachycardia disproportionate to either fever or anaemia. Listen carefully for murmurs which might provide evidence of valve disease or cardiomyopathy. Be assiduous in searching for signs of cardiac failure and do not forget to look for sacral oedema in the bed-ridden. Take the blood pressure; hypertension may be evidence of renal disease.

RS. Pleurisy is common and recurrent and is often accompanied by a friction rub but other abnormal physical findings are rare.

CNS. If abnormal, record the preoperative mental state in the notes. Note the presence of any focal lesions.

GIT. Check the weight. Anorexia, nausea and vomiting lead to weight loss. Splenomegaly is present in 15%.

Investigations

FBC. The normocytic, normochromic anaemia of chronic inflammatory disease is common and generally mild; occasionally there is an added haemolytic component. Leucopenia is the general rule. Thrombocytopaenia may be present without purpura. Clotting and prothrombin times may be prolonged due to a circulating anticoagulant which is present in 25% of cases.

U & E's, LFT's. These are normal unless there is marked renal or hepatic involvement. The serum potassium is, however, easily affected by diuretics or steroids.

CXR. There is often patchy consolidation with plate-like areas of collapse. This usually has little effect on lung function. A less frequent but more ominous finding is the 'shrinking lung' with sequential X-rays taken at intervals in full inspiration showing progressive elevation of the diaphragm. This is evidence of severe parenchymal involvement. Look for pleural and pericardial effusions. Note the heart size.

Lung function tests. These are not normally indicated unless there are specific abnormal findings when they can provide valuable baseline data. There are alterations in all lung volumes and a restrictive pattern (q.v.) with diffusion abnormalities can appear.

ECG. This can be normal or show evidence of right or left ventricular hypertrophy, pericarditis or dysrhythmias.

Preoperative preparation

If anaemic they may need a blood transfusion, but suspect a secondary cause if the Hb is less than 10 g%. Blood transfusion can exacerbate SLE. If there is renal involvement do not aim for a high preoperative haemoglobin concentration (see Chapter 7). If there are recurrent and frequent chest infections give a course of physiotherapy and antibiotics to optimize the pulmonary status.

Premedication. Unless there are specific individual contraindications, this can be of the anaesthetist's personal choice. Do not forget steroid cover if needed.

PEROPERATIVE PHASE

The main aim is to try and not exacerbate the SLE. Therefore avoid those drugs known to be triggers (penicillin, sulphonamides, hydralazine and procainamide). Think carefully before transfusing.

Regional techniques. There are no contraindications unless the clotting screen is abnormal.

Induction and maintenance. There are no particular advantages of one technique over another. If intubating, a sterile tube is wise. If there are renal or CVS problems or joint involvement (see rheumatoid arthritis) these need appropriate consideration. Renal involvement may reduce the excretion of many drugs.

POSTOPERATIVE PHASE

Continue steroid cover if needed. If there was poor preoperative ventilatory function, start physiotherapy immediately after surgery. Take care not to cause ventilatory depression. Any infection should be treated aggressively.

Ankylosing spondylitis

This is an inflammatory arthritis of the sacroiliac joints and spine leading to the ultimate ankylosis of these parts of the skeleton (bamboo spine). The hips can also be involved. The latter is the most common cause of occupational disability and often leads to prosthetic surgery. It is nine times as common in males as females and presents mainly in young men (13–40 years). Commencement over the age of 45 years is uncommon. It is rare in negroes and orientals with an incidence of up to 0.4% in adult caucasian males. There is an increased family incidence and an association with HLA B27.

PREOPERATIVE CONSIDERATIONS

History

Ask about pain in the chest which can be severe and exacerbated by breathing because of the involvement of costovertebral joints. In young men ask about limitations in sporting activities, and any changes in the onset of breathlessness. Note any comments about the reduction in the mobility of the cervical spine (e.g. unable to turn head while swimming, difficulty following the path of a squash ball from the periphery of vision). Enquire about the dyspnoea, angina and palpitations of myocardial disease. Aortic regurgitation is present in about 4% cases. Obtain a drug history because they are often on phenylbutazone, indomethacin or proprionic acid derivatives. Corticosteroid therapy may be used for iridocyclitis which occurs in 25% of cases. Radiotherapy is not commonly used now because of the risk of leukaemia.

Examination

Look specifically for mechanical problems such as neck stiffness, inability to adopt the intubating position and limited chest expansion. In severe cases note the use of the accessory muscles of respiration and look for the signs of associated fibrosing alveolitis. Always get the patient to adopt the intubating position and assess deviations from normality. Search for evidence of cardiac failure, feel for a collapsing pulse, note a low diastolic pressure and listen for aortic regurgitation (q.v.). If a local block is contemplated assess the feasibility.

Investigatons

FBC. Normochromic, normocytic anaemia should only be mild and if not, suspect a superimposed cause.
U & E's, LFT's. These should be normal.
X-rays. The extent of the ankylosis can be seen on chest and pelvic films. Atlanto-axial subluxation, although uncommon, can occur so extension and flexion views of the cervical spine are wise. On the chest X-ray apical fibrosis can resemble tuberculosis and a large left

ventricle may indicate decompensation secondary to aortic incompetence.

ECG. In 10% cases there are <u>cardiac conduction disturbances</u>, the most frequent being <u>atrioventricular block (q.v.)</u>.

Lung function tests and blood gases. These are only indicated in severe cases to assess the functional disability and to provide baseline data.

Preoperative preparation

Treat any cardiac failure, introduce the physiotherapists to the patient and if necessary treat chest infections. Unless there are specific contraindications, premedication can be of the anaesthetist's choice. Remember steroid cover if necessary.

PEROPERATIVE PHASE

Consider the possibility of a local nerve block. However, spinals, caudals or epidurals are at the best difficult and often impossible. If attempted, a <u>lateral approach</u> is recommended to minimize the passage through calcified ligaments.

Secure venous access. Always be prepared for a difficult intubation. If the neck is in fixed flexion, and even tracheostomy would be difficult or impossible, opt for awake oral or nasal intubation under local analgesia. Even if neck mobility is not as severely restricted as this, induction still presents a hazard. When general anaesthesia is chosen, a good plan is a gas or slow intravenous induction with conversion to a volatile agent in order to establish whether the airway is safe. This can be followed by a relaxant, intubation whilst breathing spontaneously or maintenance using an oral or nasopharyngeal airway. Paradoxically, although they may be exceedingly difficult to intubate, an airway can often be maintained relatively easily with the neck in the position the patient normally assumes.

For major surgery, internal jugular or subclavian catheterization for CVP monitoring may be technically difficult because of neck rigidity. A long line from an antecubital fossa is preferable.

If there is ventilatory impairment, IPPV is preferred to spontaneous ventilation; use only small doses of relaxants and ensure that they have worn off before extubation.

Do not forget that drugs such as phenylbutazone not only induce liver enzymes but also displace other drugs from their binding sites thus increasing their effective free concentration.

Position the patient carefully on the operating table, so as not to cause joint or nerve injuries.

POSTOPERATIVE PHASE

Test the adequacy of reversal of muscle relaxants by nerve stimulation (well sustained tetanus, a minimally decrementing train of four) and by clinical measurement (a large tidal volume or a good inspiratory effort). Always allow a period of satisfactory spontaneous ventilation with the tube *in situ* before extubating. Organize early chest physiotherapy and mobilize as quickly as possible to reduce the progress of ankylosis. Control of the airway should never be left to an inexperienced person before the patient is fully awake.

Marfan's syndrome

This generalized connective tissue disorder affects mainly the heart, the eye and the skeleton. It is inherited as an autosomal dominant, has variable expressivity and may be associated with older paternal age. The incidence is approximately 1 in 20000. The nature of the molecular defect is not known but collagen synthesis is impaired.

The prognosis is not good, deaths being due to cardiovascular problems. Patients may present for cardiac or ocular surgery or spinal fusion as well as with incidental illness. They are occasionally on propranolol in an attempt to retard aortic dilatation.

PREOPERATIVE CONSIDERATIONS

History

The manifestations are variable but the main symptoms are those of ocular, cardiovascular or respiratory insufficiency. 50% have subluxed lenses which may cause myopia, retinal detachment and glaucoma. 90% have incompetent aortic valves or aneurysmal dilatation of the ascending aorta. Mitral valve prolapse is also common. Shortness of breath may be due to cardiac failure, kyphoscoliosis, sternal deformity, emphysematous lungs or spontaneous pneumothorax.

Examination

The patient is usually tall and thin with long extremities. Always look in the mouth. A high arched palate coupled with crowded teeth can present an intubation problem. Concentrate on the cardiovascular and pulmonary systems to assess aortic and mitral valve disease (Chapter 1) and the degree of restricted ventilation (Chapter 2).

Investigations

FBC, U & E's. These should be normal.
ECG. This may show left ventricular hypertrophy.
CXR. This may help to evaluate aneurysmal dilation of the aorta, cardiac failure, sternal deformities, emphysematous lungs and kyphoscoliosis.

ANAESTHETIC CONSIDERATIONS

Perioperative morbidity and mortality are high. The problems are those of difficult intubation, needing a long endotracheal tube and of the cardiovascular (q.v.) and pulmonary disease (q.v.). Do not forget antibiotic prophylaxis.

Polyarteritis nodosa

This is a rare disease which is commonest in men aged 20–45 years. Approximately one third carry hepatitis B surface antigen (q.v.). There is inflammation of small and medium sized arteries with subsequent thrombosis, ischaemia and frequent muscle pains. The lesions heal by fibrosis and aneurysm formation. All organs can be affected leading to a very variable presentation.

PREOPERATIVE CONSIDERATIONS

History

Symptoms in the history include those of hypertension, angina, cardiac failure, myocardial infarction, pericarditis, acute nephritis, the nephrotic syndrome, abdominal pain, tender subcutaneous nodules, haematuria, late onset asthma, peripheral neuropathy and intracerebral thrombosis and haemorrhage. These patients take many drugs including steroids.

Examination

Concentrate on the cardiovascular, pulmonary and renal systems. Hypertension is invariable.

Investigations

FBC. The Hb is often low and leukocytosis is present in over 75% cases.
U & E's, LFT's. These are normal until the disease is very severe. There can be albuminuria and a raised urea from renal involvement.

ECG. All abnormalities are possible but remember that the first sign of cardiac involvement may be a persistent tachycardia. Examine it for ischaemic changes.

CXR. Look for signs of cardiac failure, asthma and pulmonary fibrosis.

Virology. Screen for hepatitis B carrier state.

PEROPERATIVE PHASE

Remember steroid cover where needed. Maintain the BP at preoperative levels because the presence of narrowed vessel lumens secondary to arteritis may make the tissue blood flow to organs borderline. Only use intra-arterial monitoring if it is absolutely essential because the peripheral arterial blood supply is already critical. There may be an abnormal response to suxamethonium especially if there is hepatic involvement.

POSTOPERATIVE PHASE

Ensure good oxygenation because the poor or reduced blood flow to vital organs provides a low oxygen flux (q.v.) which may be inadequate if the patient becomes hypoxic. Continue steroid cover.

Scleroderma

Although scleroderma (also called systemic sclerosis) still presents a serious prognosis, more benign syndromes and forms with localized, non-progressive lesions are being recognized. The disease, although rare is most common in middle aged women. The aetiology is unknown and against a general background of lassitude, fever and weight loss (bacterial overgrowth in atonic areas of bowel results in malabsorption), the disease is characterized by sclerosis of collagen fibres in the skin, GIT, heart, lung, kidney, locomotor system and diaphragm, leading to a variety of clinical presentations. Eighty percent of patients have Raynaud's phenomenon when exposed to the cold. Limited life expectancy is associated with cardiac, renal and pulmonary involvement.

The skin develops a non-pitting oedema and becomes smooth, waxy and tight and later thin, atrophic and pigmented and can adhere to underlying shrunken muscles. Changes are most frequent in the hands and face where it produces a mask-like expression.

PREOPERATIVE CONSIDERATIONS

History

Ask questions to reveal cardiac, renal and pulmonary involvement. Recurrent chest infections can indicate involvement of oesophageal tissues with overspill, aspiration and patchy lower lobe pneumonitis. This is often accompanied by dysphagia, oesophagitis and a 'scleroderma back'. Epistaxis may result from telangectasia of the nasopharyngeal lining and clotting abnormalities can be associated with malabsorption of fat-soluble vitamin K. Get a drug history, some patients are on steroids.

Examination

Musculoskeletal. Ask the patient to open the mouth (to check the oral aperture) and to adopt the intubating position. Involvement of the skin around the mouth may restrict lip movement and prevent adequate dental hygiene. There may be gross systemic myopathy in addition to arthritis and tendonitis.

RS. Defects in diffusing capacity appear early but may not be apparent clinically. Later pulmonary fibrosis and pulmonary hypertension can occur, progressing finally to the signs of right ventricular hypertrophy and ventilatory failure.

CVS. Raynaud's phenomenon, hypertension and left ventricular failure are common findings, dysrhythmias (often heart block) and right ventricular failure are less common and cardiomyopathy is rare.

Renal. The signs of renal failure tend to occur late together with a depressing prognosis.

Investigations

FBC. Usually there is a mild normochromic, normocytic anaemia, but there may be superimposition of iron, vitamin B_{12} and/or folate deficiencies. The ESR will normally be raised.

U & E's, LFT's. These are normal unless there is renal or hepatic involvement.

CXR. Look for cardiomegaly, pulmonary fibrosis and pulmonary hypertension. Small pleural effusions can be present.

ECG. Heart block is probably the commonest dysrhythmia. Check for ventricular hypertrophy.

Lung function tests. These are normal unless there is severe pulmonary involvement.

PEROPERATIVE PHASE

Remember steroid cover when needed. Consider the use of regional blocks. Even if normally appropriate, do not use <u>adrenaline</u> because these patients are said to be <u>hypersensitive to its vasoconstrictor</u> action. Local anaesthetics also have an anecdotal reputation of lasting for a very long time.

Site intravenous drips carefully, well away from affected hands because hand-care is so important, and away from joints. During any anaesthetic keep the peripheries warm, because <u>cold can precipitate severe ischaemia</u>.

If opting for a general anaesthetic, first prepare for a difficult intubation and be very aware of the possibility of regurgitation because of lesions in the oesophagus and stomach. It is wise to intubate on the side or during the application of cricoid pressure.

In general, there are no specific contraindications to any particular anaesthetic technique. If there is marked parenchymal lung involvement, lung compliance may be low. The patient's blood pressure is labile and they have a reduced circulating blood volume which can led to a precipitate fall in blood pressure on induction. ECG monitoring is mandatory. Halothane may exacerbate dysrhythmias. The use of <u>arterial lines in these patients is controversial</u>, one view being that no potentially thrombotic artery should be compromised when distal blood flow is already borderline.

POSTOPERATIVE PHASE

If there have been airway problems be certain an experienced person is present during recovery. Use postoperative ventilation as needed. Ensure good postoperative oxygenation and early physiotherapy, as both active and passive exercises of the hands need to be done several times a day.

Temporal arteritis

This disease, now called <u>Giant Cell Arteritis</u>, usually presents over the age of <u>60 years</u>, sometimes in the presence of <u>polymyalgia rheumatica</u>. There is a severe headache with tenderness and burning over the scalp, and very tender temporal arteries. Surgical biopsy for diagnosis (which should be done under local analgesia), is now less common and the majority are diagnosed on suspicion in the presence of a raised ESR. There can also be a systemic upset with generalized fever, weakness, arthralgia, and myalgia. The whole of the carotid system and sometimes the coronary and other arteries are involved.

The patients may be hypertensive. There is a high risk of blindness from retinal ischaemia.

It is sensible to ensure that the blood pressure stays at its pre-anaesthetic level to guarantee flow through the narrowed lumen of the ophthalmic and other end-arteries. Record any neurological deficit present prior to operation; this may be part of the general intracranial arteritis.

Anaemia is usually mild but may be severe. Steroid therapy in high doses is the rule, therefore take appropriate precautions.

Wegener's granulomatosis

This disease is characterized by a necrotizing granulomatous vasculitis involving the upper and lower respiratory tracts, and causing glomerulonephritis and variable degrees of systemic, small vessel vasculitis. The aetiology is not known.

Although it is an uncommon disorder, it is no longer thought of as extremely rare. The male to female ratio is 3:2. Presentation can be at any age but is commonest in the fourth and fifth decades.

Virtually any organ can be involved. History and examination should elicit organ system involvement but non-specific symptoms are weakness, malaise, arthralgia, anorexia and weight loss.

PREOPERATIVE CONSIDERATIONS

RS. Always ask about upper airway symptoms (paranasal sinus pain, discharge, nasal mucosal ulceration, septal perforation, otitis media). Pulmonary manifestations may present as cough, haemoptysis, chest discomfort or dyspnoea.

CVS. Involvement of the CVS is infrequent but may present as pericarditis or coronary vasculitis.

NS. Involvement of the NS, present in 20%, causes cranial neuritis, mononeuritis multiplex, or cerebral vasculitis.

Renal. Renal failure is the commonest cause of death. Look for proteinuria and haematuria.

Eye. Ocular signs occur in up to 60%. They are predominantly conjunctivitis, episcleritis or vasculitic lesions.

Drug history. Patients may be on steroids (q.v.) or cyclophosphamide, which usually induces remission.

Investigations

FBC. Mild anaemia, leukocytosis, and a raised ESR are expected. If on cyclophosphamide check for leukopenia.

CXR. This may pick up asymptomatic pulmonary infiltrates.
ECG. This may detect pericarditis, or ischaemia.
U & E's. These are important to exclude renal failure.
Blood gases. These are helpful in evaluating pulmonary involvement but should be taken very carefully to avoid arterial damage.

ANAESTHETIC CONSIDERATIONS

These depend on the degree of pulmonary and renal involvement. A strict aseptic technique for all procedures is essential, especially if on cyclophosphamide treatment. Regional analgesia is not advised if there is NS involvement. Always be careful to protect the eyes.

Intubation should be achieved gently as the granulomas bleed easily. A small tube may be needed if granulomas are present in the larynx. Avoid nasotracheal tubes and consider whether gastrostomy is preferable to nasogastric drainage.

Dermatomyositis

This rare disease forms a continuum with polymyositis. In the main, it affects women aged 40–50 years and up to one third have an underlying malignancy of the bronchus, breast, stomach or ovary. In men over 60 years presenting with this condition, approximately 60% have carcinoma of the bronchus.

There is general ill health and fever with a purple rash over the face and extremities, together with a sterile inflammation of the muscles. The onset may be acute or chronic and although the disease usually progresses gradually over weeks or months, it can pursue a more rapid, aggressive course. Striated muscle can be replaced by fibrous tissue leading to contractures. Most commonly the proximal muscles of the upper limb are tender and weak. On the CXR the lungs may have plate-like areas of collapse and/or diffuse fibrosis. Cardiomyopathy can lead to heart failure but it is rare. If the myopathy is progressive, ventilatory power is reduced and involvement of the pharyngeal and laryngeal muscles results in dysphonia and dysphagia. Intercurrent infection is common. Anaemia is rarely severe; the ESR is a poor index of disease activity.

Particular points for the anaesthetist are to beware of the risk of aspiration, to use small doses of neuromuscular blockers, to ensure adequate postoperative ventilation and, if necessary to provide steroid cover. There is a possible danger of a myasthenic response to suxamethonium. Salivary secretions accumulate quickly; endotracheal intubation is advised.

Regional anaesthesia, though not absolutely contraindicated, should be treated with respect in the presence of a myopathy.

Sjogren's syndrome

These patients (male:female 1:10) exhibit a syndrome like rheumatoid arthritis (q.v.) and, in addition, characteristically have reduced secretions from the lacrimal and salivary glands, and sometimes from bronchial, gastric and vaginal mucosa as well. Accordingly, they exhibit dry, gritty eyes, and have a dry mouth, dysphagia and frequent pulmonary infections. Dryness of the nasal mucosa may lead to recurrent epistaxis. Dependent nonthrombocytopaenic purpura may be present. Raynaud's phenomenon is present in 20%. Steroid therapy is not common.

In addition to the anaesthetic considerations of rheumatoid arthritis, there should be scrupulous care of the eyes (most require artificial tears anyway), antibiotic cover to prevent chest infections and sterile endotracheal tubes used. Drying agents are best avoided in the premedication. If the premedication is an oral prescription ensure that a sip of water is allowed.

Generous lubrication of nasogastric or nasoendotracheal tubes will help avoid causing epistaxis. Massive enlargement of parotid, submandibular and sublingual glands can make airway control and intubation difficult. Humidify postoperative oxygen.

Still's disease

Synonymous with juvenile chronic arthritis, this is a condition of chronic synovitis of childhood within which several distinct subgroups are coming to be recognized, each of which is characterized by articular and extra-articular effects and certain laboratory tests. Weight loss, poor growth and anaemia are common.

Anaesthetic considerations are similar to those of adult rheumatoid arthritis with the added problems, many of them psychological, of a chronically sick child.

CONGENITAL SKELETAL DEFORMITIES

The dwarfing syndromes

Dwarfism is dealt with as an entity in itself because of the similar problems presented, irrespective of the nature of the basic defect. It is almost always an inherited trait and it is subclassified in several ways depending upon the bone and joints involved and the relative shortening of limbs and body.

Almost all the syndromes to some degree involve mental retardation (may be difficult or unreliable history), epilepsy (q.v.), spinal deformity, hydrocephaly, congenital cardiac disease and abnormalities of the viscera. In later life there can be renal, liver and coronary heart disease. Umbilical hernias are frequent. The underlying diagnosis is very valuable so that the appropriate difficulties can be anticipated.

The problems presenting in all dwarfing syndromes are:

● Airway management may be difficult because of thick lips, a large tongue, a short neck, a distorted thorax and trachea and distorted nasal and facial bones. A hypoplastic mandible, micrognathia, cleft palate and cleft lip can all be present. It is vital to assess all these problems preoperatively, prepare for a difficult intubation, get a good assistant and probably not use relaxants to intubate until a good airway has been established. Extreme cases may warrant preoperative tracheostomy or awake intubation. An antisialogogue premedicant can be helpful but also makes bronchial secretions more viscid. Do not forget that airway management should be continued into the postoperative period until the patient is fully recovered.

If a regional block is contemplated in order to circumvent the need for intubation, bear in mind the patient's mental state and ability.

● There can be atlanto-axial instability and spinal stenosis. The former results from varying combinations of bony deformity and ligamentous laxity and can present with symptoms varying from sudden quadriplegia to progressive weakness with, or without, spasticity and hyperreflexia. The instability can often be detected on extension and flexion cervical films or suspected from the neurological history and examination. If instability is present, protect the neck very carefully as in rheumatoid arthritis (q.v.) or even use a plaster cast.

Spinal stenosis is a syndrome resulting from the pressure of the vertebral bones on the spinal column and/or cauda equina. Its presentation is variable depending on the level and the part of the cord which is compressed.

If either of these two features are present then the preoperative neurological deficit needs to be carefully documented and regional anaesthesia treated with respect. Epidural and spinal anaesthesia has an unpredictable level and effect. In periods of active demyelination suxamethonium is contraindicated.

If the spinal stenosis is above T_7 hyperreflexia (q.v.) is a potential problem.

● There may be thoracic deformity with, or without, kyphoscoliosis (q.v.) whose effects on ventilation can be anything from minimal to severe. Simple lung function tests such as vital capacity and FEV_1 when compared with the normal for age, sex and height can indicate the gravity of impairment and the magnitude of the ventilatory reserve over the resting conditions. If there is any doubt, consider a period of postoperative ventilation until all neuromuscular blockers have worn off. Beware of the use of postoperative opioids with their concomitant ventilatory depression.

Craniofacial and mandibulofacial dysostoses and fibrous dysplasias

These comprise a mixed bag of syndromes with abnormalities of the face, skull and cervical spine which are not usually associated with small stature. Each case presents slightly differently, with varying problems of mouth opening, intubation, mask fit, visualization of larynx, large tongue and small or absent nasal route for tubes. There can be associated visceral abnormalities.

Assess the airway preoperatively and prepare for a difficult intubation. A spontaneous breathing technique is best until the anaesthetist is confident that a good airway can be maintained. Ensure that the surgeon is capable of performing a tracheostomy and that he is ready to do so, if called upon in an emergency. Extend skilled airway management into the postoperative period.

GOUT AND HYPERURICAEMIA

Gout is a clinically recognizable disease resulting from the deposition of crystals derived from hyperuricaemic body fluids causing acute arthritis, tophi, renal disease and urolithiasis. Although all patients with gout have hyperuricaemia, hyperuricaemia can occur without clinical gout. The incidence of gout in adult males is 0.5%, and in adult females is 0.08%. The incidence of asymptomatic hyperuricaemia is 6%.

Clinical gout is usually classified into primary, resulting from an inborn error of purine metabolism, and secondary, due to either decreased excretion of uric acid or increased production of uric acid. 10% of all clinical gout is associated with myeloproliferative and lymphoproliferative disorders, which cause increased purine turnover (e.g. polycythaemia rubra vera, myelofibrosis, myeloid leukaemia, multiple myeloma, Hodgkins disease). Other rapidly progressing malignancies and chronic haemolytic anaemia may also be responsible.

Drug-induced gout can follow treatment with thiazide diuretics and salicylates.

Chronic renal failure, although often associated with hyperuricaemia, rarely causes clinical gout.

PREOPERATIVE CONSIDERATIONS

History

Ask about the onset of the disease. If it is chronic or recurrent and familial, it is usually primary gout. If the condition has progressed to chronic tophaceous gout, note the association with renal disease (q.v.) and renal stones and ask about symptoms of this (polyuria, nocturia, anorexia, nausea, vomiting, fatigue, dysuria, haematuria and oedema). If the disease is of relatively recent onset, consider secondary causes.

Ask about the symptoms of hypertension, obesity, coronary artery disease, heart failure and diabetes mellitus (recurrent urinary tract infections, vaginitis), all of which have a higher incidence in people with hypercuricaemia and gout when they are compared with an age-matched group in the general public.

The drug history is important and it is vital to make arrangements to give the drugs parenterally postoperatively if the GIT is likely to be out of action for a while.

Examination

CVS. Look for signs of hypertension (q.v.), heart failure (q.v.) and oedema.
Musculoskeletal. Check joint movements, the condition of the skin, the position of tophi, and make sure that the temporomandibular joint is not restricted. Gout spares the axial skeleton and the cervical spine is usually normal.

Investigations

FBC. If anaemia is present, look for a further cause such as renal failure or drug-induced GIT blood loss. Look at a blood film for evidence of myeloproliferative or lymphoproliferative disease.
U & E's. These should be normal unless there is renal failure or unless the patient is on diuretics when the serum potassium can be low.
LFT's. There should be no abnormality.
CXR. Look for an enlarged heart and signs of cardiac failure.
ECG. Gout only rarely affects the conducting system. When it does, it causes heart block and dysrhythmias.

PEROPERATIVE PHASE

Since emotional strain can precipitate an acute attack of gout, an anxiolytic premedication is advisable. Ensure good hydration. It is good practice to establish an intravenous infusion during the preoperative fasting period to enhance the excretion of urate.

Induction and maintenance of anaesthesia can be with a wide variety of agents (but *not* methoxyflurane, which worsens hyperuricaemia). The only deviation from normal are the preparations required for a difficult intubation if there is temporomandibular arthritis. Colchicine is itself a weak anaesthetic and can potentiate the central depressant effects of barbiturates, anaesthetics and analgesics.

POSTOPERATIVE PHASE

Maintain a high fluid load (> 3500 cc/day) preferably via the oral route, since this is less likely to precipitate cardiac failure. If a diuretic is necessary because of the fluid retention following surgery, spironolactone is probably the best choice because the thiazides and frusemide induce hyperuricaemia. Gouty arthritis, precipitated by surgery, usually occurs towards the end of the first postoperative week. This can be a particular problem for those patients maintained on oral agents who cannot take tablets in the postoperative period and it should be remembered that an intravenous preparation of colchicine is available.

Avoid salicylates for postoperative analgesia because they block the uricosuric effect of probenecid and sulphinpyrazone.

PAGET'S DISEASE

This is a common condition in the middle aged and elderly with an incidence of 1% at 50 years, rising to 10% at over 70 years. Males are affected more frequently than females, and the disease is only clinically important in a minority of patients. On X-ray there is an increased incidence of osteoblastic and osteoclastic activity as indicated by areas of bone formation and increased density, alternating with areas of rarefaction. The disease which is usually widespread in the skeleton but painless can, on occasions, be quite the reverse. Deafness may occur but bony deformities are only present in advanced disease. Fractures present after only minor trauma but usually heal normally.

When Paget's disease involves more than 30–40% of the skeleton there is a significant increase in cardiac output (due to hypervascularity of active osteolytic bone lesions), which may lead to cardiac enlargement and high output cardiac failure.

The serum alkaline phosphatase is usually greatly increased but there is hypercalcaemia only if the patient is immobile. The lesions are most commonly found in the axial skeleton and long bones, but have been recorded everywhere.

Patients can be on no treatment, calcitonin, steroids or salicylates.

Anaesthetic considerations tend to revolve around the axial skeleton. The cervical spine should be X-rayed in flexion and extension, and all pre-existing neurological signs noted. Think about the possibilities of vertebral stenosis with cord compression and basilar invagination of the cerebellum. During all procedures respect the neck, and move it and pad it carefully.

OSTEOPOROSIS AND OSTEOMALACIA

These are two chronic diseases of bone. They both weaken the bone but their causation and pathology are different. Osteoporosis occurs when the rate of bone destruction exceeds the rate of bone formation. Osteomalacia, (which means softening of bone) results from a failure to lay down calcium and phosphorous in an adequate bone matrix. Histologically the difference is immediately obvious, but bone biopsy is virtually never undertaken.

Osteoporosis

In Western civilizations this is by far the more common of the two. Its distribution can be local (due to immobility of limbs, bed rest etc.) or general. Seen radiologically it presents as a loss of bone density with a reduction in the number and size of trabeculae and thinning of the bone cortex. The vertebral bodies become concave in their upper and lower surfaces (cod-fish vertebrae).

Clinical presentation is usually because of a fracture, principally of the wrist, femur or vertebrae. The majority of cases have no known cause and the incidence increases with age. Rarely, and often in a younger age group, osteoporosis can be associated with Cushing's syndrome, thyrotoxicosis, acromegaly, reduction in sex hormones, rheumatoid arthritis, long-standing hepatic disease, chronic alcoholism and protein malnutrition. The commonest iatrogenic cause is steroid therapy.

Persistent pain is not a common feature and when present it is principally due to fractures with, or without, associated nerve compression. Serum calcium, phosphate and alkaline phosphatase are all normal.

Osteomalacia

This usually results from a deficiency of Vitamin D causing inadequate mineralization of bone. The clinical presentation differs in adults and children.

Adults. Bone pains and bone tenderness are frequently present and persistent. There is often muscular weakness of the lower limb and symptoms of malabsorption. Spontaneous fractures and tetany are rare.

Juveniles. Because of the effect on growth plates there are deformities in the legs, chest and skull with hypotonia and weakness.

In both adults and juveniles there are reduced serum calcium and phosphorus levels with an increase in the serum alkaline phosphatase. Radiological examination shows rarefactions of bone and translucent bands (pseudofractures or Looser's zones) which are usually bilateral and at points of compressive stress. They are described in the medial cortex of the upper femur, the pelvic rami, ribs and axillary borders of the scapulae. In rickets, the distal epiphysis of the radius is cupped (champagne sign).

The cause is frequently a reduced intake of Vitamin D, either from the diet or from manufacture in the skin. It occurs commonly from malabsorption in coeliac disease and after extensive surgery to the GIT. Chronic renal disorders can fail to convert Vitamin D to its active form. Long-term anticonvulsant therapy induces liver enzymes which in turn increases the catabolism of Vitamin D, thereby reducing the effect of an ingested dose.

Treatment is principally that of the underlying disorder and then the use of Vitamin D supplements and adequate minerals in the diet. The response to treatment is good.

Anaesthetic considerations

The main anaesthetic considerations for both these bone disorders is the protection of the fragile bones particularly in lifting and positioning. Any underlying disease or coexistent abnormalities such as uraemia, anaemia, clotting deficiencies or malnutrition need the appropriate management.

Within the above limitations, there are no specific contraindications to any anaesthetic technique. Encourage early postoperative mobilization.

OSTEOARTHROSIS

Traditionally, this has been classified into primary generalized osteoarthrosis which occurs as a familial trait in middle aged females with a predilection for the terminal interphalangeal joint (Heberden's nodes) and secondary osteoarthrosis due to congenital, traumatic, metabolic or inflammatory causes. A more modern definition is a 'disease causing an alteration in hyaline cartilage'. New bone is laid down at the edges of the joints resulting in osteophyte formation. Bony ankylosis never occurs, though limitation of movement may be very marked. The affected joints have pain, stiffness, swelling, deformity and loss of function. It is regarded as a 'normal' response to ageing and on radiographic assessment, it is present somewhere in 90% of the population by the age of 40 years.

The axial skeleton, hips and knees are the joints most commonly affected. Morning stiffness is mild compared to rheumatoid arthritis. Pain tends to intensify when the joint is used and is relieved by rest. Muscular wasting is usually present surrounding the affected joint. Only a minority of sufferers have severe symptoms but surgery is often required (arthrodesis, arthroplasty, osteotomy or joint replacement) for symptomatic improvement.

The disease is not commonly associated with any serious background pathology but a drug history is important because many patients are on anti-inflammatory drugs such as salicylates and phenylbutazone.

Characteristic anaesthetic problems are difficulties with curling the patient up to do spinal or epidural blocks and getting the legs into the lithotomy position. The latter can be a particular problem in urological and gynaecological procedures. The legs should always be moved simultaneously and never be forced into position. If there is cervical involvement, hyperextension and hyperflexion of the neck must be avoided and care taken when maintaining an airway and intubating the patient. If prolonged immobility is anticipated consider the use of subcutaneous heparin to avoid deep vein thrombosis.

UNUSUAL ARTHROPATHIES

From time to time patients are presented for anaesthesia for joint aspiration or from some other reason who have a co-existing incidental arthropathy of obscure cause. This can be due to infection, endocrine and metabolic disorders, neoplasia or a blood dyscrasia.

Viral

Rubella. A polyarthritis follows the rash by one to seven days. The virus is transmitted in nasopharyngeal secretions which may still carry live virus during the arthralgic phase. Avoid contact with staff in early pregnancy.

Mumps. This polyarthritis is usually obvious from the history. The virus is transmitted by inhalation of affected particles from saliva for approximately six days after the clinical onset of parotitis.

Hepatitis B. Malaise, fever, anorexia and a rash together with arthritis of the hands, wrists, knees, ankles and shoulders can last for up to four weeks, remitting when the jaundice develops. There is usually a tender liver and abnormal liver function tests. The virus is transmitted via blood and saliva and can enter the body through the conjunctiva. If this disease is suspected, urgent virology is mandatory with appropriate warnings on the blood sample.

Bacterial

Gonococcal and tuberculous arthritis are increasing in incidence. The latter is much more common in the elderly and immigrants, in whom a chest X-ray is indicated.

Salmonella arthritis commonly resembles rheumatic fever. Although the diagnosis is usually well established, it should be remembered that sufferers can continue to excrete bacilli in the faeces, urine and bile for over a year and occasionally become indefinite carriers.

Endocrine

Arthropathies are occasionally seen as presenting features of acromegaly, hypothyroidism and hyperparathyroidism.

Metabolic

Arthropathies can occur in haemochromatosis, hyperlipidaemia and Wilson's disease. Pyrophosphate arthropathy usually affects the knees of elderly people and is important because of its association with hyperparathyroidism, haemochromatosis and diabetes mellitus.

Malignancy

Arthritis can occur with almost any type of malignancy but most commonly does so with carcinoma of bronchus, prostate or breast. It may precede the other signs and symptoms of malignancy. With hypertrophic pulmonary osteoarthropathy there is burning pain in the fingers, wrists and shins with recurrent effusions. Finger clubbing can be present and radiology shows periosteitis of the shafts of the affected bone. Symptoms suggestive of this syndrome demand a preoperative chest X-ray and clinical examination of the breast or prostate gland.

FURTHER READING

Birkinshaw, K.J. (1975) Anaesthesia in a patient with an unstable neck. *Anaesthesia*, **30**, 46–9.

Christophidis, N. & Huskisson, E.C. (1982) Misleading symptoms and signs of cervical spine subluxation in rheumatoid arthritis. *Br. Med. J.*, **285**, 364–5.

Jayson, M.I.V. (1984) Systemic sclerosis: a collagen or microvascular disease? *Br. Med. J.*, **288**, 1855–7.

Kafer, E.R. (1980) Respiratory and cardiovascular functions in scoliosis and the principles of anesthetic management. *Anesthesiology*, **52**, 339–51.

Lake, C.L. (1978) Anesthesia and Wegener's Granulomatosis: Case report and review of the literature. *Anesth. Analg.*, **57**, 353–9.

McConkey, B. (1982) Rheumatoid cervical myelopathy. *Br. Med. J.*, **284**, 1731–2.

Pyeritz, R.E. & McKusick, V.A. (1979) The Marfan Syndrome: diagnosis and management. *N. Engl. J. Med.*, **300**, 772–7.

Sinclair, J.R. & Mason, R.A. (1984) Ankylosing spondylitis: The case for awake intubation. *Anaesthesia*, **39**, 3–11.

Verghese, C. (1984) Anaesthesia in Marfan's Syndrome. *Anaesthesia*, **39**, 917–22.

Walts, L.F., Finerman, G. & Wyatt, G.M. (1975) Anaesthesia for dwarfs and other patients of pathological small stature. *Can. Anaesth. Soc. J.*, **22**, 703–9.

9/Haematology

Anaemia
Physiology
The clinical setting
Hypochromic anaemia
Macrocytic anaemia
Normochromic-normocytic
   anaemia
Haemolytic anaemia

**Anaesthetic considerations of
   common anaemias**
   Preoperative considerations
   Peroperative phase
   Postoperative phase

**Problems and hazards of blood
transfusion**

Jehovah's Witnesses

Haemoglobinopathies

Bone marrow failure

Bleeding disorders

Polycythaemia

Multiple myeloma

Haemochromatosis

ANAEMIA

Anaemia is not a disease in itself, but a feature of many underlying conditions which may, or may not, be related to the necessity of surgery. It can be defined as a diminished oxygen carrying capacity of the blood due to a reduction in the number of red cells, or in their haemoglobin (Hb) content, in the presence of a normal blood volume. The usual classification of anaemias is based on aetiology:
• Blood loss. This is by far the commonest cause in western society resulting from the p's (piles, peptic ulcer, periods, pain killers, parturition, polyps). The two common routes of loss are the GIT and per vaginam. In chronic form, the net loss of blood induces an iron deficient state.
• Decreased red cell survival.
• red cell abnormalities (spherocytosis, haemoglobinopathies)
• splenomegaly
• toxins
• Red cell production failure.
• reduced number of stem cells (aplastic anaemias)
• reduced manufacturing capacity (marrow infiltrates)
• shortage of manufacturing components (Vitamin B_{12}, folate, iron)
• bone marrow 'depression' (anaemia of chronic diseases, e.g. rheumatoid arthritis, chronic renal failure).

Additional classifications are those based on red cell morphology and appearance (microcytic, macrocytic, hypochromic, normocytic, normochromic).

Physiology

The oxygen tensions and carrying capacities of normal arterial and mixed venous blood are given in Table 9.1. The Hb is assumed to be 15 g%.

Table 9.1. The oxygen characteristics of normal arterial and mixed venous blood.

	Arterial blood	Mixed venous blood
PO_2 (mmHg (kPa))	100 (13.3)	40 (5.3)
Oxygen attached to Hb per 100 mls of blood (mls)	20	15
Oxygen in solution per 100 mls of blood (mls)	0.3	0.15

For anaesthetic purposes it is best not to think about anaemia purely in terms of the haemoglobin concentration, but in terms of the amount of oxygen available to the tissues and the way in which the body compensates to maximize this.

The comparison of a normal man (Hb = 15 g%) and a man made acutely anaemic by loss of blood and transfusion of clear fluid so that his Hb is 7.5 g% is shown in Fig. 9.1. To deliver 5 ml of O_2 per 100 ml of blood, normal man moves from A (arterial point) to B (mixed

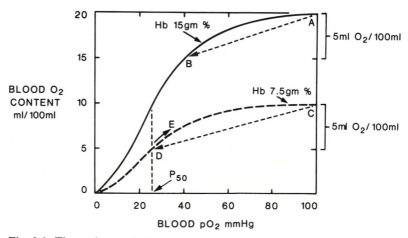

Fig. 9.1. The oxyhaemoglobin dissociation curve in a normal man and in a man made acutely anaemic. See text for details.

venous point) and still has 15 ml O_2 per 100 ml blood remaining. The anaemic man, despite full oxygenation to a PaO_2 of 100 mmHg (13.3 kPa) starts with only 10 ml of O_2 per 100 ml of blood at C (arterial point) and moves to D (mixed venous point) with a mixed venous PO_2 ($P_{\bar{v}}O_2$) of 26 mmHg (3.5 kPa) and a reserve of only 5 ml O_2 per 100 ml of blood. Tissue PO_2 is closely related to the $P_{\bar{v}}O_2$ and hence anaemia can produce tissue hypoxia, an effect which is intensified if there are high oxygen requirements (e.g. shivering, pyrexia, hypermetabolism, sepsis). In order to prevent tissue hypoxia the body decreases the amount of oxygen released per 100 ml of blood and effectively moves the mixed venous point to E. It achieves this by reducing the transit time through the capillaries. This is done by increasing tissue blood flow. Hence anaemic patients often have a high cardiac output. The ability to compensate with an increased cardiac output depends upon the health of the underlying cardiovascular system.

A corollary of the above arguments is that decreases of cardiac output during anaesthesia should be avoided in the anaemic patient, and that those techniques known to reduce cardiac output (e.g. deliberate hypotension by myocardial depression) are positively contraindicated. In addition, although the PaO_2 confirms the adequacy of lung oxygenation, the $P_{\bar{v}}O_2$ is a valuable measure of the adequacy of cardiac output and tissue oxygenation. It is therefore not unreasonable to measure the $P_{\bar{v}}O_2$ preoperatively, and to use it as a guide during major operations. The lowest $P_{\bar{v}}O_2$ compatible with life is approximately 20 mmHg (2.7 kPa).

The quantity of oxygen released to the tissues is also affected by the shape and the position of the oxygen dissociation curve which can be moved to the right or to the left (Fig. 9.2). Shifts in this curve are described by the changes in P_{50} (the PO_2 at 50% saturation). Despite the changes in right and left shift, if lung function is normal, when blood leaves the lungs it always carries approximately the same quantity of oxygen at a PaO_2 of 100 mmHg (13.3 kPa). This can be described by point F. However, to release 5 ml of O_2 per 100 ml blood the curve with the right shift has accomplished it at point G when the $P_{\bar{v}}O_2$ is 50 mmHg (6.7 kPa) whereas the curve with the left shift has had to fall to a $P_{\bar{v}}O_2$ of 25 mmHg (3.3 kPa) at point H. Thus right shifts allow oxygen delivery to the tissues to occur more easily and at a higher tissue PO_2 (decreased Hb affinity for O_2). Left shifts do the reverse.

Because the venous point is on the steep part of the oxygen dissociation curve, even moderate changes in the P_{50} have a considerable effect on the amount of oxygen which can be released to the tissues. If the PaO_2 is 100 mmHg (13.3 kPa) and the $P_{\bar{v}}O_2$ is 40 mmHg (5.3

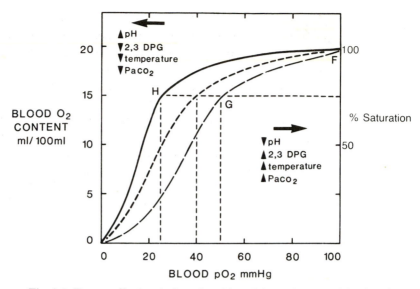

Fig. 9.2. Factors affecting the lateral position of the oxyhaemoglobin dissociation curve. See text for details.

kPa), with a P_{50} of 26 mmHg (3.5 kPa), 25% of the oxygen carried is released to the tissues. If the P_{50} increases to 35 mmHg (4.7 kPa), 40% of the oxygen carried will be released.

Factors which affect the P_{50} are temperature, pH, intracellular 2,3-diphosphoglycerate (2,3-DPG), the composition of intracellular enzymes and the type of haemoglobin. Changes in the $PaCO_2$, base excess and fixed acid mainly exert their effect on the P_{50} by alterations in pH. The proportionate effect that temperature and pH have over the physiological range is shown in Tables 9.2(a) and 9.2(b). From this the detrimental effects of the excessive use of bicarbonate, hyperventilation and hypothermia can be estimated.

Within the erythrocyte, apart from the level of haemoglobin, it is the intracellular concentration of 2,3-DPG which has the greatest effect on the delivery of oxygen to the tissues via the changes it induces in the P_{50}. The levels of 2,3-DPG are increased in all forms of

Table 9.2 (a) The effect of temperature on the P_{50}.
(b) The effect of pH on the P_{50}.

(a) Temperature °C	40	37	34
P_{50} mmHg (kPa)	29 (3.9)	26 (3.5)	21 (2.8)
(b) pH (H⁺ nmol/litre)	7.7 (20)	7.4 (40)	7.1 (80)
P_{50} mmHg (kPa)	18 (2.4)	26 (3.5)	37.5 (5.0)

anaemia. With a normal haemoglobin molecule, at a haemoglobin concentration of 8 g%, the P_{50} can be increased by anything up to a value of 33 mmHg (4.4 kPa). This compensation takes days to develop fully. This ability with a high 2,3-DPG to deliver oxygen to the tissues more easily means that in chronic anaemias there is little increase in cardiac output until the Hb has fallen to less than 9 g%. Below this level any increase in oxygen demand can only be met by an increased tissue blood flow.

Intracellular enzyme abnormalities (which are rare), have changes in 2,3-DPG associated with them. The range of P_{50}'s found is represented by pyruvate kinase deficiency (high 2,3-DPG, $P_{50} = 38$ mmHg (5.1 kPa)) and hexokinase deficiency (low 2,3-DPG, $P_{50} = 19$ mmHg (2.5 kPa)).

Abnormal haemoglobins also affect the P_{50}, partly by associated changes in 2,3-DPG. That of greatest clinical importance is sickle cell anaemia. Depending upon the severity of the disease the P_{50} can lie anywhere up to 46 mmHg (6.1 kPa).

It is of interest to note that changes in pH and temperature (which can be varied therapeutically and inadvertently during anaesthesia) have an immediate effect on the P_{50} whereas, 2,3-DPG levels take hours or days to exert their effect.

A useful summary is to think of the equation

$$\begin{array}{llll}
\text{Delivery of oxygen} & = \text{Cardiac} \times & \text{ml oxygen carried} \times & \text{fraction of oxygen} \\
\text{to tissues per unit} & \text{output} & \text{per unit volume} & \text{content released} \\
\text{time} & & \text{of arterial blood} & \text{to tissues}
\end{array}$$

$$\begin{bmatrix} \text{Depends on PaO}_2 \\ \text{and Hb level} \\ \text{(height of oxygen} \\ \text{dissociation curve)} \end{bmatrix} \begin{bmatrix} \text{Depends on the P}_{50} \\ \text{(lateral position of} \\ \text{oxygen dissociation} \\ \text{curve)} \end{bmatrix}$$

It should be noted that a fractional reduction in any one factor is *multiplied* by the fractional reduction in another.

The clinical setting

A proportion of patients presenting for surgery with anaemia will already have been investigated and be on appropriate treatment. In some instances the cause of the anaemia may be the reason for their operation (e.g. peptic ulceration). In others, anaemia may be discovered incidentally during the routine preoperative assessment. When this occurs it is essential to look beyond the immediate needs of surgery and to search for evidence of the aetiology.

History

A mild chronic anaemia may be totally asymptomatic. Symptoms common to all anaemias are rather non-specific and include tiredness, lassitude, dyspnoea (especially on exertion), dizziness, fainting, irritability and difficulty in concentrating. With severe anaemia (<8 g%) the compensatory increase in cardiac output may be sensed by the patient and is often described as 'palpitations'. This situation can precipitate the symptoms of angina and heart failure in the elderly and in those with coronary heart disease.

Questioning is necessary about:

Blood loss. This may be from menstruation, haemorrhoids or peptic ulcer, or be associated with pregnancy. Ask about indigestion and melaena.

Drugs. Salicylates cause occult blood loss, anticonvulsants may cause folate deficiency and cytotoxic agents or chloramphenicol cause bone marrow depression.

Previous surgery. Malabsorption, colitis or absence of intrinsic factor may be the cause.

Diet. Alcoholics can have folate deficiency. The elderly or vagrant might have insufficient dietary iron, folate or Vitamin C. Vegans may have Vitamin B_{12} deficiency. Do not overlook the possibility of carcinoma causing anorexia and weight loss.

Examination

The characteristic finding is pallor which gives a poor guide to the Hb level. The two commonest sites to examine for it are the conjunctiva and the palmar creases. When the latter are as pale as the surrounding skin, the haemoglobin is usually less than 7 g%. There may be signs of an increased cardiac output (tachycardia with a wide pulse pressure and a systolic ejection murmur) or cardiac failure. Glossitis and stomatitis are found in several anaemias. Koilonychia occurs in iron deficiency and swallowing is, on very rare occasions, affected by the presence of a post cricoid web. Mild jaundice can indicate excessive red cell destruction.

Neck lymph nodes might be enlarged in leukaemia, reticuloses or in those with secondary deposits. The abdomen may reveal splenomegaly, hepatomegaly or neoplasms of the stomach, colon or uterus.

Vitamin B_{12} deficiency is occasionally associated with mental disturbances and subacute combined degeneration of the cord (symmetrical paraesthesia with loss of proprioceptive and vibration senses).

306

Look for the signs of associated chronic diseases (e.g. chronic renal failure, connective tissue disorders).

Investigations

A full blood count and film is necessary to confirm the diagnosis and define the type of anaemia. Normal adult reference values are shown in Table 9.3. If further tests are required by the haematologist (bone marrow, serum folate, Vitamin B_{12}, iron, iron binding capacity, ferritin) they should be done before transfusion or other treatment (e.g. Vitamin B_{12} injections). All negroes must be screened for sickle cell disease.

The haemoglobin level varies throughout life. It is approximately 20 g% at birth falling to 15 g% at 1 month, reaching a low of 10 g% at three months and steadily returning to adult values at 2–5 years.

Table 9.3. Normal haematological values.

	Males	Females
Haemoglobin (g/dl)	14–18	12–16
Packed cell volume	0.42–0.55	0.36–0.48
Red cell count ($\times 10^{12}$/litre)	4.8–6.5	4.1–5.5
Mean corpuscular haemoglobin (pg)	27–32	27–32
Mean corpuscular volume (fl)	76–96	76–96
Mean corpuscular haemoglobin concentration (g/dl)	30–35	30–35
Reticulocytes (%)	0.2–2.0	0.2–2.0
White cell count ($\times 10^{9}$/litre)	4.0–11.0	4.0–11.0
Platelets ($\times 10^{9}$/litre)	150–400	150–400

Hypochromic anaemia

This indicates that a shortage of iron is present in the cell manufacturing machinery and the commonest cause is chronic blood loss. The cells have a low mean corpuscular volume (MCV), appear small and pale on a film, the serum iron is low or low-normal (normal = 9–29 μmol/litre) and the iron binding capacity is high (normal 45–72 μmol/litre). When the cause of the blood loss is identified and cured, treatment with oral iron (ferrous sulphate 200 mg tds) increases the haemoglobin concentration by 2 g% in three weeks. Failure of response to oral iron occurs in patients who do not take their tablets, in those who continue to bleed, and in those who have connective tissue disorders, chronic infections, chronic renal failure, malabsorption or sideroblastic anaemia (the marrow stores are full of iron which cannot be utilized).

For patients unable to absorb iron or who are poorly compliant, an intravenous iron infusion (1 g of iron) is given.

307

Macrocytic anaemia

This is caused by impaired DNA synthesis whose function is needed for the maturation and reduction in size of the reticulocyte as it is gradually changed to the erythrocyte. It is most commonly caused by Vitamin B_{12} or folic acid deficiency. Both produce a megaloblastic marrow.

With Vitamin B_{12} deficiency the serum level is low (normal 103–517 pmol/litre). It takes a prolonged period to become manifest clinically because the body stores are sufficient for 3–6 years. Hence there is adequate time for physiological compensation and mild disease is frequently asymptomatic. The causes of Vitamin B_{12} deficiency are poor diet, increased needs (e.g. in pregnancy, neoplastic disease or hyperthyroidism) and impaired absorption. The latter may be due to lack of intrinsic factor in the stomach (e.g. gastric cell atrophy or gastric resection) or to ileal resection, coeliac disease, intestinal lymphoma or parasitic disease. Treatment is by intramuscular Vitamin B_{12}.

Folic acid is the commonest dietary vitamin deficiency and the body stores are sufficient only for three months. Both the serum folate (normal 4–20 nmol/litre) and red cell folate (normal 340–1020 nmol/litre) are decreased. It occurs in any disease impairing intestinal absorption and is found in many severely ill patients, pregnant women and the elderly who do not eat green vegetables. Phenytoin and other barbiturates used to control epilepsy can affect folate absorption sufficiently to produce a macrocytosis, but this is rarely accompanied by a marked fall in haemoglobin concentration. Treatment is by oral folic acid.

Other points of importance in macrocytic anaemia are:
- If the marrow is required for diagnosis it must be taken prior to treatment since the megaloblastic changes disappear within 24 hours of the start of treatment.
- Patients with a macrocytic anaemia (especially one due to Vitamin B_{12} deficiency) have a high circulating blood volume and are therefore at great risk of developing congestive cardiac failure if they are overtransfused.
- Once treatment has started reticulocytes flood into the circulation. This, paradoxically, increases the average MCV for up to one week before they are all converted into mature erythrocytes. The anaemia should be corrected in 1–2 months although symptomatic improvement occurs soon after starting treatment.
- If folic acid is administered in the presence of a Vitamin B_{12} deficiency, mental disturbances and the symptoms of subacute combined degeneration of the cord may be precipitated or intensified.

Induction. This should be preceded by preoxygenation and the induction agent should be given slowly to minimize cardiovascular disturbances. If a crash induction is essential, an arterial line inserted before induction will allow the most rapid detection and correction of blood pressure and heart rate changes.

Maintenance. Never forget that cyanosis is a very late sign in the anaemic and that its absence does not imply adequate oxygenation. Arterial samples for blood gas analysis are advisable in long cases. Beware the possibility of awareness if the oxygen concentration is raised to 50% in nitrous oxide. In theory, nitrous oxide is a bad anaesthetic to use with macrocytic anaemia because of its effect on the bone marrow.

Spontaneous ventilation with its high physiological dead space (see Chapter 2) is suitable only for short procedures. To overcome hypoxia secondary to hypoventilation, raise the oxygen content of the inspired gases to 50%. High concentrations of volatile agents depress ventilation and myocardial performance, both of which are essential for the maintenance of oxygen flux. The resultant change in blood gas status to mild respiratory acidosis does not, however, impair oxygen delivery to the tissues. Pay meticulous attention to airway control and if there are difficulties, intubate earlier rather than later.

Controlled ventilation is to be preferred for longer operations. Ventilate to normocapnia: alkalosis impairs oxygen delivery (see Fig. 9.2 and Table 9.2(b)), and hypocapnia reduces cardiac output (Chapter 1).

Remember that a mild tachycardia and a wide pulse pressure may be physiological and not a sign of light anaesthesia. On the other hand, these compensatory mechanisms might be obtunded by anaesthetic agents. Adequate tissue perfusion can be judged clinically by blanching the ear lobes, nose or forehead with pressure and watching the pallor disappear and quantitatively by measuring the $P_{\bar{v}}O_2$ (see 'Physiology').

Keep the patient as warm as possible by using a warming blanket, maintaining a high theatre temperature, and heating all IV fluids. Intraoperative blood loss should be replaced promptly by packed cells or whole blood. Falls in systemic blood pressure and cardiac output produced by venous pooling secondary to adverse posturing can be a problem. Positioning of the patient in such instances needs prior discussion with the surgeon so that postural effects can be minimized.

POSTOPERATIVE PHASE

Extubate the patient only when there are signs of powerful venti-latory effort. The first 12–24 hours should be spent in a recovery or high dependency area where the patient's ventilation can be moni-tored and oxygen enriched air given from a facemask. Anaemic patients are put at great risk by the factors producing postoperative hypoxia. If shivering occurs, give 100% oxygen over the acute period since the oxygen requirement may increase to over four times the resting level. It should be emphasized to the nursing staff that hypoxia may not manifest itself as cyanosis but is more likely to result in confusion and drowsiness.

The elderly are at an increased risk of developing pulmonary oedema in the postoperative period if they have been transfused.

Check the haemoglobin postoperatively and adjust the intravenous fluid regimen to suit.

THE PROBLEMS AND HAZARDS OF BLOOD TRANSFUSION

The first reference to an attempt at human blood transfusion was in 1492 when blood was taken from three young fit men and given to Pope Innocent VII. Sadly, all four died. Today, things have im-proved and the total incidence of all reactions is less than 5%, and the majority of these are mild. Not least of the causes of serious reactions is human error, in giving the patient blood intended for someone else. Most donor blood is now fractionated to obtain specific compo-nents. The use of these is described in 'bleeding disorders'.

Characteristics of stored blood

In the UK, citrate-phosphate-dextrose (CPD) is the most widely used storage medium and it is the properties of CPD blood that are described below. (Acid-citrate-dextrose (ACD) blood differs in that there is a lower red cell survival rate, and the ATP and 2,3-DPG levels fall more rapidly, but there are less microaggregates formed during the first 10 days.)

Each unit of blood contains approximately 450 ml of blood and 60 ml of CPD solution and is stored at 4–6°C. Concentrated red cells are prepared from this when requested.

A pack of blood is stored upright and is not issued unless there is a clear line of demarcation between the sedimented cells and the supernatant plasma, which should be straw coloured and free from visible signs of haemolysis. Haemolysis is recognized as a reddish

314

purple discolouration in the plasma immediately above the cell layer which gradually spreads upwards. A fat layer on the surface of the plasma is unimportant.

Apart from a prolonged storage time, haemolysis can also be caused both by freezing and by attempts at rapid warming (e.g. putting blood bags on radiators). Warming should only be done by the use of warming coils in water baths at 37°C or in specially designed microwave ovens.

Minimize the time that blood is out of the refrigerator or insulated box before transfusion. If this period exceeds 30 minutes (unless the blood is wanted for transfusion almost immediately), it should not be returned for storage at 4–6°C for future use. The temporary warming allows chance contaminating bacteria to multiply and blood so affected may cause a severe or fatal reaction.

Red cells. The viability of red blood cells falls to 80% after 21 days storage. The fall in ATP is gradual but the 2,3-DPG concentration remains constant for seven days then begins to fall. Both these factors shift the O_2 dissociation curve to the left (the P_{50} is approximately 20 mmHg (2.7 kPa) after three weeks storage) and inhibit oxygen release at tissue level. It takes 24–48 hours after transfusion for the deficit to be corrected.

Electrolytes. There is a rise in serum sodium by up to 20 mmol/litre. The potassium concentration gradually rises to 20 mmol/litre after 21 days storage. When transfused, re-entry of the potassium into the red cells occurs with warming and clinical hyperkalaemia is very rare. The lactate and ammonia concentration gradually increase and the pH falls to 6.5 after 21 days.

White cells. Neutrophils lose all phagocytic activity after 48 hours storage but a few lymphocytes survive for 21 days.

Platelets. There are no platelets viable after 24 hours storage.

Coagulation factors. The concentration of factors V and VIII is reduced to 10% after 24 hours storage. Factor IX and X concentrations are less than 10% by 7 days.

Complications of transfusion

Febrile reactions. These are separated into unimportant (temperature below 38°C and no other signs) and significant (temperature over 38°C with rigors and/or other systemic symptoms). If the former occurs, the transfusion can continue under a careful watch and an antipyretic (e.g. aspirin) may produce symptomatic relief of the pyrexia. If the temperature rises above 38°C the transfusion should be stopped.

The cause is thought to be endogenous pyrogens in the transfused blood, or pyrogens which are produced by a reaction between the patient's serum antibodies and antigens on donor white cells and platelets. These antibodies may have been formed as a result of previous transfusions or pregnancy. If severe, subsequent reactions in the same patient can be minimized or avoided by the transfusion of washed red cells, which are leukocyte and platelet deficient.

Allergic reactions. Correctly crossmatched blood in up to 2% of cases initiates an allergic reaction which is presumed to be due to incompatible plasma proteins which react with recipient white cells. This is usually first seen as erythema along the path of the infusion vein and can develop into urticaria over other parts of the body. There is usually a very mild pyrexia with no disturbance of blood pressure or heart rate and an absence of constitutional symptoms. Such cases can be treated by slowing the transfusion, observing carefully and giving chlorpheniramine (Piriton) 10 mg IV.

More serious reactions may cause bronchospasm and angioneurotic oedema. Rarely anaphylaxis occurs. These cases obviously require the transfusion to be stopped and supportive measures to be instituted.

Haemolytic reactions. Principally, these result from lysis of donor cells by incompatibilities in recipient serum. A haemolytic reaction, similar to that following the transfusion of incompatible blood, may follow the transfusion of out-dated blood, or blood which has been haemolysed by freezing, overheating or infection. The reaction, which is mediated by complement, can become apparent after only a few millilitres or after a whole unit has been transfused. In general, the smaller the amount of donor blood required as a trigger, the more severe the outcome.

Symptoms vary from case to case. Usually there is a rapidly developing febrile reaction with dyspnoea, headache and a sense of impending doom. There are rigors, restlessness and lumbar and substernal pain. Hypotension may develop with peripheral circulatory collapse. Subsequent haemolysis produces haemoglobinuria with jaundice appearing hours or days later. Disseminated intravascular coagulation (DIC) may be precipitated.

Once suspected, stop the transfusion and send donor and patient blood back to the laboratory for urgent recrossmatching and Coombs testing. (In Coomb's test, antiserum is added to either the patient's blood or to their plasma which has been mixed with red cells of known antigenicity. A positive result indicates an immune haemolytic process.) The main danger is acute renal failure from haemoglobin deposition. Treatment is circulatory support with an emphasis on high urine output. This may need assistance with mannitol.

The majority of cases (which are now rare) present during the transfusion of the offending blood but others present several hours later. Occasionally they may only be detected by a Coombs test performed because of an unexplained jaundice occurring several days after transfusion.

Transmission of donor infections. Hepatitis B and syphylis are screened for. Brucellosis, toxoplasmosis and trypanosomiasis can be transmitted. Cytomegalovirus and Epstein–Barr viruses transmit easily in fresh blood but are inactivated after a few days at 4°C.

Transfusion of infected blood. This is fortunately very rare. It carries a mortality of 50–100%. Presentation and treatment is as for a haemolytic reaction. If it is suspected, take blood cultures and start non-nephrotoxic broad spectrum antibiotics immediately.

Citrate toxicity. Signs of citrate toxicity are muscle tremors, circulatory depression and ECG changes of hypocalcaemia (prolonged Q-T interval). The effects of citrate are countered by mobilization of calcium from bone and by metabolism by the liver. The warm adult, with a normally functioning liver, can tolerate the administration of one unit of warmed blood every 5 minutes. This may not be the case in the sick, especially if there is liver disease, hypotension, hypothermia or low liver blood flow. Since calcium administration increases myocardial irritability and can cause ventricular ectopic activity and even ventricular tachycardia, it should ideally only be given if there are ECG signs of hypocalcaemia or hyperkalaemia. In practice, however, a common 'rule of thumb' is to give 10 ml of calcium gluconate with every four units of blood but there seems little logical basis for this.

Metabolic acidosis. The acid load of stored blood is up to 40 mmol/litre and its pH is approximately 6.7. The routine use of alkalinizing solution is not, however, recommended. An induced alkalaemia further impairs oxygen delivery at tissue level (see Fig. 9.2), creates an additional sodium load and reduces the ionized calcium level. The acidosis is mainly due to citric and lactic acid generated during storage and these are rapidly metabolized over the first 24 hours.

317

Coagulation difficulties. Massive transfusion of blood (approximately 10 units in a previously fit adult) can lead to a dilutional coagulopathy. The survival times of platelets and clotting factors are given above and it can be seen that unless the transfused blood is very fresh, which is unusual, the levels of activity will be well below normal.

The onset of a dilutional coagulopathy is suggested intraoperatively by oozing, rather like DIC. A quick check is to take 10 ml of fresh blood into a plain glass tube and put the tube into the water bath being used to heat the transfusion fluids. It should clot within 10 minutes. A normal result can, however, be obtained in the face of borderline coagulation factor levels and platelet deficiency. After a full coagulation screen, appropriate therapy with fresh frozen plasma (FFP) and platelets should follow. The amount of calcium required to facilitate clotting is so small that supplements are never needed for this purpose.

The likely requirement of FFP is 1 unit for every 5–6 units of blood transfused but, if there is any doubt, recheck the coagulation screen. Bleeding due to thrombocytopenia commonly occurs 8–12 hours after massive blood transfusion. If the count is below 50 000, platelet infusions are definitely indicated and one unit can be expected to raise the count by 5000–10 000.

Transfusion reactions under anaesthesia

These are very difficult to both detect and treat with confidence. It is important always to be aware of the possibility of their occurrence. Useful points are:
- Monitor the patient's temperature before and during transfusion. If it rises at all (since it usually falls with time during surgery) a febrile reaction may be occurring.
- Try and have the limb with the intravenous infusion visible and look for wheals along the vein. Occasionally glance at other parts of the body for urticaria. The ventilator pressure may increase because of bronchospasm.
- So many haemodynamic changes occur during surgery that, without the benefit of the conscious patient's symptoms, the physiological deterioration of a haemolytic reaction may be completely misinterpreted. However, if it is suspected, it should be treated as present until the laboratory fails to confirm it.
- Haemoglobinuria is an early sign of a haemolytic reaction. Spurious false positive results can occur if the catheter balloon is traumatizing the bladder wall.

JEHOVAH'S WITNESSES

Jehovah's Witnesses, by their own choice, in principle refuse to accept blood products from any other person because they believe that it is against the law of God. When faced with the possibility of death without transfusion some do, but the majority do not, change their mind. This is a difficult situation to handle in the emergency setting (e.g. childbirth, major injuries) and it is wise for a junior anaesthetist to contact the consultant on call. It is best if a plan is agreed before surgery between the patient, his relatives and the senior surgeon and anaesthetist in charge of the case. Although autologous transfusion is possible, it is not usually available and colloid and crystalloid solutions are all that can be offered.

For elective operations there is the possibility of the patient donating his own blood and having it stored in liquid nitrogen until the time of surgery. Even this course is often refused because their belief is that the blood must be continually moving.

Children pose a special problem. On the one hand the anaesthetist may feel that a young child must be protected from the beliefs of its parents: on the other, if the child does receive blood, his family may theoretically refuse to take him back. Conflicts should be dealt with as described under consent (Chapter 10). In all cases a special consent form should be signed.

HAEMOGLOBINOPATHIES

These are disease states created by the failure of production of a particular haemoglobin chain or by the production of an abnormal haemoglobin. Over 350 structurally different human haemoglobin variants have been discovered, but less than one third of these have any clinical significance. They are often called by the place with which they are linked, either by incidence or molecular analysis. The abnormality in about 90% is the incorrect placement of a single amino acid in the globin chains.

Some variants are unstable and may cause haemolysis (e.g. Hb Bristol, Hb Hammersmith, Hb Koln), some have a high oxygen affinity but pose no anaesthetic problem (e.g. Hb Chesapeake, Hb Kempsey, Hb Malmo, Hb Yakima) and others causes methaemoglobinaemia (e.g. Hb M of Hyde Park, Boston, Iowa, Saskatoon, Milwaukee). The latter cause patients to look cyanosed and hence their skin colour is no guide to arterial hypoxaemia. The only two common haemoglobinopathies are sickle cell disease and thalassaemia.

The sickle cell syndromes

Theoretical background. The globin of haemoglobin consists of four polypeptide chains and it is abnormalities in these which produce the haemoglobinopathies. There are three normal human haemoglobins, each having two pairs of chains.

- HbF. This is foetal haemoglobin which is almost totally replaced by normal adult haemoglobin by the age of 6 months. It has a P_{50} of 19 mmHg (2.5 kPa) and is comprised of 2 alpha and 2 gamma chains.
- HbA. 98% of adult haemoglobin is HbA. It has 2 alpha and 2 beta chains.
- HbA_2. 2% of adult haemoglobin is HbA_2, which has 2 alpha and 2 delta chains.

Because alpha chains are present and necessary in all forms of haemoglobin, structurally significant alpha chain abnormalities tend to be very serious and usually incompatible with life. Beta chain abnormalities can, however, be countered by continued production of gamma and delta chains.

The two commonest errors in the beta chains are those described as Hb S and Hb C. Both produce haemolytic anaemia in homozygotes but that due to Hb C is less severe. The abnormal genes can occur alone, or together, in any one individual and can, in some instances, be combined with a component of thalassaemia (q.v.).

The genes for the beta chains of Hb S and Hb C are allelic to the genes for normal beta chains. Thus, if only one chromosome carries the abnormal gene and its pair carries the normal gene (heterozygotes) then 25–40% of the individual's haemoglobin will be abnormal. If both carry the abnormal gene then all the haemoglobin will be abnormal (homozygotes). Inheritance is by classical Mendelian genetics and is transmitted by, and affects, both sexes.

It is thought that Hb S confers a biological advantage against malaria. It is most common in negro populations but is occasionally found (especially as the trait, Hb AS) in Southern Italians, Greeks, Indians and half-castes. The sickle cell trait (HbAS) is found in 10% of UK negroes. Sickle cell anaemia (HbSS) is found in 0.25% of UK negroes and double heterozygote states (HbSC or HbS-thalassaemia) are found in 0.04% of UK negroes.

In the deoxygenated state, HbS crystallizes forming tactoids. These distort the cell membrane and produce the characteristic sickle shape. These altered cells initiate capillary and venous thrombosis which can progress to infarction. They are also removed prematurely from the circulation by the spleen. This results in anaemia and a high reticulocyte count as the marrow attempts to compensate.

The ease with which sickling occurs depends upon the percentage of deoxygenated HbS in the red cell, the blood pH, the presence of other abnormal haemoglobins and coincident infection.

PREOPERATIVE CONSIDERATIONS

Patients with sickle cell trait (HbAS) are asymptomatic and have no abnormal physical findings. Detection therefore depends on routine screening of the population at risk. The sickledex test is positive but their Hb is usually over 11 g%. Haemoglobin electrophoresis for the exact genotype takes 24 hours and should be done before elective surgery. If the sickle trait is found, it does not incur a high anaesthetic risk but sickling might occur under extreme conditions.

In contrast to the more common HbAS, patients with HbSC may also be asymptomatic, sickledex positive and have a normal haemoglobin concentration. They, however, have a high propensity to sickle. In urgent situations, where electrophoresis results are unavailable, it is therefore essential to treat all patients who are sickledex positive (even with a high haemoglobin) as being at risk of sickling. Knowledge of the sickle state may also affect the surgical procedure undertaken, influence decisions on day case surgery, help in the diagnosis of postoperative complications, reassure the anaesthetist, have medico-legal implications, and determine the need for management in a high dependency area.

Patients who are homozygous for HbS have sickle cell anaemia with 95% of their haemoglobin as HbS and 5% as HbF. They all give a history since childhood of 'crises' with bone and joint pains. Some have neurological damage from cerebral infarction. Vascular occlusions in the spleen can mimic an acute abdomen. There is often lymphadenopathy with an enlarged liver and spleen, jaundice and the clinical signs of anaemia (Hb usually 5–8 g%). The heart may be enlarged. Infarction of the renal medulla with haematuria is common. Survival beyond 30 years is unlikely.

The crises which occur are principally of two types. Firstly, sequestration crises are caused when there is a sudden increase in the number of sickled red cells. This may be provoked by hypoxia, acidaemia, cold peripheries, infection, trauma (including surgery), pyrexia and pregnancy. Secondly, aplastic crises occur when the bone marrow is unable to keep pace with the high rate of red cell destruction, usually during a viral infection.

Patients with HbS-thalassaemia have decreased production of normal beta chains but HbS synthesis is unimpaired. They have approximately 75% of their haemoglobin as HbS, 20% as HbF and 5% as HbA_2. They are at great risk of sickling. The clinical picture is similar to homozygous sickle cell disease.

321

The haemoglobin concentration in any one patient with homozygous sickle cell disease varies by up to 3 g%, so the timing of
elective surgery is important and *must* be done with the consultation
of a haematologist. It is a field where there are continuing changes in
recommendation. The objective is to raise the concentration of HbA
to 40% before surgery, but transfusion carries the risk of bone
marrow suppression. On occasions, repeat transfusion or exchange
transfusions are used. The optimum haemoglobin is approximately
10 g%. Above this, both the frequency and the severity of crises intensify, possibly from increased blood viscosity. Transfused blood
must be warmed to 37°C and be as fresh as possible.

Any co-existing infection needs vigorous treatment with antibiotics. Do not allow patients to become dehydrated.

Most premedicants are suitable but avoid ventilatory depression
with its risk of hypoxia and respiratory acidosis.

PEROPERATIVE PHASE

There is no evidence that any one anaesthetic drug or technique is
superior to any other. Many specific treatments have been suggested
to prevent sickling. These include sodium bicarbonate, urea, pro-
mazine, megestrolacetate, warfarin, cyanate, carbamyl phosphate,
dextran and aspirin. None of these is of proven value and the
mainstay of prevention of crises is avoidance of all factors which predispose to sickling (hypoxia, hypotension, dehydration, acidosis,
hypothermia) and taking the precautions essential to any case of
anaemia (see above). Although sickle cell trait (HbAS) patients are
much less likely to sickle than HbSS, HbSC or HbS-thalassaemia, it
is sensible to treat them with the same care during the perioperative
period. Whatever anaesthetic technique is chosen, it is essential to
keep the patient well hydrated, well oxygenated and warm. Check
the theatre temperature, warm all infusion fluids, and put a warming
blanket on the operating table. Humidify the inspired gases. A temperature probe is useful in long operations. Give blood replacement
as required up to a maximum estimated haemoglobin of 10 g%.

Whether regional or general anaesthesia is chosen, factors predisposing to sickling must be avoided. The use of tourniquets with their
consequent stasis, acidaemia and hypoxia can be disastrous. Bier's
blocks are therefore contraindicated. Local anaesthetic field blocks
should not be done with adrenaline containing solutions.

Sympathetic blockade secondary to regional anaesthesia can produce falls in blood pressure, cardiac output and tissue perfusion. In
the areas not affected by blockade there is a compensatory vasoconstriction. The first line treatment is the infusion of warm intravenous fluids, augmented by atropine if there is a bradycardia.

Vasoconstrictors, although raising central blood pressure can reduce peripheral tissue blood flow. Give supplementary oxygen on a facemask.

Prior to general anaesthesia always preoxygenate the patient. Give the induction agent slowly and never tolerate a poor airway. If necessary, intubate earlier rather than later. Keep the F_IO_2 at 50%. Cyanosis is doubly difficult to detect in a negro who is also anaemic. High concentrations of halothane for long periods are contraindicated because of ventilatory and myocardial depression and postoperative shivering. If maintenance is by IPPV, then ventilate to normocapnia. Acidosis predisposes to sickling and alkalosis reduces oxygen delivery to the tissues. For long operations, as well as maintaining the PaO_2, it is valuable to monitor the $P_{\bar{v}}O_2$ since this is a better index of cardiac output and tissue PO_2 (see earlier). The preoperative baseline $P_{\bar{v}}O_2$, with an F_IO_2 of 21%, is the minimum acceptable intraoperatively. Lower values require an appropriate correction to the cardiac output.

POSTOPERATIVE PHASE

Patients who only possess the trait can, after an appropriate stay in the recovery area, be returned to the general ward or be allowed to go home.

Others (HbSS, HbSC, HbS-thalassaemia) need nursing in a high dependency area for at least 24–48 hours and should receive oxygen supplementation for the first 24 hours. They must be kept warm and well hydrated with a good circulating blood volume. Encourage early mobilization to promote tissue circulation and prevent thrombosis. Adequate analgesia is required to prevent the vasoconstrictive reaction to pain (and impaired diaphragmatic movement with an upper abdominal incision) but guard against excessive ventilatory depression.

After major operations prophylactic antibiotic cover is advisable to prevent pulmonary infections which have a higher incidence than usual.

Crises can occur in the postoperative period and may be heralded by odd, unexpected aches and pains. These are obviously difficult to detect after major surgery and a high index of suspicion is required. Close co-operation must be maintained with the haematologist because the treatment of a crisis in a postoperative patient is a complex and individual matter. If severe bone pains occur, patients are anticoagulated to try and prevent the inevitable pulmonary embolus.

323

The thalassaemias

The composition of normal haemoglobin is described above. The thalassaemias is a collective term used to describe a group of inherited disorders which are characterized by a reduced rate, or absence, of synthesis of one of the normal adult protein chains and a compensatory production of HbF. The abnormalities are found in negroes, Asians and Mediterranean peoples.

Heterozygous patients (described as alpha minor or beta minor) present a variable picture and may be completely asymptomatic. If they have anaemia, it is mild and they present no special anaesthetic problems unless they are also heterozygous for HbS (see above).

Homozygous alpha thalassaemias are incompatible with life and result in foetal or neonatal death.

Homozygous beta thalassaemia (also known as Cooley's anaemia, Mediterranean anaemia or beta thalassaemia major) is the commonest severe abnormality seen in clinical practice. Patients may have life-threatening anaemia from early childhood and only very rarely survive to adulthood.

Increased bone marrow activity with ineffective erythropoesis results in cephalofacial deformities and thinning of cortical bone. There is frontal bossing and overgrowth of the maxilla can make laryngoscopy and the application of a facemask difficult. Be careful not to produce iatrogenic fractures. Spinal cord compression has been recorded secondary to vertebral expansion from haematopoeisis. Hepato-splenomegaly is inevitable and hepatic malfunction may be sufficient to cause a prolongation of the prothrombin time. Iron overload (due to increased GIT absorption and repeated transfusion) leads to functional abnormalities of the liver, endocrine system and heart (supraventricular dysrhythmias, congestive cardiac failure, pericarditis). These should be treated as described in the appropriate sections.

The anaesthetic implications are related to the severity of the anaemia (see earlier) and preoperative blood transfusion may be required. Some patients have thrombocytopenia secondary to the enlarged spleen.

BONE MARROW FAILURE

The leukaemias

These are a group of disorders of unknown aetiology. Abnormal white cells accumulate in the bone marrow and replace normal marrow cells leading to anaemia, granulocytopenia and thrombocytopenia. They present with the clinical symptoms and signs of anaemia, infection and bleeding. To a lesser extent other organs are infiltrated (e.g. testis, liver, brain, lymph nodes) but this does not usually lead to organ failure.

The leukaemias are classified according to their morphology and their chronicity. Untreated acute leukaemias survive only months whereas chronic leukaemias evolve slowly over years. Advances in treatment of acute leukaemias, particularly in children, have resulted in greatly improved survival. Treatment is with a variety of cytotoxic regimens tailored to the individual leukaemia. These drugs also depress the production of normal cells. During this time the patient will require intensive supportive care to prevent overwhelming infection, anaemia and bleeding. For some patients the whole body is irradiated to produce an aplastic anaemia, which is then treated by bone marrow transplantation.

Children frequently require anaesthetics during treatment for bone marrow aspirations, the administration of intrathecal cytotoxics and for irradiation treatment (see Chapter 12).

Whilst it is important to be aware of the type of leukaemia and its prognosis, the clinical presentation, principles of treatment and anaesthetic implications are similar to those of any cause of bone marrow failure (see below).

Aplastic anaemia

Aplastic anaemia is bone marrow failure resulting in decreased production of red cells, platelets and granulocytes. Causes include autoimmune mechanisms, dose-related drug reactions (e.g. antineoplastic drugs, chloramphenicol, ionizing radiation), idiosyncratic drug reactions (e.g. chloramphenicol, gold, phenylbutazone, phenothiazines, barbiturates), hepatitis and other viral infections. In severe disease the mortality is 50% within 4 months but a small proportion (10–20%) recover completely.

Some patients are treated with steroids in an effort to decrease capillary fragility. Other treatments are supportive (preventing infection by isolation, blood and platelet transfusions) whilst hoping for spontaneous recovery. Transplantation of histocompatible donor bone marrow improves long-term survival to 75% provided it is done early, before the patient is sensitized to the transplantation antigens from blood transfusion. Transplanted bone marrow (which is given intravenously) takes 2–4 weeks to become functional and during this time the patient will be on immunosuppressive therapy to prevent rejection. Patients often require parenteral feeding as part of their general support and the anaesthetist's help is sought to insert central venous cannulae. Unless the patient is a child (which is uncommon) this should be accomplished under local analgesia. See below for the anaesthetic implications of aplastic anaemia, which are those of bone marrow failure.

Anaesthetic considerations of bone marrow failure

PREOPERATIVE CONSIDERATIONS

The most important features to assess are the degree of anaemia, the presence of infection and the tendency to bleed. The problems of the anaemia *per se* are related to its severity and have already been discussed. Establish whether bone marrow transplantation is being considered because this will affect preoperative transfusion. If you decide to correct the anaemia, do so in consultation with a haematologist and use packed red cells which should be as fresh as possible.

Search for any overt signs of infection, particularly if there is a fever. Remember that pus will not form in the absence of granulocytes. Look especially for chest and throat infections. Make sure that swabs and blood cultures have been taken, note the sensitivity of the organism and treat with the appropriate antibacterials. If no organism has been isolated and it seems likely that there is some infection, use broad spectrum antibacterials on the advice of the microbiologist (e.g. gentamicin and carbenicillin). In specialized units with cell separators, it may be possible to transfuse donor granulocytes.

Avoid IM injections. Thombocytopenia is a problem with any surgical procedure, including central vein cannulation. Ensure that the platelet count (done that day) is over 50000. If necessary transfuse platelet concentrate. Other coagulation problems are dealt with more fully later. They are best corrected prior to surgery (usually with FFP) in consultation with a haematologist.

In leukaemic patients, check that the lymphadenopathy is not causing pressure symptoms or displacement of vital structures (e.g. trachea). The psychological approach is especially important for those likely to require repeat anaesthetics and where possible it is helpful to have the same anaesthetist on each occasion.

PEROPERATIVE PHASE

Take all the precautions outlined under anaemia and bleeding disorders. Intraoperative bleeding which is not surgical should be controlled with transfusions of platelets, FFP and fresh blood.

Be scrupulous in cleanliness and sterility. Use a disposable sterile endotracheal tube with a low pressure cuff.

If asked to give IV cytotoxic therapy, inject the drugs through a central line or fast running drip.

POSTOPERATIVE PHASE

Return the patient to his isolation ward as soon as possible. It is often best to recover them there, thus avoiding exposure to infection in the recovery area. Therefore it is most important that the patient, if extubated, breathes well and is able to maintain an airway unaided during transit. If there is any doubt extubate the patient in the isolation unit. Chest infections are a major cause of mortality. Aggressive physiotherapy is essential. Granulocyte transfusions may be given. Watch for continued bleeding and transfuse appropriately.

BLEEDING DISORDERS

General management

Each bleeding disorder requires the management appropriate to the individual deficiencies and should be done in consultation with the haematologist. The assessment and general principles are common to them all. Refer to the relevant section below for specific management.

On examination look for overt signs of bleeding (ecchymoses, haematomas, petechiae). Examine joints for contractures (especially in haemophiliacs), thinking about potential problems in positioning the patient.

Before any surgery always ascertain the value of a recent haemoglobin and the activity of relevant clotting factors. If already subjected to multiple transfusions of blood or blood products verify the hepatitis carrier state. Ensure that there is blood and appropriate products available, even for minor surgery.

Be gentle with all handling of the patient. Avoid intramuscular injections both in premedication and for postoperative analgesia. Always secure good venous access (which may not be easy) and do not cause unnecesaary trauma. Do not attempt subclavian or internal jugular catheterization before the clotting deficiency has been corrected. Be especially gentle with any manipulation (e.g. nasogastric, nasotracheal or orotracheal intubation) and avoid the nasal route where possible. If this is unavoidable, contract the mucosa with a vasoconstricting spray.

Local anaesthetic techniques are mostly best avoided because of the dangers of bleeding. Do not use aspirin because it depresses platelet aggregation and accentuates bleeding. Blood loss needs to be monitored closely for many days.

Haemophilia

This is an inherited bleeding disorder due to deficiency of Factor VIII, the antihaemophiliac factor (AHG). It is transmitted as sex-linked recessive; the disease is usually only manifest in the male (incidence 1 in 10 000), the female being the carrier. Thirty percent of haemophiliacs have no family history. All treated haemophiliacs should be screened for hepatitis B.

Laboratory investigation reveals a prolonged clotting time, partial thromboplastin time and thromboplastin generation test. Prothrombin time, platelet numbers and function, fibrinogen, bleeding time and tests of capillary integrity are all normal.

Factor VIII levels must be measured before surgery. Severe haemophiliacs with spontaneous bleeding have no AHG activity. Those with 1–5% AHG activity will have severe bleeding after only minor injury and those with 5–25% activity will bleed severely after surgery. One hundred percent activity is normal; at least 30% AHG activity is needed for surgery but the aim is to provide 70–80% activity for safety.

Factor VIII may be replaced with FFP (100 mls provides 100 units AHG and when thawed has a half-life of 4–8 hours), cryoprecipitate (4 mls provides 100 units AHG which has a half-life of 10–12 hours when thawed), Cohn fraction or AHG rich fibrinogen (100 ml provides 100 units AHG and is reconstituted with water), or glycine-precipitated factor VIII (15 mls provides 100 units AHG). Since the loading dose immediately before surgery should be approximately 50 units/kg, cryoprecipitate has the advantage of being the smallest infused volume.

Postoperatively, monitor Factor VIII levels and expect to give approximately half the loading dose 12 hourly. Continue this for at least 10 days postoperatively, but longer in the presence of wound dehiscence or infection. If it is not possible to measure Factor VIII, the partial thromboplastin time is a helpful guide. Epsilon-aminocaproic acid (24 g per day for a 70 kg adult, orally for 7 days) is helpful after dental extractions because it reduces salivary plasmin which would otherwise dissolve clots.

Christmas disease

This disease, also known as Haemophilia B, is an inherited sex-linked deficiency of Factor IX. As well as the patient's personal history of bleeding (which is similar to the haemophiliac) ask about the bleeding in relatives. This gives a guide to the severity of the disease. Manage the patient in a similar manner to one with haemophilia, using either FFP or Factor IX concentrate. Maintain Factor IX levels above 30%. Its half-life is 20 hours.

Von Willebrand's disease

This inherited disorder is due to abnormal capillaries and the deficiency of a plasma protein required for the formation of platelet aggregates. Inheritance is autosomal dominant but, inexplicably, is observed more frequently in females. Although the laboratory findings are variable most patients have a prolonged bleeding time and abnormal Factor VIII–Von Willebrand protein. Oral, gastrointestinal and uterine bleeding are common but joint haemorrhage is not. The severity of bleeding declines with age. The bleeding disorder is corrected with cryoprecipitate (but not the more highly purified factor concentrates, e.g. glycine-precipitated AHG because there is less active protein) several hours before surgery. The patient is then managed in a similar manner to a haemophiliac.

Thrombocytopenia

Thrombocytopenia is normally defined as a platelet count of under $100\,000$ mm^3. There is an approximate relationship between the platelet count and the severity of bleeding, but bleeding can be aggravated by a sudden drop in the platelet count, infection or anaemia.

Look for signs of spontaneous bleeding (petechiae, purpuric spots or confluent ecchymoses) in the skin and mucous membranes. Bleeding due to trauma occurs immediately, might respond to local pressure and usually stops within 48 hours. The causes of thrombocytopenia are listed in Table 9.4. Where possible, establish the cause and remove it (particularly drugs). The patient may be on steroids (idiopathic thrombocytopenic purpura) or present for splenectomy.

For surgery, ensure that the platelet count is above $50\,000$. If not, transfuse ABO compatible platelets (ideally within 6 hours of collection and certainly within 24 hours). In the absence of antibody, 1 unit of platelets will elevate the count by $5000–10\,000$ per mm^3. Never give them through a blood filter.

Table 9.4. Causes of thrombocytopenia.

1. Decreased production	— marrow infiltration (malignancy, myelofibrosis)
	— marrow hypoplasia (radiation, drugs, viruses, chemicals)
	— congenital (Fanconi's pancytopenia, rubella)
	— hereditary (autosomal dominant)
2. Increased destruction	— drugs (e.g. acetazolamide, chlorpropamide, sulphonamides, phenytoin, methyldopa)
	— idiopathic thrombocytopenic purpura
3. Increased consumption	— thrombotic thrombocytopenic purpura
	— disseminated intravascular coagulation
	— haemolytic uraemic syndrome
4. Sequestration	— hypersplenism
5. Dilutional	— massive blood transfusion

Disseminated intravascular coagulation (DIC)

This term covers a spectrum of conditions which result from a self-generating activation of the clotting system. The effects are deposition of thrombi and damage to the walls of the microcirculation, the consumption of platelets and clotting factors by this process, the overactivation of the fibrinolytic system in response, and the consequent inability of the body to produce any form of adequate haemostasis.

The syndrome always accompanies another serious condition. The commonest of these are shock, sepsis, trauma, burns and obstetric complications. ARDS often develops as well.

Diagnosis. The clinical picture is characterized by bleeding from incisions, wounds and intravascular cannulae sites, frequently accompanied by cyanosis and a shock-like picture. Diagnosis is confirmed by haematological tests showing reductions in platelets, clotting factors and fibrinogen. The clotting time, prothrombin time and partial thromboplastin time are all prolonged.

Treatment. The most vital aspect of treatment is to arrest and reverse the underlying pathology which led to the development of the DIC. If this is not done the coagulopathy progresses inexorably.

To assist in this recovery, and to enable the patient to survive the acute crisis, infusions of platelets, FFP and fibrinogen may be necessary. These should be given in consultation with a haematologist who will, on the basis of clotting factor titres, platelet count etc., be able to advise on the best dosage and regimen. The use of anticoagulants is very controversial.

POLYCYTHAEMIA

This is principally an overproduction of erythrocytes with a high haematocrit but there may be a concomitant increase in granulocytes and thrombocytes. Where the cause is unknown, it is called polycythaemia rubra vera (PRV). Alternatively, it can develop because of increased erythropoeitin production secondary to hypoxia or certain neoplasms (e.g. hypernephroma). The peak incidence of PRV is between 50 and 65 years. It affects males slightly more commonly than females and rarely there is a positive family history.

PREOPERATIVE PHASE

History

Common complaints are headaches, dizziness, vertigo, visual disturbances, tinnitus, syncope and pruritus. Thrombotic episodes are due to increased viscosity, vascular stasis and high platelet levels. There may be haemorrhage, particularly from the nose or secondary to peptic ulceration. This results from vascular distension, defective platelet function and interference with clot formation by excess red cells in the fibrin mesh. Exercise tolerance is often limited by shortness of breath, angina or claudication.

Ascertain the current treatment. If phlebotomy is being used find out when it was last done and whether the patient is due for a repeat venesection. Treatment with radioactive phosphorus (^{32}P) leads to a 15% incidence of leukaemia. Myelosuppression may also be achieved with radiation, melphalan, busulphan and chlorambucil, in which case the white cell and platelet counts may be low.

Examination

Suspect the condition in plethoric patients with a ruddy cyanosis. Look for any underlying cardiac or pulmonary cause of hypoxia. Check that increased blood viscosity and volume has not precipitated heart failure. Associated hypertension is common. Assess splenomegaly. This may be massive and impair breathing.

Investigations

FBC. The haemoglobin concentration is frequently over 18 g% and the haematocrit is correspondingly raised. Cells are normochromic and normocytic unless there is a superimposed iron deficiency. The ESR is low. The white cell count is normally moderately raised, as is the platelet count in more than half the patients with PRV. Platelet

331

adhesiveness may be defective but this investigation does not help in the perioperative management. Confirmation of a high red cell mass is done using Cr-labelled autologous red blood cells. In the absence of this investigation haemotocrits greater than 60% are likely to be due to erythrocytosis.

Blood gases. Blood gas estimation is mandatory to establish whether the polycythaemia is primary or secondary to hypoxia.

Preoperative preparation

Establish whether the polycythaemia is primary or secondary. If it is secondary to hypoxia, oxygen supply to the tissues is enhanced despite the increased viscosity and the haemoglobin concentration needs to be maintained. Refer to Chapters 1 or 2 if a cardiac or pulmonary cause is known.

Untreated patients with PRV for elective surgery should be postponed until the condition is well controlled by phlebotomy or myelosuppression. Preoperative phlebotomy is also important in reducing the operative mortality 4–5 fold for emergency surgery. Prevent vascular instability in the acute situation by exchanging blood loss with a plasma expander.

PEROPERATIVE PHASE

When inducing anaesthesia, remember that the circulation time may be prolonged and hence that an overdose might occur. Polycythaemic patients become cyanosed easily. Always ensure good oxygenation. Maintain the cardiac output as well as possible. Keep the patient well hydrated. Pneumatic leggings help to prevent sluggish blood flow. Dextran 70 or subcutanous heparin assist in preventing DVT. Be prepared for the patient to bleed more than usual. This may need treatment with either FFP or platelet concentrate.

POSTOPERATIVE PHASE

Continue oxygen therapy on the ward. Mobilize early.

MULTIPLE MYELOMA

Multiple myeloma is a disseminated malignancy of plasma cells that may be associated with bone destruction, bone marrow failure, hypercalcaemia, renal failure (see Chapter 7) and recurrent infections. The median age of onset is 60 years and males are affected

332

slightly more frequently than females. The annual incidence of the disease is 3 per 100 000 of the population. Diagnosis is confirmed by finding Bence Jones protein on urine or serum electrophoresis.

Hypercalcaemia is treated with prednisolone and phosphate. Keep the patient well hydrated. Bone destruction may result in pathological fractures. Identify these before operation and always handle the patient carefully. Because 5% of patients have extradural plasmacytomas arising from a vertebra, spinal or extradural block it is probably best avoided. Paraplegia from this cause requires acute decompression. Consider prophylactic antibiotics and warn the physiotherapist of any rib fractures. Check the platelet count because it may be low. Prophylaxis against postoperative DVT is wise.

HAEMOCHROMATOSIS

This is a rare disorder (1 in 10 000 population) which occurs principally in males and has a weak inherited tendency. The basic flaw is the failure of the gastrointestinal tract to inhibit the uptake of iron and thereby regulate the amount in the body stores. After the accummulation of an excess of 15 to 20 grams of iron, symptoms begin to appear. Many patients give a history of a high alcohol intake and women with a heavy menstrual loss tend to have the onset of the disease delayed. The excess iron is deposited predominantly in the liver, resulting in cirrhosis (q.v.) and disordered liver function tests. Portal hypertension occurs late. Iron is also deposited in all other body tissues leading to the classical presenting triad of diabetes mellitus (q.v.), cirrhosis and skin pigmentation (bronze diabetes). There may be symptoms of congestive cardiac failure (q.v.) and less commonly cardiac arrhythmias (q.v.).

Medical management of the condition is by regular phlebotomy.

Anaesthetic management is that of the individual complications of the disorder. Excess blood transfusion is obviously detrimental.

FURTHER READING

Adams, A.P. & Hahn, C.E.W. (1982) *Principles and Practice of Blood Gas Analysis.* 2nd edn. Churchill Livingstone.

Alberti, K.G.M.M., Darley, J.H., Emerson, P.M. *et al.* (1972) 2,3-DPG and tissue oxygenation in uncontrolled diabetes mellitus. *Lancet*, **ii**, 391–5.

Astrup, P., Engol, K., Severinghaus, J.W. *et al.* (1965) The influence of temperature and pH on the dissociation curve of oxyhemoglobin of human blood. *Scand. J. Clin. Lab. Invest.*, **17**, 515–23.

Bruce-Churatt, L.J. (1984) Infection, immunity and blood transfusion. *Br. Med. J.*, **288**, 1782–3.

Carter, R.F., McArdle, B. & Morritt, G.M. (1981) Autologous transfusion of mediastinal drainage blood. A report of its use following open heart surgery. *Anaesthesia*, **36**, 54–9.

Clarke, J.M.F. (1982) Surgery in Jehovah's Witnesses. *Br. J. Hosp. Med.*, **27**, 497–500.

Davies, S.C. & Hewitt, P.E. (1984) Sickle Cell Disease. *Br. J. Hosp. Med.*, **31**, 440–4.

Editorial (1981) Post transfusion hepatitis. *Br. Med. J.*, **283**, 1–2.

Filshie, J., Pollock, A.N., Hughes, R.G. *et al.* (1984) The anaesthetic management of bone marrow harvest for transplantation. *Anaesthesia*, **39**, 480–4.

Harris, T.J.B., Parikh, N.R., Rao, Y.K. *et al.* (1983) Exsanguination in a Jehovah's Witness. *Anaesthesia*, **38**, 989–92.

Machin, S.J. (1979) The problems of blood transfusion. *Br. J. Hosp. Med.*, **21**, 294–300.

Marshall, M. & Bird, T. (1983) *Blood Loss and Replacement*. Edward Arnold Ltd., London.

Oski, F.A., Marshall, B.E., Cohen, P.J. *et al.* (1971) Exercise with anaemia: the role of the left shifted or right shifted oxygen-hemoglobin equilibrium curve. *Ann. Int. Med.*, **74**, 44–6.

Rudowski, W.J. (1980) Evaluation of modern plasma expanders and blood substitutes. *Br. J. Hosp. Med.*, **23**, 389–97.

Samaja, M. & Winslow, R.M. (1979) The separate effects of H and 2,3-DPG on the oxygen equilibrium curve of human blood. *Br. J. Haematology*, **41**, 373–81.

Searle, J.F. (1973) Anaesthesia in sickle cell states. *Anaesthesia*, **28**, 48–58.

Shapell, S.D. & Lenfant, C.J.M. (1972) Adaptive genetic and iatrogenic alterations of the oxyhemoglobin-dissociation curve. *Anesthesiology*, **37**, 127–39.

10/Psychiatry

The problem of consent

Drugs
Tricyclic antidepressants
Monoamine oxidase inhibitors
Phenothiazines
Butyrophenones
Lithium

Mental disorders
Affective disorders
Mental subnormality
Down's syndrome
Neurosis
Schizophrenia
Organic cerebral syndromes
Eating disorders

Drug abuse
Drug abusers
Drugs which produce psychological
dependence only:
    amphetamines
    cocaine
    marijuana
    LSD
Drugs which produce psychological
and physical dependence:
    barbiturates
    opioids
    alcohol

THE PROBLEM OF CONSENT

Psychiatric patients frequently present problems when consent is required for surgery. Failure to obtain consent from a patient prior to the most minor examination may theoretically lead to a civil action for trespass, assault or battery or to a criminal trial for common, aggravated or indecent assault, depending upon the circumstances.

Consent may be 'implied' or 'express'. Implied consent assumes that when the patient presents himself to a doctor he has already tacitly agreed to some sort of limited examination. This is normally taken to mean nothing more advanced that inspection, palpation, percussion and auscultation. Any other procedure (e.g. blood tests, endoscopy, radiology, rectal and vaginal examinations) requires express consent.

Express consent means exactly what it says. The patient gives his consent expressly for a well defined procedure to be undertaken after a full explanation of its objectives. This consent may be oral or written; both are of equal validity if adequately witnessed. Written consent has the advantage of permanence and easy proof, which may be important in subsequent litigation.

Consent for any medical or dental procedure can only be given by conscious, mentally sound adults. This implies that it must be obtained before premedicant drugs are given. An adult for these purposes is anyone over 16 years old. Below this age, consent should be obtained from the parent or guardian. This can give rise to problems when, for instance, a minor wishes to have a therapeutic abortion without her parent's knowledge. Nonetheless it is strongly advised to obtain parental consent.

Difficulties arise because of psychiatric illness when an adult of unsound mind is unable to give consent for surgery on either himself or on a dependent under the age of consent. A mentally deficient adult is in a similar situation to a minor. Permission is obtained from the closest possible relative or, in their absence, from the officer (who need not be medical) of the institution in which they live. There must be good evidence for the abnormal mental state of the patient. It is only reasonable that the surgeon and anaesthetist satisfy themselves of this in their assessment, before proceeding to surgery without express consent. Occasionally, in exceptional circumstances, a patient may be put under the jurisdiction of a court of protection for the administration of all their affairs, and court officers may then give consent for an operation.

Certified mental patients who are compulsorily detained, can give consent if it is considered that they comprehend what is intended. If not, the medical officer in charge should sign the consent since the relatives have no legal standing under these circumstances.

When a minor is prevented from receiving treatment considered to be of benefit to him, because the adult guardian holds peculiar beliefs or is mentally defective, there are two courses of action for the doctor. He can seek the assistance of the Children's Officer of the Local Authority who may, with a magistrate, convene an emergency court at the bedside. The magistrate may then authorize the removal of the child's custody from the parents to a 'fit person' (usually the Children's Officer) who is then able to authorize the operation or treatment. This procedure is very rarely used and a directive from the Minister of Health in 1961 advised its abandonment. Instead, he recommended that the doctor involved should get a written supporting opinion from a colleague that the patient's life is in danger without the proposed line of treatment, and he should then go ahead provided that he is competent to accomplish the task.

In true emergency, life-threatening situations the treatment of the mentally defective is similar to that of the previously normal (e.g. the unconscious). If rapid consent cannot be obtained from a relative, guardian, or medical officer, the operating team act as 'agents of necessity', and proceed as they think fit. In so doing, it is assumed that a normal, adult patient finding himself in this situation would give his willing consent.

In general the concept of consent, with all its varied implications is a matter of common sense. In the final analysis no court will litigate (at least not in this country) against a doctor who has acted reasonably, and in the patient's best interests throughout, provided that he was competent to undertake the procedures carried out.

DRUGS

Many of the drugs used in psychiatric illness have important implications for the anaesthetist.

Tricyclic antidepressants

These drugs are used to treat many psychiatric symptoms including depression, phobic anxiety, other psychosomatic disorders and as an adjunct in the treatment of chronic pain. The commonest members of this large group of compounds are amitriptyline and imipramine. They work by blocking the uptake of noradrenaline and serotonin at sympathetic nerve endings, but in addition they have strong anti-muscarinic actions which may contribute to their beneficial actions. The therapeutic effects take 2–3 weeks to develop and after stopping therapy the serum level decreases by 50% in 2–3 days.

There are two schools of thought about continuing therapy until the time of surgery. Patients on tricyclics have a similar, if not more dramatic, hypertensive response to direct and indirect sympathomimetic amines as those taking monoamine oxidase inhibitors (MAOI's). In view of this dangerous interaction some authorities advise stopping all tricyclics 2 weeks before elective surgery. Others continue them because of the risks of rebound depression. If they are not stopped, the altered response to drugs must be anticipated. Sympathomimetic amines need avoiding (especially adrenaline). If a hypertensive crisis develops, alpha-adrenoceptor blockade (phentolamine, chlorpromazine) or vasodilation with sodium nitroprusside is effective. When treating hypotension secondary to vasodilatation, felypressin and methoxamine do not interact adversely with tricyclics. Theoretically it seems wise not to use anaesthetic drugs with sympathomimetic effects (e.g. ketamine).

Side effects of tricyclic therapy are sedation and anticholinergic features (dry mouth, blurred vision, constipation, urinary retention). Omit centrally acting anticholinergics (atropine, hyoscine) in premedication and anaesthesia because the additive effect may precipitate confusion and delirium (especially in the elderly). Glycopyrrolate is a better choice if a drying agent is thought necessary.

Animal experiments and isolated reports in humans suggest that patients on tricyclic therapy are more sensitive to narcotic analgesics and barbiturates so the dose of these should be reduced until the response is observed. In therapeutic doses, the tricyclic antidepressants depress cardiac conduction and may produce dysrhythmias, especially if there is underlying cardiac disease. This is less of a problem with the tetracyclic antidepressants. Perioperative continuous ECG monitoring is therefore essential. The threshold for ventricular ectopic activity is decreased, especially in the presence of halothane, and treatment with IV lignocaine may be needed. Blood pressure monitoring is important because orthostatic hypotension is frequent. Enflurane can have an additive epileptogenic effect with tricyclics.

Monoamine oxidase inhibitors

These antidepressant drugs (e.g. phenelzine, isocarboxazid, tranylcypromine) are usually only used when the response to tricyclics has not been favourable. Thus, they are encountered less frequently. MAOI's have less sedative and less anticholinergic effects than tricyclics but orthostatic hypotension is common. They enjoy an infamous reputation in their interaction with anaesthesia.

MAOI's prevent the breakdown of noradrenaline, serotonin and dopamine. In the brain this produces the antidepressant effect but it also means that there is increased noradrenaline available in peripheral nerve endings. Tyramine (found in cheese, broad beans, avocado pears, some wines and other foodstuffs), a precursor of noradrenaline, increases the build up and release of noradrenaline because of monoamine oxidase inhibition. Like indirect sympathomimetic drugs, tyramine can precipitate severe hypertension and the patient has to be obsessional in avoiding tyramine ingestion.

Where appropriate, it is desirable to discontinue MAOI's for at least 2 weeks, and preferably 3 weeks, before surgery. Elective surgery should thus be planned in conjunction with psychiatic advice in case of a suicidal tendency. If it is not appropriate to stop MAOI therapy, as in emergencies, agents which may precipitate a hypertensive crisis must be avoided. Because of increased noradrenaline stores the biggest danger of unpredictable changes in blood pressure is with indirect acting sympathomimetic agents (e.g. ephedrine, metaraminol, amphetamine-like psychostimulants). Direct acting sympathomimetics, including adrenaline and noradrenaline, are largely destroyed by catechol-o-methyl transferase (COMT). Although still dangerous these produce fewer unexpected hypertensive problems. If a hypertensive crisis does develop it can be treated with alpha-adrenoceptor blockade (phentolamine) or by vasodilation with sodium nitroprusside.

Also important, although not common, is the interaction with pethidine. Agitation, restlessness, hypertension, rigidity, convulsions and hyperpyrexia may result. The primary narcotic effects of pethidine may also be potentiated causing coma, depressed ventilation and hypotension. Morphine and dihydrocodeine appear to be safe. Adequate analgesia is important to prevent excess sympathetic drive as a result of pain.

The anaesthetic technique ought to avoid causing endogenous release of sympathomimetic amines (e.g. light anaesthesia, hypercarbia, ketamine). Patients may also be sensitive to barbiturates and the action of almost all CNS depressants is potentiated.

Phenothiazines

The phenothiazines are a group of about 25 clinically used drugs of which the prototype is chlorpromazine. To a greater or lesser degree they all have antipsychotic, antiemetic, antihistamine and sedative properties. The most prominent effect determines the clinical use of the drug. Chlorpromazine is described here because it is the commonest.

It causes a return towards normality in the psychotic but dysphoria in normals. This is attributed to an antidopaminergic effect which can result in extrapyramidal symptoms (see Parkinsonism). Even in small doses, vigilance and psychomotor ability are impaired which may mitigate against treatment on a day case basis. Side effects which should be sought preoperatively are rare hypersensitivity reactions resulting in obstructive jaundice and blood dyscrasias. Dermatological reactions occur in up to 5% of patients.

Interactions with other drugs are common, several of which are important in anaesthesia. The analgesic, ventilatory depressant and sedative effects of narcotics are potentiated leading to decreased narcotic requirements. The predominant effect on the CVS is alpha-adrenoceptor blockade and hypotension is to be expected. The consequent vasodilatation increases heat loss and together with a central effect on the temperature regulating system usually leads to an intraoperative fall in body temperature. The hypotensive effect of halothane is enhanced. The sedative effect reduces the dose of barbiturate required to induce anaesthesia, and prolongs the sleeping time. Because of dopamine receptor blockade, effects of exogenous dopamine are attenuated. The antiemetic effect is on the chemoreceptor trigger zone, hence it does not prevent vomiting due to gastric irritation or bowel obstruction.

Although chlorpromazine is only weakly anticholinergic, it can have additive effects with atropine or hyoscine which may precipitate ileus, urinary retention or restlessness and confusion. Glycopyrrolate is therefore preferable as an antisialogogue, especially in the elderly.

Butyrophenones

The two main drugs in this class are haloperidol and droperidol. Only haloperidol is used as a potent antipsychotic in psychiatry. Droperidol is used in neurolept anaesthesia.

Haloperidol causes more specific dopamine blockade than chlorpromazine but the alpha-adrenoceptor blockade is less. In other respects, the interactions with anaesthetic drugs are similar to those of chlorpromazine.

Lithium

Lithium carbonate is predominantly used as a chronic medication to stabilize mood in manic-depressive patients. It differs from all the other psychotropic drugs in having no discernible effect in normal people. It is thought to act by inhibiting the release and increasing the uptake of noradrenaline, and by increasing serotonin synthesis in the CNS.

The therapeutic level is close to the toxic level. Plasma concentrations are monitored and kept below 1.5 mmol/litre. Above this, side effects increase greatly in incidence and severity. Chronic side effects are nephrogenic diabetes insipidus with polyuria and polydipsia (which disappears when lithium is stopped), a low free thyroxine (but most patients remain euthyroid), and a benign and reversible depression of the T wave unrelated to sodium or potassium depletion. Allergic dermatitis and vasculitis may occur, and the white blood cell count can rise up to $14000/mm^3$.

Lithium treatment should only be given to patients with a normal sodium intake and even then, in certain circumstances (e.g. excessive sweating from manual work in the summer) the dosage may need to be reduced.

Before anaesthesia, a recent serum level should be checked and the last two doses omitted (it is normally taken 3 or 4 times daily). This is important because acute intoxication can easily occur in the perioperative period. Toxicity is characterized by vomiting, profuse diarrhoea, ataxia, dysarthria, focal neurological signs and ultimately coma and convulsions. There may be cardiac arrhythmias and hypotension.

The main route of excretion of lithium is via the kidney where it interacts with sodium. If the sodium intake is lowered, or sodium excretion is enhanced by loop diuretics, severe intoxication may ensue. This may be precipitated by the preoperative fast if the lithium level is at the upper end of the therapeutic range. In order to prevent toxicity patients should have a *saline* infusion at a rate to keep up with sodium losses, before surgery. In a similar manner, established intoxication can be treated by saline infusion and the excretion of lithium may be enhanced by osmotic diuretics.

Lithium potentiates the effects of depolarizing and non-depolarizing muscle relaxants, and of all anaesthetic agents. Reduced dosages of drugs should therefore be given until their effect is assessed.

Postoperatively, the fluid balance considerations are equally important and if the GIT is in action, thirst must be satisfied and an adequate sodium content put in the diet.

MENTAL DISORDERS

Affective disorders

These are all characterized by a primary disturbance of mood with altered behaviour and changes in energy, sleep, appetite and weight. The extremes are intense excitement and elation (mania and hypomania) and severe depression. Depression can arise *do novo* with no apparent cause (endogenous), be secondary to psychic trauma (reactive), or follow physical illnesses, surgery and the prescription of certain drugs (reserpine, methyldopa, sulphonamides, barbiturates, the contraceptive pill). The overall incidence is about 2%. The patient always has a depressed mood and may have retarded physical and mental activity. Occasionally, delusional ideas, altered perception and a lack of insight are prominent. History taking can be tedious and unreliable. If the depression is chronic there may be cachexia (q.v.), obesity (q.v.), or evidence of alcohol (q.v.) or drug abuse (q.v.).

Physical illnesses particularly associated with depression are hypothyroidism (q.v.), parkinsonism (q.v.), pernicious anaemia (q.v.) and carcinoma of lung or prostate. Consequently it is reasonable for all depressed people, especially those in middle age or older, to have their drug therapy reviewed and to have some investigations (e.g. FBC, U & E's, LFT's, thyroid function tests, acid phosphatase and CXR) performed.

The major implication for the anaesthetist is that of the antidepressant drugs prescribed above. The patient is usually passive, accepting whatever treatment is recommended but he is not prepared to contribute to his recovery. A firm hand is often required with regard to physiotherapy and mobilization. Encouragement from relatives may help.

Mania and hypomania are much less common than depression and are only rarely attributable to an organic cause. The major differential diagnosis is that of drug abuse with amphetamines and hallucinogens such as LSD. The anaesthetic problems are related to the patients drugs (e.g. lithium).

Mental subnormality

The majority of subnormals are normal variants, but some have the condition as part of a broader syndrome, the features of which may affect anaesthetic management. Consequently, all such patients need a thorough examinaton of the CVS and RS. Usually they have been investigated at length by the paediatricians. If they have been diagnosed as a named syndrome, then check on the implications of this.

Communication difficulties are very similar to those of paediatric anaesthesia. If the patient is adult, he is much stronger than a child and interpersonal skills play a vital role in dealing with these patients.

The preoperative visit is best made when the parent or guardian is with the patient. This enables the relevant history to be obtained (both medical and psychological), the consent for surgery to be signed (q.v.), advice to be taken regarding fears or phobias (e.g. masks, needles, trolleys) and the most likely way to gain cooperation to be discussed. The patient will also recognize the anaesthetist and form some sort of trust.

Make an assessment of their mental age and explain what is going to happen in language appropriate to that age. The patient may ask very direct questions which ought not to be evaded but answered according to their understanding. If the mental age is below 4 years explanations are not likely to help.

Heavy oral or intramuscular premedication may be of benefit but each patient needs individual assessment. Time the arrival in the anaesthetic room to cause the patient minimal waiting. Sensible parents can provide invaluable help at induction by reassurance, but their presence can be detrimental if they are frightened. Concessions may have to be made regarding the donning or removing of clothing (remember false teeth) and posture (e.g. sitting, or even standing) for induction of anaesthesia. Ensure that there is adequate help with lifting. Whether anaesthesia is induced by gas or an IV technique has to be assessed individually, but both may call for exceptional skills and expert, firm assistants for successful management. On occasion forceful restraint, or IM ketamine is required. Always be prepared for a possible difficult intubation.

The presence of parents, guardian or a familiar comfort object can help to avoid disturbances in the postoperative period. Always remember that the patient may not vocalize pain.

342

Down's syndrome

Down's syndrome (mongolism) is a chromosome abnormality (Trisomy 21) which is more likely to occur with older maternal age. Although it only accounts for 1% of mentally defectives, its associated medical conditions (congenital heart disease (q.v.), duodenal, anal or choanal atresia, leukaemia (q.v.)) mean that they frequently present for anaesthesia. Dental care often requires general anaesthesia. There is a high mortality from the disease in early childhood but many now survive to adulthood.

Mongols have characteristic abnormalities in the anatomy of the face and skull. The mid-facial structures are crowded, the tongue is large and the jaw is small. Nasal passages are constricted. All these features predispose to difficult intubation and airway management. Mongols are affected more than usual by ventilatory depressant drugs. Their eyes are very sensitive to atropine but this is not a problem with the normal systemic doses. Extubation stridor occurs frequently and may require nursing in a humidified atmosphere.

Neurosis

Neuroses are the commonest psychiatric disorders seen, and represent up to 20% of all general practitioner consultations. They are diseases in which the personality remains intact and contact with reality is preserved. The symptoms are subjective, persistent and troublesome and are associated with malaise, an inability to cope and feelings of anxiety. Neurosis is frequently seen in surgical patients simply because it is so common in the general public.

Many patients are on anxiolytic (benzodiazepines usually), or antidepressant drugs. Normally they are very anxious and a heavy sedative premedication and reassurance are advisable. Anaesthetically they cause few problems. Occasionally those obsessed with regular purgations have chronic electrolyte alterations. Phobias (e.g. claustrophobia, agaraphobia, needle phobia) need sympathetic and imaginative but *firm* management.

Schizrenia

The incidence of schizophrenia in the general population is 0.8% but it is considerably higher in close relatives of schizophrenics. It is a syndrome of personality change and other symptoms which tends to start in early adult life and which can lead to a dramatic disintegration of the personality. Some symptoms are cardinal (e.g. primary delusions, thought disorders, hallucinations) and others are less specific (loss of drive, blunted emotions, lack of interpersonal contact, stereotyped movements). The presentation and progress of the disease are classically divided into simple, hebephrenic, paranoid and catatonic.

The anaesthetist's problems are those of the underlying disease requiring surgery, difficult history taking, drug therapy, the patient's loss of contact with reality, and the possibility of becoming the object of a paranoid delusion.

Organic cerebral syndromes

These are of great importance to the anaesthetist and should always be suspected when there is an abnormal mental state. Their aetiology may affect anaesthesia and they may be curable.

Organic cerebral syndromes are caused by dysfunction at the cellular level resulting from ischaemia, toxins, inflammation, tumour or trauma. The lesion may be reversible, permanent but stationary, or progressive. They present with a mixture of intellectual impairment, memory loss, change in personality and confusion. Focal neurological signs may be present. The causes are listed in Table 10.1.

It is therefore essential, if an organic cerebral syndrome is suspected, to have a thorough preoperative work up. Its presence, especially in the elderly, is easily missed.

Table 10.1. Causes of organic cerebral syndromes

Broad group	Examples and notes
Drugs	Alcohol, barbiturates, steroids, any psychotropic medication.
Infections	Meningitis, encephalitis, any systemic infection causing a high fever. Neurosyphilis is now rare.
Electrolyte disturbances	GIT disturbances in the elderly. After GI and GU surgery.
Hypoxia	Especially in the elderly, e.g. from chest infections, LVF.
Intracerebral	Abscess, tumour, trauma (especially subdural haematoma in the elderly).
Cardiovascular	Intracerebral arterioslcerosis, low cardiac output, severe anaemia.
System failure	Renal or hepatic failure. Hypothyroidism, Cushing's syndrome, Addison's disease, nonketoacidotic diabetic coma.
Recognized dementia	Senile dementia, Alzheimer's disease, Pick's disease, Huntington's chorea.
Toxic	Carbon monoxide, heavy metals (all are rare).

The history is usually impossible to obtain except from relatives. On examination, look for the presence of right and left ventricular failure, cyanosis, hepatomegaly and chest infection.

Direct investigations to any abnormalities elicited in the history and examination. Tests which may be indicated are FBC, U & E's, LFT's, thyroid function tests, arterial blood gases, ECG, CXR, urine and serum screening for the presence of drugs and CAT scanning. If there are no signs of raised intracranial pressure, a lumbar puncture may be done. In an emergency, LFT's and thyroid function tests will not be available since they are assayed in batches.

Anaesthetic management is that of any underlying disease found. Both before, and especially after, surgery these patients can pose major ward problems. Frequently because of their antisocial activities they tend to be ignored by the ward staff who request sedation to keep them quiet. The patient cannot grasp what is happening and the environment appears strange and frightening. He often misinterprets events around him and may suffer both delusions and hallucinations which leave him tearful and terrified. This leads to over activity, objectionable behaviour, and episodes such as attempts to leave the ward or refuse medication. Drips and catheters are pulled out and oxygen masks are thrown away. The clouding of consciousness is always worse at night when the visual cues are less clear.

Sometimes calm nurses and doctors are all that is required. On other occasions there is so much activity on the ward that constant stimuli unsettle the patient. At times it may become essential to sedate the patient for his own benefit. This should never be done without first ensuring that he is not hypoglycaemic or hypoxic, that he is not hypotensive or in heart failure, that he has no electrolyte imbalance, and that he has not had a pulmonary embolus.

Eating disorders

Eating disorders occur predominantly in teenage and young adult women (male:female = 1:10). Their incidence is increasing.

Anorexia nervosa is a state of self-induced weight loss far beyond that accepted as normal dieting. Some investigators require a loss of 25% of the original body weight to confirm the diagnosis. The current incidence is up to 1% of the schoolgirl population aged 16–18 years. Amenorrhoea is a constant feature.

Severe cases, in general, have the same problems as those with malnutrition (q.v.). Vomiting or purging can produce electrolyte abnormalities. Iron deficiency anaemia is common. A CXR is helpful because there is an increased incidence of tuberculosis secondary to reduced immune competence.

Bulimia nervosa is a less common abnormality characterized by episodic gluttony followed by self-induced purgation and vomiting. The main anaesthetic hazard is any resultant electrolyte disturbance. The patients are usually of normal weight, but in a minority the condition can overlap with (and may be regarded as an unusual form of) anorexia nervosa.

DRUG ABUSERS

Drug abuse means taking a drug in a way that exceeds its proper medical or social use. Drug dependence is the development of a state in which the person has to continue taking the drug because he needs its mental effects (psychological dependence) or because he becomes ill if he stops (physical dependence). Often these are interrelated.

Many classifications of the types and degree of dependence are described. For our purposes it is simpler and sufficient to classify the problem as in Table 10.2.

Table 10.2. Drugs causing physical and psychological dependence

Type of drug	Physical dependence	Psychological dependence
Central stimulants/euphoriants (e.g. amphetamines, cocaine) Hallucinogens (e.g. LSD, marijuana, mescaline)	None	Considerable
Opioids (e.g. heroin, morphine)	Severe, often not dose related	Very strong
Alcohol, barbiturates	Severe, often dose related	Very strong

PREOPERATIVE CONSIDERATIONS

History

The *known* addict is usually frank and cooperative about his drug problem. Take a thorough drug history, ascertaining the type of drug, the usual dosage (tolerance occurs to many drugs), when he had his last dose and what drugs he has had since being in hospital. Check whether he is currently drug dependent. Ask about the source of drug and whether he is registered with an addiction centre or psychiatrist. Contact them to verify the story as extreme cases may fake physical illness so as to obtain drugs. If he is a 'new addict', engage the help of a doctor working with addicts at an early stage.

Drug addiction is much commoner in young adults, therefore have a high index of suspicion in the 15–40 year olds who behave oddly, and particularly if there is evidence of venepuncture. Surgery is often related to the drug abuse, e.g. infection from unsterile needles, burns from falling asleep with a lighted cigarette, crashing a car etc.

Examination

Always look carefully for signs of infection (due to general debility or infected needles), especially those of endocarditis and pulmonary infection. Look for jaundice. The high incidence (over 80%) of hepatitis B in those who use injected drugs means that all patients should be assumed to be carriers until proven otherwise.

Assess the patient neurologically. Rarely, with narcotic addicts, a transverse myelitis occurs which would contraindicate spinal anaesthesia.

Investigations

FBC. There may be a mild anaemia due to general debility.
CXR. Look for signs of infection.
LFT's. The hepatitis carrier state must be identified. Liver function is frequently deranged.

Treatment

Withdrawal from drugs needs to be carried out in hospital under the supervision of a psychiatrist. Unfortunately the treatment of addicts is frequently unsuccessful, with recurrent returns to old habits. This high relapse rate has been blamed on both the intrinsic psychiatric makeup of the patient, and on his environment which exposes him to temptation.

Physical dependence has developed when the presence of the drug in the body is required for normal cellular metabolism. Therefore withdrawal, of necessity, produces physiological symptoms (anxiety, irritability, sweating, lacrimation, mydriasis, tremors, piloerection, nausea, vomiting, abdominal cramps, diarrhoea, muscle spasms) which may be so severe as to be life-threatening (e.g. fits after barbiturate or alcohol withdrawal).

Those drugs which do not produce physical dependence do not precipitate physical withdrawal symptoms when stopped, but they can produce a desperate craving. There is, however, no physiological risk in their sudden cessation.

Preoperative preparation

It is generally agreed that the perioperative period is not the time to withdraw drugs which cause physical dependence. For elective operations, the possibility of deferring surgery until withdrawal is complete should be discussed. The patient may welcome this help and should be referred to a suitable psychiatrist. If the patient declines this offer, or if surgery is urgent, the maintenance dose of the drugs which cause physical dependence, (e.g. opioids, barbiturates) should be continued and may be used as part of the premedication.

The particular implications of individual drugs are now considered.

Drugs which produce psychological dependence only

Amphetamines

These are sympathomimetic agents which, when taken orally or IV produce a feeling of mental euphoria, power and increased physical ability. The chronic user presents for a wide range of procedures, but those acutely intoxicated can present with trauma secondary to the results of intoxication.

Acute intoxication can range from mild restlessness and irritability through a hypomanic state to convulsions and coma. There is a tachycardia, hypertension, flushing, headaches, pyrexia, nausea and vomiting. Appetite and thirst are suppressed leading to superimposed dehydration and ketosis. Ventricular arrhythmias are common.

Preoperative management consists of counteracting the mental hyperactivity with sedation (diazepam, chlorpromazine), correcting dehydration (do U & E's, replace losses appropriately), blocking the peripheral effects of sympathomimetic activity (propranolol, practolol) and treating dysrhythmias and hypertension as they occur. With hyperactivity, local anaesthetic techniques may not be suitable unless combined with light general anaesthesia. Postoperatively, the patient should be heavily sedated in a high dependency unit.

The chronic user has depleted body stores of noradrenaline and in many ways behaves as if he is alpha-adrenoceptor blocked, with hypotension and somnolence. The response to indirectly acting sympathomimetics is reduced but the response to direct acting drugs (noradrenaline, adrenaline, isporenaline) is normal and these can be used to maintain cardiac output if necessary.

Cocaine

Cocaine, taken as a nasal snuff, is currently increasing in its frequency of abuse. It was used by Sherlock Holmes to the chagrin of Dr Watson.

Although structurally dissimilar, its effects are sympathomimetic and similar to those of the amphetamines. Peripherally it prevents the re-uptake of noradrenaline and acts centrally as a CNS stimulant.

The management is essentially the same as that of amphetamine abuse.

Marijuana

The physiological effects secondary to marijuana are usually mild with a slight tachycardia, a dry mouth and sedation. Troublesome mental disturbances usually respond to benzodiazepines and sympathomimetic activity can be controlled with beta-adrenoceptor blockade. There is said to be an increased incidence of bronchitis and asthma in chronic users.

There are no special anaesthetic considerations except that marijuana intensifies the ventilatory depression of narcotics. Very severe cases should be treated symptomatically along the guidelines for amphetamines.

LSD

LSD is almost devoid of all peripheral actions, working exclusively in the CNS. In addition to its actions as a hallucinogen, it also has intrinsic analgesic properties, 0.1 mg of LSD being equivalent to 100 mg pethidine. Tolerance occurs rapidly and in normal patients this dose would produce a strong psychedelic experience.

In overdosage, LSD produces a central sympathomimetic picture (tachycardia, hypertension, dilated pupils, muscle tremors, increased reflexes, occasionally seizures) without peripheral sympathomimetic vasoconstriction. Ventilatory depression may occur. These physiological changes should be treated symptomatically. The presentation is dominated by anxiety and panic. A calm light environment helps, but often drugs (e.g. diazepam, chlorpromazine) are needed. Nurse in a high dependency area.

Analgesic requirements can be reduced in the presence of active LSD. LSD possesses *in vitro* anticholinesterase activity but there are no reports indicating whether or not it has a clinical effect on suxamethonium and ester-linked anaesthetics.

There have been several reports from centres which deal regularly with addicts indicating that surgery and general anaesthesia can produce 'flashbacks'. These are hallucinations, usually unpleasant, in people who have stopped taking the drug several months previously. They should be suspected if odd behaviour occurs in the postoperative period. Diazepam is a suitable treatment.

Drugs which produce psychological and physical dependence

Barbiturates

An acute overdosage of barbiturate fits the textbook description. Provided treatment is given early enough, unconsciousness, hypotension, ventilatory depression and hypothermia respond to supportive measures and the patient recovers once the drug has been metabolized.

Chronic barbiturate abuse has a more variable presentation. In those maintained on a stable dose (e.g. sleeping pills) for years, there may be little suggestion that anything is wrong. However, any increase in this maintenance dose can produce signs of intoxication (apprehension, sluggish physical and mental activity, slow speech, faulty judgement, emotional lability). Provided the patient is on a good diet, little damage to any organ system accompanies chronic barbiturate addiction or intoxication.

Tolerance to barbiturates develops within a few days of regular usage, the most prominent feature being a reduction in sedation after approximately one week. This is obviously important for epileptics needing phenobarbitone. Both an increase in drug metabolism (from enzyme induction in the liver) and a pharmacodynamic tolerance (with adaptation of nervous tissue to the presence of the drug) have been described. Despite the phenomenon of tolerance, the lethal dose of barbiturates is almost the same in both normals and addicts. This implies that a chronic addict is at great risk from a superimposed overdose. There is cross tolerance between most of the barbiturates.

As discussed earlier, chronic barbiturate abusers are in danger of experiencing a physical withdrawal syndrome, the severity and duration of which are variable but which can, in the worst instances lead to life-threatening fits. For this reason the drugs should be continued in the perioperative period. Cross tolerance to, and rapid metabolism of, other drugs must be anticipated. Isolated reports in the literature suggest that this is very variable and patients must be treated individually. When inducing anaesthesia in a chronic taker of barbiturates, a large dose of thiopentone or methohexitone is usually required and the serum level may well approach the lethal range. However, since the major cause of death is ventilatory depression, this can be avoided by artificial ventilation, continued if necessary into the postoperative period. A non-barbiturate induction agent appears preferable.

This group of patients are at risk from the toxic metabolites of other drugs because of liver enzyme induction. In particular, repeat anaesthetics with halothane or single anaesthetics with methoxy-flurane are contraindicated. The two volatile agents of choice are probably isoflurane (because so little is metabolized) and ether (metabolized to CO_2 and water).

Opioids

Narcotic addicts pose considerable problems. Many are hepatitis B positive, in poor general health, and malnourished. They undertake a variety of occupations (prostitution, theft etc.) in addition to normal employment in order to obtain funds to buy their 'fix'. Many are unable to hold a regular job down. They have a high incidence of sepsis, phlebitis, skin disorders, liver disease, incidental trauma and chest infections. Two serious complications are tetanus and endocarditis.

There is a remarkable degree of tolerance which develops to the analgesic, ventilatory depressant, sedative, euphoric and emetic effects. Some addicts build up to regular daily dosages of several grams of morphine or heroin (diamorphine). In contrast to the barbiturates, the lethal dose is greatly increased with chronic usage, although tolerance is not absolute and there is always a dose capable of producing death from ventilatory depression. The regular dosage of drug should be maintained perioperatively.

Withdrawal symptoms are as described earlier. Although unpleasant, they are never life-threatening *per se.* If patients have undertaken their own withdrawal (which lasts 7–10 days) they may present as dehydrated, hypotensive and shocked with acid-base disturbances due to failure to take in food and drink.

Obtaining venous access can be a problem for the anaesthetist. It is not uncommon to have to resort to subclavian or internal jugular venous catheterizaton or to a cutdown. The anaesthetic technique should *not* include partial or pure narcotic antagonist drugs (e.g. pentazocine, buprenorphine, naloxone etc.) because they will precipitate withdrawal symptoms.

Intraoperative hypotension, not due to hypovolaemia or anaesthetic overdose has been attributed in isolated reports to a poor adrenal reaction to stress and to failure to maintain the addictive levels of narcotic.

Postoperatively, addicts present considerable difficulties in the control of pain. One solution is to continue their daily maintenance dose and use regional blockade until minor analgesics are sufficient. Alternatively, their narcotic dosage can be increased, or a second opioid added. Pethidine has the reputation of giving good analgesia to morphine addicts. These decisions are best taken in consultation with the psychiatrist in charge of the patient. Patients who have their opioid dosage increased are still at risk of developing ventilatory depression and this must be explained to the nursing staff. An obvious possibility is that the patient will keep asking for higher and higher doses.

A problem rarely mentioned in the literature is that of the reformed addict. It would seem sensible to treat him as a normal person but not to prescribe opioid agonist drugs at any stage, instead substituting pentazocine, buprenorphine or a regional block. The reduced sensitivity to CO_2 which addicts are said to possess may persist for many months.

Alcohol

Alcoholism is an increasingly serious social problem. There is no accurate way to establish the total number of alcohol dependent people because it is freely available for purchase. However, approximately 10% of the adult UK population are teetotal, and 66% of women and 75% of men drink regularly. The number of heavy drinkers in the UK (over 80 g alcohol/day in men and over 40 g/day in women) at the last estimation in the late 1970s was 2 million. About one third of these are problem drinkers of whom 10% are so dependent on alcohol that they suffer withdrawal symptoms when they stop drinking. Only a minority present the typical picture of the 'skid-row' alcoholic, so the great majority are able to maintain full employment and pass unnoticed. One third of patients in hospital have been found to be heavy drinkers. The potential for patients having withdrawal symptoms in the perioperative period is therefore considerable.

The key to success is a high index of suspicion, but even then detection can be difficult. Relatively few people are honest about their alcohol intake. A heavy drinker may appear anywhere in the range from normal to that of a person with a bloated face, telangectasia, acne, blood-shot eyes, tophi, awful gums, gynaecomastia, pot belly with striae, tremulous fingers, dupuytren's contracture, bruises, an odd history of faints, mental symptoms and signs, and peripheral neuropathy. There is an accompanying peripheral vasodilatation with a bounding pulse. Oesophagitis, gastritis, pancreatitis, cirrhosis, cardiomyopathy, pneumonia, tuberculosis, gout and bone demineralization all have a high associated incidence.

Although there are many abnormal investigations and tests in patients with alcoholism they are all due to secondary organ damage and are therefore non-specific. Diagnosis can be confirmed by a random sample (e.g. in outpatients) for blood alcohol. With no signs of inebriation a blood alcohol level of over 80 mg% is suggestive, and of over 150 mg% is diagnostic, of alcohol dependence.

The known alcohol dependent patient should continue his usual daily consumption throughout the period in hospital. The patient who does not admit his dependence is likely to take alcohol normally before surgery, but may develop withdrawal symptoms in the postoperative period.

Anaesthetic considerations are firstly those of associated disorders secondary to alcoholism (see above) and secondly, those due to the effect of alcohol *per se*. The effect of alcohol itself depends upon whether or not the patient is intoxicated. As a general rule, all acutely intoxicated patients (whether alcohol dependent or not) are sensitive to, and require reduced dosages of, narcotics, sedatives and hypnotics. The danger with normal doses is severe ventilatory depression.

On the other hand, chronic alcohol abusers who are sober, on their usual intake, and whose cellular machinery is for them working normally, exhibit cross tolerance to many sedative, hypnotic and anaesthetic agents, but not to opioids. The action of opioids is potentiated thereby increasing the risk of ventilatory depression. All types of anaesthesia have been employed with success, providing there is no particular contraindication (e.g. no spinals with peripheral neuropathy), but two recurring problems emerge. Firstly, the induction is always more stormy than normal and requires large doses of both IV and volatile agents. Secondly, maintenance with a volatile agent requires greater concentrations than in the non-alcoholic.

The first suspicion of alcohol dependence may only occur in the postoperative period. Withdrawal symptoms vary from mild irritability and uncooperative behaviour to the fully developed unmistakable delirium tremens. Minor degrees should be suspected if there is confusion, disorientation, nausea, anxiety or sweating. Withdrawal can be fatal because of convulsions. Hallucinations can be so vivid that the person, if not physically robust, can develop nervous and physical exhaustion and cardiovascular collapse. The withdrawal syndrome can be treated with alcohol, chlormethiazole or chlordiazepoxide. It is best done in conjunction with a psychiatrist.

FURTHER READING

Alcohol Problems (1982) A collection of papers published by the *Br. Med. Ass.*
Cullen, B.F. & Miller, M.G. (1979) Drug interactions and anaesthesia: a review. *Anesth. Analg.*, **58**, 413–23.
Fairburn, C.G. (1983) Bulimia nervosa. *Br. J. Hosp. Med.*, **29**, 537–42.
Havdala, H.S., Borison, R.L. & Diamond, B.I. (1979) Potential hazards and applications of lithium in anesthesiology. *Anesthesiology*, **50**, 534–7.

Janowsky, E.C., Risch, S.C. & Janowsky, D.S. (1981) Psychotropic agents. *In:* Ty Smith, N., Miller, E.D. & Corbascio, A.N. (eds.), *Drug Interactions in Anesthesia*. Lea & Febiger. 177–95.

Jefferson, J.W. (1975) A review of the cardiovascular effects and toxicity of tricyclic antidepressants. *Psychosom. Med.*, **37**, 160–79.

Jenkins, L.C. (1972) Anaesthetic problems due to drug abuse and dependence. *Can. Anaesth. Soc. J.*, **19**, 461–77.

Kerry, R.J., Ludlow, J.M. & Owen, G. (1980) Diuretics are dangerous with lithium. *Br. Med. J.*, **iii**, 371.

Knight, B. (1982) *Legal Aspects of Medical Practice*. 3rd edn. Churchill Livingstone. 32–7.

Norkans, G., Frosner, G., Hermodsson, S. & Iwarson, S. (1980) Multiple hepatitis attacks in drug addicts. *J. Am. Med. Ass.* **242**, 1056–8.

Pfeffer, J.M. (1981) Management of the acutely disturbed patient on the general ward. *Br. J. Hosp. Med.*, **26**, 73–8.

Sjoqvist, F. (1965) Psychotropic Drugs (2): Interaction between monoamine oxidase (MAO) inhibitors and other substances. *Proc. R. Soc. Med.*, **58**, 967–78.

St Haxholdt, O., Krintel, J.J. & Johannson, G. (1984) Pre-operative alcohol infusion: the need for analgesic supplementation in chronic alcoholics. *Anaesthesia*, **39**, 240–5.

Ty Smith, N. (1981) Sedatives and hypnotics. *In:* Ty Smith, N., Miller, E.D. & Corbascio, A.D. (eds), *Drug Interactions In Anesthesia*. Lea & Febiger. 197–210.

11/Anaesthesia and old age

The pattern of ageing
Cardiovascular system
Pulmonary system
Nervous system
Gastrointestinal system
Metabolic & endocrine systems
Locomotor system
Renal function
Mental function
Handling of drugs

Anaesthetic management
Preoperative considerations
Peroperative phase
Postoperative phase

THE PATTERN OF AGEING

The definition of the age at which one becomes 'geriatric' is arbitrary, but it is usually taken as 65 years. These people now number some 14% of the population of which approximately 35% are over 75 years. There are many theories of ageing ranging from 'self destructing genes' to purely environmental causes. A popular theory is that of a gradual, random accumulation of genetic errors controlling protein synthesis, with superimposed environmental factors and disease processes.

In the main, normal ageing can be described as a gradual erosion of all the body's margins of safety coupled with a decreasing ability to adapt.

One of the main problems, both in general and hospital practice is that of late presentation. Probably one of the reasons why the elderly are so reluctant to report illness or disability to their doctor is that they themselves attribute their physical deterioration to old age. Symptomatology is often much less florid than in the young as exampled by the 'silent infarct'.

Cardiovascular system

The heart. The ageing heart has a decrease in both the size and the number of active myocardial fibres and an increase in the amount of epicardial fat. Stroke volume, resting heart rate, maximum possible heart rate, and resting cardiac output all decrease. This increases the

arm-brain circulation time. The ability to respond to increased demands is slowed and the effect of catecholamines is diminished. This
automatically produces a reduced exercise tolerance and cardiac
reserve. The conducting system from the S-A node to the ventricles
can become involved in a fibrous replacement, producing several
types of conduction disturbance (q.v.).

The incidence of valvular lesions increases with age, the most
commonly affected being the mitral valve. Degenerative changes,
either in the valve ring itself or the papillary muscles may cause
mitral incompetence. In contrast, aortic valve lesions caused by ageing are relatively unimportant to valve function and produce the systolic ejection murmur of aortic sclerosis. It is therefore important to
distinguish this from the pansystolic murmur of mitral incompetence.

The incidence of coronary artery disease increases with age but
may not always produce angina. Instead it can present as an infarct,
with breathlessness, or an ankle swelling. Many elderly patients have
quite advanced disease but their exercise tolerance is so reduced by
other factors (e.g. arthritis) that they never provoke an anginal
attack.

Approximately half the geriatric patients presenting with right or
left heart failure have coronary artery disease. The others have valve
disease, hypertension, thyrotoxicosis, anaemia and dysrhythmias.

Peripheral CVS. As the major vessels age, there is a progressive
structural deterioration with destruction of the intima, reduction in
smooth muscle and loss of elastin. The result is a fibrotic, calcified,
ulcerated, inelastic distributing system. The corollary of this is that
the response to the injection of a given volume of fluid into the
arterial system is a much higher systolic blood pressure than would
be seen in younger people. In the past this was called the 'benign systolic hypertension of the aged' to distinguish it from essential hypertension which has an associated rise in diastolic pressure secondary
to arteriolar hypertrophy. A reasonable working rule in the elderly is
that the systolic blood pressure should not exceed (100+age in years)
mmHg. Whether antihypertensive treatment is indicated is
controversial.

Small vessel disease is also more common in old age but claudication is often undetected because of low mobility.

The haemoglobin level remains constant throughout adult life and
anaemia should be investigated and treated as in Chapter 9.

Pulmonary system

There is a progressive deterioration with age in both the quality and the efficiency of the lung parenchyma and in the strength and mobility of the muscles and skeletal structures which provide the inspiratory and expiratory movement. Because of this, a person aged 70 years has a vital capacity which is 70% and a residual volume which is 120% of that of a young adult. The functional residual capacity (FRC) remains static, or only increases minimally with age, thus implying a reduction in the expiratory reserve volume.

The lung volume at which small basal airways begin to close during expiration increases with age. This is thought to be secondary to a deterioration in the interbronchiolar 'guy ropes' which maintain airway patency. In normal people, the closing capacity becomes equal to the FRC at approximately 45 years in the supine position and at about 65 years in the upright position. Once the closing capacity exceeds the FRC, during normal tidal breathing a certain amount of air trapping will occur, resulting in the shunting of pulmonary blood through underventilated alveoli. This is now thought to be one of the major determinants of the dependence of PaO_2 on both age and position (see Chapter 2). This oxygen transfer defect is intensified by the head down position. The physiological dead space to tidal volume ratio is increased but there is also an increase in the anatomical dead space due to dilatation of the trachea and upper airways. These both decrease efficient gas exchange. The elderly will often tolerate a larger size endotracheal tube than anticipated because of the tracheal dilatation.

Reductions in muscle strength and elasticity and early airways closure cause a fall in the FEV_1 and the ability to produce an effective cough. The FEV_1/VC ratio is approximately 70% at 70 years. This is assumed to be the reason (together with airways closure) for the frequent occurrence of hypostatic pneumonia ('the old man's friend') in the bed ridden and postoperative elderly.

Nervous system

The human nervous system is thought to degenerate in two ways. Firstly, there is a physiological deterioration in the functioning of nerve cells. The weight of the brain decreases linearly with age such that at 80 years it is approximately 80% of that of the young adult. There is a loss of myelin and a reduction in the number of synapses and nerve fibres in well demarcated tracts. The surface of the cortex shrinks from the dura and the sulci become wider and deeper. The rate of synthesis of neurotransmitters declines. These changes can cause a reduction in sensory and motor abilities and impair intellectual function (especially short term memory). Conduction velocity in peripheral nerves is slowed and the number of active motor neurones decreases. In the special senses, the eye develops cataracts and presbyopia, the ear often suffers from presbycusis (perceptive deafness) and tinnitus from degeneration of the hair cells in the organ of Corti, and loss of the sense of taste and smell can produce disinterest in food leading to anorexia, weight loss and depression.

Secondly, it is now well established that lack of sensory stimulation can intensify and accelerate deterioration in a functional sense. This may be due to physiological deprivation (e.g. cataracts, nerve deafness), physical and social conditions or ill health. It has been suggested that man has an inborn need to be stimulated and to maintain mobility. This requirement has been termed kinosephilia.

Superimposed upon this background are genuine physical insults such as cerebrovascular disease, repeated transient ischaemic attacks, hypoxia from poor pulmonary function and inappropriate use of drugs.

The effect on anaesthesia of all these changes is a reduction in the concentrations of volatile agents (MAC), and dosages of narcotics, muscle relaxants and local anaesthetics required to produce a satisfactory result. A given dose of epidural local anaesthetic results in a higher block than usual. This is thought to be due partly to an increased sensitivity to the drug and partly to an increased spread up and down the epidural space because of inelasticity and blocked intervertebral foramina. In young adulthood 1.5 mls of local anaesthetic given epidurally in the lumbar region blocks one spinal segment: by 80 years only half this quantity is required.

The sympathetic nervous system also suffers a deterioration manifested by decreased compensation to blood volume changes. Postural hypotension is common and the response to a reduction in circulating fluid volume is only mild vasoconstriction and a mild tachycardia. Hence the blood pressure falls early during blood loss.

Gastrointestinal system

Although these changes are relatively minor they are nonetheless important. Loss of appetite, poverty and poor dentition lead to malnutrition.

The mucosa throughout the GIT atrophies with reduced production of gastric acid. Smooth muscle activity decreases causing reduced peristalsis, delayed gastric emptying and constipation. Hiatus hernia is also more common. There is little literature assessing these effects on the absorption of food and drugs.

In the healthy elderly, liver function tests should all be normal except that decreased albumin production may reduce the plasma concentration by 20%. Liver blood flow is thought to decrease with age which limits the clearance of many drugs. The effect of age on microsomal enzymes is uncertain. The incidence of cholelithiasis approaches 40% by the eighth decade.

Metabolic and endocrine systems

The geriatric patient gradually loses his lean body mass and hence has reduced muscle power. Basal metabolic rate (BMR) is decreased by 20% as a consequence.

The ability to maintain the body temperature constant in the face of changing environmental conditions is diminished. Atrophy of sweat glands and the inability to vasodilate reduces the ability to cool. Conversely a reduced capacity for vasoconstriction and a reduced BMR allows hypothermia to occur easily.

The pituitary and parathyroid glands gradually decrease in weight but maintain their function well. The secretion of cortisol is reduced but this is matched by reduced disposal and excretion rates. The circadian variation and responsiveness to ACTH are unaltered. Mineralocorticoid activity is reduced (aldosterone secretion by 50%) which makes the elderly very vulnerable to sodium loss during acute illness.

Thyroid disorders are common and are frequently unrecognized. Both over and undersecretion of thyroid hormones can present atypically.

Glucose intolerance is almost universal in the elderly. It is due both to decreased sensitivity of the pancreatic beta cells to serum glucose and also to a reduced insulin secretion. However, less than 20% can be described as diabetic and the majority respond well to weight loss (if appropriate), diet and oral hypoglycaemics. Often diabetes is occult and only becomes apparent in the stress of surgery or intercurrent illness. The renal threshold for sugar is notoriously unpredictable in the elderly and so urine testing is not a reliable guide to the presence or absence of hyperglycaemia.

Locomotor system

This deteriorates because of both nervous system (q.v.) and skeletal system problems, the movements being slower, weaker, less co-ordinated and harder to correct. Muscles waste and shrink and there is a decrease in the number of muscle fibres as age advances. They are replaced by inelastic fibrous tissue. Body height is lost. Consequent joint contractures are unusual but do occur, and in rare cases have led to starvation because of the inability to feed.

Collagen loss is a common feature with senile atrophy of the skin, loss of subcutaneous tissue, and a reduction in the strength and stability of ligaments and tendons. Pot bellies and inguinal hernias become more frequent. The intervertebral discs reduce in thickness.

Senile osteoporosis (common in women) increases in severity with age and can present as bone pain, bone tenderness or fractures. The mechanism is poorly understood but is related to the menopause in women. Pathological fractures are easily produced.

Renal function

The kidney maintains its morphological and functional properties until the age of approximately 40 years. After this age the weight of the kidneys falls, the cortex losing more than the medulla. The resting renal blood flow and glomerular filtration rate (GFR) diminish and the secretory and reabsorptive capacities of the tubules are impaired (NB glucose). The GFR at 70 years is approximately 60% of that of the young adult and the blood urea on a normal diet approximately doubles to 20 mmol/litre.

This reduction in renal capability causes little problem until the system is stressed. The poor tubular function means that the water conserving ability is not good and dehydration occurs easily, producing a sudden rise in serum urea. This is compounded in many old people by an inadequate water intake in response to thirst. Because of the poor concentrating ability, the only way to ensure rapid clearance of drugs and substances which depend on renal excretion is to increase the urine volume. If this is done therapeutically it must be in the presence of an adequate fluid load or renal damage might occur.

Despite the fall in GFR with age, there is no rise in serum creatinine even though creatinine clearance parallels GFR. This is because as the BMR and muscle mass decrease, the creatinine load is reduced. Therefore, any increase in the serum creatinine points to a greater than anticipated impairment of renal function.

Even so, renal reserves are still considerable and able to handle most illnesses. Prostatic hypertrophy is common in elderly males and frequently causes postoperative urinary retention.

Mental function

Psychiatric problems associated with ageing are all too frequently overlooked. Deafness and poor sight may reduce the mental ability to interpret questions, the patient saying simply 'yes' or 'no' rather than taking the trouble to grasp and answer the questions properly. There may also be genuine acute or chronic brain failure. The former is non-specific, frequently appears with illness, might follow an anaesthetic and might be reversible. Chronic brain failure may be appreciated by the patient who finds his intellectual impairment both puzzling and distressing. Thankfully, the dement is usually unaware of his condition, but he gives an unreliable history. Many are able to function adequately both socially and physically until they are removed from their well known surroundings. About 15% of all those over 75 years suffer from chronic brain failure. If it is identified preoperatively, some investigations are worthwhile because there may be a reversible component of another chronic underlying disease (hypothyroidism, hyperthyroidism, pernicious anaemia, neoplasia, diabetes mellitus, chronic infection. See also Chapter 10).

Functional disorders are also common in the elderly with excessively sad, anxious, cheerful, hostile or suspicious moods. Depression is often overlooked because the classic presenting features may be absent. It may be endogenous or reactive (e.g. recent bereavement, chronic pain) and if it is identified it is worth treating. Depression often deteriorates postoperatively producing little cooperation with physiotherapists and nurses, the patient repeatedly wishing 'it was all over'.

Common concomitants of senile depression are hypochondriasis and paranoid states, the patient expressing exaggerated fears of a delusional type. Some patients may be unable to give informed consent (see Chapter 10).

Handling of drugs

It is well known empirically that old people handle and respond to many drugs in a different way to the young adult. The most frequently quoted example is that of diazepam which has an elimination half-life of 20 hours at 20 years and 85 hours at 80 years. The actual basis for these differences is not always understood in detail. Some of the possible reasons are outlined below, but it must be emphasized that in general, the elderly require a reduced dose of drug to produce a given effect, and that the same dose given to a number of elderly people produces a wide variation in response. The rule is therefore, small incremental doses to a level sufficient to achieve the desired pharmacodynamic response, and the assumption (for safety) that the clearance of the drug will be impaired.

Pharmacokinetics

Clearance. With age the GFR decreases and the ability of the tubules to modify the filtrate is impaired. This causes serious reductions in the clearance of most drugs including curare, gallamine, digoxin, lithium, and most antibiotics. The renal clearance of pancuronium in a 75 year old is approximately half that of a 20 year old.

There is also a reduction in the rate of drug metabolism by the liver which is thought to be due to a combination of decreased hepatic blood flow and decreased enzyme activity. Propranolol is the most commonly quoted example of a drug which can achieve unexpectedly high plasma concentrations in the elderly because of decreased hepatic blood flow.

Volume of distribution. After the age of 65 years, whatever the previous level of obesity, there is atrophy of subcutaneous fat. There is also a 10–20% reduction of body water and muscle mass. Distribution of drugs into fat soluble and water soluble compartments is therefore very variable and a dose based on body weight alone can produce unpredictable results.

The concentration of active drug is also affected by protein binding and both the albumin and globulin levels change with age. The classic example of this is pethidine, whose bound fraction is halved between the ages of 30 years and 75 years.

The increased proportion of unbound drug implies that greater quantities and concentrations of the drug are presented to the liver and kidney. Consequently, although a higher serum concentration is achieved with a given dose, the effective duration of pharmacodynamic action may be reduced.

In general, features which produce an extension of the elimination half-life make the geriatric patient very susceptible to accumulation from repeated doses (e.g. digoxin).

Pharmacodynamics

The pharmacodynamic effect of a given serum concentration of a drug depends both on the number of receptors and the magnitude of their response. Evidence in this area is conflicting. The receptor response to non-depolarizing muscle relaxants given on a body weight basis has been regarded as independent of age for many years. On the other hand, decreases in both adrenergic and cholinergic receptor density and sensitivity have been invoked to explain attentuated responses to catecholamines, sympathetic nervous system activity and atropine.

ANAESTHETIC MANAGEMENT

PREOPERATIVE CONSIDERATIONS

History

Taking an adequate history can be difficult because of the problems associated with ageing. When hearing is impaired, if the doctor sits in a good light, speaks slowly, loudly and with good mouth movements, conversation is usually greatly improved. Many patients unconsciously develop a facility for lip reading over the years. In a patient who is feeble minded, the history must be obtained from relatives. With a patient of sound mind, probe into his normal life style, his ability to climb stairs, his eating and his drinking habits, and his general health. Ask specifically about symptoms associated with heart disease, chest disease, diabetes, anaemia and thyroid function (q.v.). Often it is very difficult to separate pathology from normal 'wear and tear'. Frequency and nocturia secondary to prostatic hypertrophy may predict postoperative urinary retention. Ask about falls at home. These are not usually due to external hazards but reflect instability associated with impaired general health. Although a remedial cause may not be found, it may alert the anaesthetist to an increased risk of surgery for the patient. Make an assessment of the patient's biological (as opposed to chronological) age.

Many patients present on existing medications. These can both indicate the presence of certain underlying conditions (which the patient may not be aware of) and give a warning of possible drug interactions. Of particular danger in the elderly is the combination of digoxin and diuretics. Beta-adrenoceptor blockers may attentuate an already compromised autonomic nervous system.

Multiple pathology is exceedingly common. Worsening of one pathology may hasten the deterioration of others.

Examination

Examine the cardiovascular and pulmonary systems and treat any abnormalities as described in previous chapters (q.v.).

Neurological deficits should be recorded in the case notes, and if a stroke was recent remember the dangers of suxamethonium (q.v.). Assess the ability to move all joints, especially those in the neck and the jaw. Get the patient to put their head back to test for vertebrobasilar disease. Check the condition of the skin and review the possible drip sites.

Get the person to lie flat. He may not have done so for many years, and if he is unable to, spontaneous breathing in the supine or head down position is an unsuitable anaesthetic technique.

363

Dehydration is common in the sick elderly and presents with postural hypotension, dry mucosal surfaces and oliguria. They often have poor tissue turgor anyway.

Always look at the teeth. Solitary, fragile pegs can make intubation unusually awkward.

Investigations

The question of what preoperative investigations are appropriate in the elderly is often discussed. Apart from those suggested by the history and examination the following are probably satisfactory for a 'normal' elderly patient.

FBC. 20% of 'normals' in this age group have anaemia whose cause should be elicited.
U & E's. The elderly are often on diuretics, or have occult renal disease.
Blood sugar. Occult diabetes mellitus is common.
ECG. There is a high incidence of conduction defects, signs of ischaemia and hypertrophy.
CXR. This is useful as a baseline, particularly for major surgery. It not infrequently reveals occult pathology such as tuberculosis, pneumonia, tumours (primary or secondary) or an enlarged heart.
Serum thyroxine. Up to 5% of the over 65's have abnormal results.

Remember that many elderly patients are very anxious and frightened in a strange environment. A short time explaining the procedure is usually appreciated. It is important that the patient (and, or relatives) is aware of the reason for, and the anticipated benefit of, surgery. Many of these patients do have short term memory loss and despite explanations on the ward may arrive in the anaesthetic room completely unaware of what is to happen to them.

PEROPERATIVE PHASE

Pre-existing conditions should be treated as outlined in the appropriate chapters (q.v.). Gentleness and speed of operating with minimal exposure of tissues and careful haemostasis are the hallmarks of a successful outcome. Therefore be sure the surgeon is ready. Always take great care with venous cannulation as the veins are very fragile.

Premedication. The choice is obviously personal and it is frequently best omitted. Many psychotropic drugs have unpredictable effects and both hyoscine and atropine can cause confusion or unwanted tachydysrhythmias.

General or regional?

The argument as to which is best for the elderly has continued for many years. Papers have appeared supporting both techniques whilst others have claimed no difference, concentrating instead on the preoperative condition and the skill of the anaesthetist. In many instances it may be the postoperative care which is the crucial factor determining the outcome of surgery.

Regional. For success, the selection of patients is vital. They must be mentally lucid, able to lie flat for the appropriate period, be well motivated, understand what is involved, and be able to adopt the position necessary for the block to be performed.

Often it is possible to combine a regional block with a light narcosis with Entonox. Doing this, problems can arise when the patency of the airway is lost but the patient is not deep enough to accept an airway. There are only two solutions: allow the patient to wake up or deepen anaesthesia and insert an airway.

The commonest form of regional anaesthesia for operations below the umbilicus is either spinal or epidural block. An inability to flex the vertebral column and the presence of calcified ligaments may make the lateral or oblique approach easier and more successful than the midline approach. To be pleasant for the patient the lateral approach does require the liberal use of local anaesthetic around the lamina to anaesthetize the periostium, which is often scraped by the needle.

The reduced volume of local anaesthetic necessary for epidural anaesthesia has been described above. With intrathecal block the level of anaesthesia is effectively independent of age. With both techniques, the effect of a given dose is said to last longer because of reduced tissue washout by elderly spinal vessels.

The major complication of spinal and extradural block is hypotension, the degree of which is said to increase with age for a given level of block. Possibly this is due to a reduction in inherent vascular tone with age. Because of the dangers of fluid overload after the block has worn off it is reasonable to limit IV fluid loading to 500 mls and then to use small incremental doses of vasoconstrictors if necessary. If hypotension is associated with a bradycardia, ephedrine is the drug of choice, if it is not methoxamine is appropriate. It is important not to overshoot and produce a tachycardia associated with hypertension, thus increasing myocardial work sufficiently to cause myocardial ischaemia. The action of both these drugs IV is only a few minutes and repeat IV or IM doses are normally required.

General anaesthesia. There have been many papers published recording successful results with many different anaesthetic drug combinations. The obvious conclusion is that it is the care with which the anaesthetic is given which is more important than the agents chosen.

Induction. Pre-oxygenation is important in increasing the margin of safety. The circulation time in the elderly is much longer than in the young, and time must be allowed for incremental doses of drugs to work before others are given, otherwise gross overdosage is a real possibility. In the very decrepit, gas induction has been favoured by some authors but others have succeeded just as well with very slow IV induction.

Maintenance. Spontaneous ventilation can have several problems and is often only suitable for short procedures. In the edentulous with stiff necks, airway control can be very awkward. It can be difficult to get a good fit with a facemask and it can at times be advantageous to keep the dentures in. A nasopharyngeal airway often helps, but not infrequently intubation is necessary. Problems related to the use of volatile agents are cardiovascular depression (with hypotension and an increased tendency to dysrhythmias), ventilatory depression (increased $PaCO_2$ and reduced PaO_2, because of a reduced tidal volume and a high closing volume), and delayed recovery. A bonus claimed by some is that because the $PaCO_2$ rises, so does cerebral blood flow, thereby off-setting the effects of low blood pressure on cerebral perfusion.

IPPV is the method favoured for longer operations. Frequently, no relaxant is necessary either for intubation or ventilation. If a relaxant is needed, the required dose of a non-depolarizing agent is reduced and it has an extended duration of action. Intubating those at risk of inhalation of gastric contents requires the same 'crash induction' procedure as in the young. It is better to give a dose of suxamethonium rather than 'wait and see' if it is necessary.

The low basal metabolic rate and the reduced CO_2 production imply that it is very easy to hyperventilate the elderly and to drive their $PaCO_2$ to very low levels. This is dangerous both from its effect on the myocardium (low contractility and hypotension) and in decreasing cerebral blood flow. Monitoring end-tidal CO_2 is ideal, but intermittent blood gases (venous is adequate for CO_2 alone) are satisfactory. To maintain normocapnia often requires very low minute (and tidal) volumes. This can produce a lower PaO_2 than expected from the F_IO_2. Airway closure occurs and there is a danger of post-operative pneumonia. The solution is either to add inspired CO_2 and increase the minute volume when using a minute volume divider, or to employ some sort of partial rebreathing circuit with a large tidal volume.

Pay meticulous attention to body temperature and make every effort to keep the patient warm. This may require a warming blanket, warm IV fluids, humidified gases and having the theatre temperature higher than the surgeon would like it.

Induced hypotension in the elderly is a controversial subject. There have now been several reports suggesting that as a means of reducing intraoperative blood loss it is both effective and safe. Other authors have cautioned against it because of the risks of cerebral and myocardial ischaemia. With an awake patient monitored on a CM5 lead both these problems can probably be detected early. Whether this gives sufficient time to completely reverse them is not recorded. In the unconscious patient although the CM5 ECG lead can monitor the left ventricle, there is no convenient or reliable monitor of cerebral perfusion. Clinically, some would say that if the ear lobes were pink and well perfused then so is the brain. However, it is the practice of the authors to maintain the intraoperative blood pressure in the preoperative range ($\pm$ 30 mmHg) since this is known to be both adequate and safe for the patient.

The use of opioid supplements is standard practice. The quantity of drug required to produce a pharmacodynamic effect is often surprisingly low and the aged usually, (as a rule of thumb) only need half that required by a young adult.

Reversal of neuromuscular blockade can pose a problem because of atropine and its effect on the cardiovascular and central nervous systems. If atracurium is being used (this may in time prove to be the drug of choice) waiting for spontaneous reversal is feasible, but with the other non-depolarizing agents, glycopyrrolate may be a better choice than atropine.

Prior to reversal, if there are copious secretions a thorough bronchial toilet can improve pulmonary function in the immediate post-operative period until the patient is able to co-operate with the physiotherapist. If the ventilatory movements are incoordinated and weak, there should be no hesitation in proceeding to a period of post-operative ventilation. Once this decision has been made it is often best to continue overnight and aim to extubate early the next morning.

POSTOPERATIVE PHASE

In many ways this is the most important period of care. It is useless to expend effort on pre and intraoperative technique and to neglect the postoperative needs. Often the phrase is heard 'well they've had their chance, lets send them back'. This thoughtlessness is nonsense; if the surgery is worth doing, then good postoperative care is vital to success. Admittedly this is a difficult area because many specialized units have arbitrary age limits for intensive therapy. The best solution is to discuss the postoperative course *before* surgery with everyone involved and establish what will happen to the patient postoperatively. Often a good compromise is to have them 'specialled' in full view of the nursing station on a surgical ward. Always put the patient into a warm bed.

Regional blocks. The elderly often request to 'sit up' so that they can 'breathe better'. As local anaesthetics are metabolized, motor and sensory function can return whilst an autonomic block persists. Therefore, always beware of the postural fall in blood pressure when sitting these patients up. Propped up in bed, their cerebral perfusion cannot benefit from the physiological fall to the ground. It is imperative that nursing staff are alert to this possibility and do not attribute postoperative confusion secondary to cerebral ischaemia as the effects of surgery and anaesthesia upon old age.

General anaesthesia. Convention says that old people take longer to recover consciousness. This may be due to an effect at cellular level, a relative overdose or failure of the serum level to fall rapidly because of changes in the pharmacokinetic and pharmacodynamic properties of drugs. The clearance of neuromuscular blockers and opioids is reduced and both these groups of drugs can contribute to hypoxia (and therefore delayed recovery) by reducing alveolar ventilation. Think also of the possibility of hypoglycaemia or a cerebrovascular accident as causes of prolonged unconsciousness.

The ECG and blood pressure need monitoring in the first few postoperative hours. It is important that any hypotension is investigated and treated promptly. The usual causes are lack of circulating fluid volume, left ventricular failure, or hypoxia. Clinical examination and perusal of the anaesthetic chart can usually identify which it is. As with regional blockade, always be careful of hypotension occurring in the sitting position because of the consequent cerebral ischaemia. Giving steroids empirically to a hypotensive patient (assuming them to be Addisonian) *is not* a first line of management.

For postoperative analgesia (as outlined above), the elderly usually need less opioids than the young. After their administration it is essential that the ventilation is monitored. Epidurals (both local and opioid) have been used with success but can be difficult technically to insert and may be unpredictable in extent (see above).

One of the most common complications is postoperative atelectasis and chest infection, which can be reduced in incidence by physiotherapy. Early mobilization helps to prevent the development of DVT's.

A frequently missed cause of confusion in the elderly male is postoperative urinary retention. If possible, he should be got out of bed, or sat on the edge of the bed regularly and offered a bottle. This requires two assistants in case a faint occurs. With those who have to remain in bed, catheterization is often inevitable.

FURTHER READING

Adams, G. (1977) The process of ageing. In: *Essentials of Geriatric Medicine.* Oxford University Press. 1–11.

Bromage, P.R. (1969) Ageing and epidural dose requirements. *Br. J. Anaesth.,* **41**, 1016–22.

Castleden, C.M., Kaye, C.M. & Parsons, R.L. (1975) The effect of age on plasma levels of propranolol and practolol in man. *Br. J. Clin. Pharmacol.,* **2**, 303–6.

Chan, K., Kendall, M.J., Mitchard, M. *et al.* (1975) The effect of ageing on plasma pethidine concentration. *Br. J. Clin. Pharmacol.,* **2**, 297–302.

Exton-Smith, A.N. (1978) Disturbances of autonomic regulation. *In*: Isaacs, B. (ed.), *Recent Advances in Geriatric Medicine.*Churchill Livingstone. 85–100.

James, O.F.W. (1982) Drugs and the ageing liver. *In*: Evans, J.G. & Caird, F.I. (eds), *Advanced Geriatric Medicine 2*. Pitman. 100–10.

Klotz, U., Avant, G.R., Hoyumpa, A. *et al.* (1975) The effects of age and liver disease on the disposition and elimination of diazepam in adult man. *J. Clin. Invest.,* **55**, 347–59.

McKenzie, P.J., Wishart, H.Y. & Smith, G. (1984) Long term outcome after repair of fractured neck of femur. *Br. J. Anaesth.,* **56**, 581–5.

McLeod, K., Hull, C.J. & Watson, M.J. (1979) Effects of ageing on the pharmacokinetics of pancuronium. *Br. J. Anaesth.,* **51**, 435–8.

Mellemgaard, K. (1966) The alveolar-arterial oxygen difference: its size and components in normal man. *Acta Physiol. Scand.,* **67**, 10–20.

Overstall, P.W. (1978) Falls in the elderly-epidemiology, aetiology and management. *In*: Isaacs, B. (ed.), *Recent Advances in Geriatric Medicine.*Churchill Livingstone. 61–72.

Pfeffer, J.M. (1981) Management of the acutely disturbed patient on the general ward. *Br. J. Hosp. Med.,* 73–8.

Pontoppidan, H. & Beecher, H.K. (1960) Progressive loss of protective reflexes in the airway with the advance of age. *J. Am. Med. Ass.,* **174**, 2209–13.

Quasha, A.L., Eger, E.I. & Tinker, J.H. (1980) Determination and applications of MAC. *Anesthesiology*, **53**, 315–34.

Richey, D.P. & Bender, A.D. (1977) Pharmacokinetic consequences of aging. *Ann. Rev. Pharmacol. Toxicol.,* **17**, 49–65.

Sewell, I.A. (1979) Surgery for the elderly: Part 1. *Hospital Update*, Sept., 791–812.

Sewell, I.A. (1979) Surgery for the elderly: Part 2 *Hospital Update*, Oct., 889–921.

Seymour, D.G. & Pringle, R. (1983) Post-operative complications in the elderly surgical patient. *Gerontology*, **29**, 262–70.

Sharrock, N.E. (1978) Epidural anesthetic dose responses in patients 20 to 80 years old. *Anesthesiology*, **49**, 425–8.

Tornebrandt, K. & Fletcher, R. (1982) Pre-operative chest x-rays in elderly patients. *Anaesthesia*, **37**, 901–2.

Wickstrom, I., Hohnberg, I. & Stefansson, T. (1982) Survival of female geriatric patients after hip fracture surgery: A comparison of 5 anesthetic methods. *Acta. Anaesthesiol. Scand.*, **26**, 607–14.

12/Miscellaneous conditions

Deafness

Blindness

The common cold

Migraine

Epidermolysis bullosa

Porphyria

Pregnancy
First trimester
Second trimester
Third trimester
The puerperium

Acquired immune deficiency
syndrome (AIDS)

Radiotherapy

Chemotherapy

Deafness

The social definition of deafness is a degree of hearing loss whereby everyday auditory communication is almost impossible. Hearing level can be defined by the difference in decibels (dB) between the faintest pure tone that the patient can hear and the normal reference level of the standard. Normal conversation is impaired at a 40 dB hearing loss and is inhibited almost completely at an 80 dB loss.

The types of hearing loss are classified as conductive, sensorineural and central, depending on the anatomical site of pathology.

Conductive deafness may be caused by impacted wax in the external canal, otitis media, otosclerosis, trauma or congenital malformations of the external and middle ear. Hearing is better with louder speech.

Sensorineural deafness results from lesions of the cochlea and/or the auditory division of the eighth cranial nerve. This may be congenital (e.g. rubella), hereditary, infective (labrinthitis), or secondary to trauma, drugs (e.g. antibiotics), tumour (acoustic neuroma, vestibular schwannoma) or occlusive vascular disease. A subacute, relapsing form is seen in Menière's syndrome where there is functional hearing loss accompanied by tinnitus and vertigo. Hearing in sensorineural deafness is improved by a quiet background but not by increasing the loudness of speech.

Central hearing disorders result from lesions of the central auditory pathways which may be due to pontomedullary infarction or multiple sclerosis. Speech is best heard when clearly spoken in a quiet environment.

History taking can obviously be extremely difficult but, optimize speech and environment according to the type of deafness. Speak slowly and clearly in full view of the patient who may be able to lip read to a degree. Enlist the help of relatives to obtain a history and to explain sympathetically what is going to happen. Determine which ear is the better of the two. If there is any ambiguity write down any important questions or explanations.

If the patient's hearing is improved with an aid ensure that this is worn to the anaesthetic room. It should be removed gently once the patient is asleep and kept in a safe place, with the batteries switched off, until it is needed again in the recovery ward. Local anaesthetics with the patient awake, are relatively contraindicated when the patient is so deaf that explanation is difficult, both because of possible poor co-operation from the patient and because of hindering the surgeon by constant shouting. Warn the recovery staff that the patient will not be woken by the usual spoken voice.

Blindness

The statutory definition for the purposes of registration as a blind person under the National Assistance Act (1948) is that the person is 'so blind as to be unable to perform any work for which eyesight is essential'. This takes into account both visual activity and field of vision. In the UK there are 200 000 people on the blind or partially sighted register but it has been estimated that there are three times this number who are not actually registered.

The commonest causes of blindness are senile macular degeneration, glaucoma, cataract, diabetic retinopathy and myopic degeneration. Anaesthetic considerations are those of the underlying condition (e.g. old age, diabetes mellitus), familiarizing with surroundings and sympathetic explanation of all procedures. The consent form should be formally witnessed and a mark will suffice for signature.

The common cold

In the broadest sense, the common cold refers to any undifferentiated upper or mild lower respiratory tract infection which may be characterized by sneezing, rhinorrhoea, nasal congestion, sore throat, cough and mild malaise. Fever is absent. Rhinoviruses are the commonest cause and are spread by droplet infection.

The incidence of the common cold is highest (6–12 per year) in pre-school children. Parents with young children have approximately 6 colds per year whereas other adults have 2 or 3 per year.

The infection is self-limiting and bacterial complications are uncommon. Although there is no hard data on the influence of surgery and anaesthesia on the likelihood of complications, it seems wisest to postpone major elective operations. Significant nasal obstruction may make airway management difficult, and fever may suggest bacterial complications or a mistaken diagnosis. For some emergency surgery local anaesthesia may be preferable, but if general anaesthesia is required endotracheal intubation is usually necessary for airway management. Nasal intubation should be avoided if possible; the inflamed mucosa bleeds easily and freely.

Migraine

Migrainous headaches affect up to 5% of the population. The headache is periodic, unilateral and throbbing and may be preceded by aura and accompanied by photophobia, ocular pain, visual disturbances, nausea and vomiting. Ergot preparations taken early may abort an attack. Migraine patients tend to be intelligent and know their diagnosis.

The attacks may be precipitated by ingestion of certain foods, anxiety or hunger. The latter two mean that they may be provoked perioperatively. A sedative, anxiolytic premedication, adequate hydration and normoglycaemia with intravenous dextrose infusion and a prophylactic antiemetic all help to prevent an attack.

Epidermolysis bullosa

This rare hereditary disorder of the skin affects 1 in 300 000 of the population. Bullae are formed in response to even minor trauma or lateral shearing forces to the skin. Mucous membranes are also susceptible and oesophageal strictures may occur. Survival beyond the second decade is unusual.

In general assessment look for signs of malnutrition and anaemia (q.v.). Electrolyte imbalance may be present in severe cases. Steroid therapy (q.v.) is not infrequent. Assess the airway; the tongue may be deformed causing a difficult intubation.

The most important anaesthetic implication is avoiding all trauma to skin and mucous membranes. The anaesthetic mask should be covered in soft cotton wadding, and lubricated with a gel containing hydrocortisone. Introduce and secure an endotracheal tube carefully, using a well lubricated laryngoscope and low pressure cuffed tube. Avoid oral airways and nasal tubes. Profuse bleeding from the buccal and soft palate may occur and the patient with an oesophageal stricture is more likely to regurgitate.

Venepuncture may be difficult and any IV site should be wrapped carefully. Avoid skin trauma when placing or removing ECG electrodes. Pad the sphygmomanometer cuff or use intra-arterial monitoring for major surgery. Throughout surgery, all pressure points should be well protected.

The incidence of porphyria is increased in epidermolysis bullosa and therefore barbiturates may be best avoided. Ketamine may be useful, especially if muscle relaxation is not required. Regional anaesthesia is often not possible because of infected bullae and local infiltration may cause sloughing.

Porphyria

BIOCHEMISTRY

The term porphyria is used to describe any of a group of disturbances of porphyrin metabolism which are characterized by a marked increase in the formation and excretion of porphyrins or their precursors. The disease can vary in severity from the harmless to the life-threatening and it may be genetically inherited or directly acquired.

Porphyrins are the basis of the respiratory pigments of animals and plants. They are cyclic compounds formed from four pyrrole rings which complex easily with metallic ions. The haem of haemoglobin is an iron porphyrin. The manufacture of haem (100 mg/day in the liver, 300 mg/day in the bone marrow and erythrocytes) commences with a condensation of glycine and succinyl Coenzyme A. There are then several enzyme-dependent steps before the final product. If one enzyme is overactive, or another fails to convert the substrate supplied to it, then excess metabolic intermediates and/or porphyrins enter the blood, urine (uroporphyrins) or faeces (coproporphyrins).

The exact mechanism which explains the overproduction of porphyrins and/or their precursors has not yet been definitely identified. One theory is that the activity of aminolevulinic acid synthetase (the rate controlling enzyme in porphyrin synthesis) is controlled by a repressor gene. In porphyria, this repressor gene is thought to be either abnormal or only partially effective (genetic form) or adversely affected by toxins, drugs, alcohol, liver disease or blood dyscrasias (acquired form). The two effects can occur together or enzyme-inducing drugs (especially the barbiturates) can enhance the activity of aminolevulinic acid synthetase, possibly producing 'crises'.

SYMPTOMS

Abnormalities of porphyrin metabolism present clinically in a variety of ways. There are two major groups of symptoms which can exist singly or in combination.

The cutaneous manifestations are seen in areas heavily exposed to sunlight and there is a wide variation in the degree of exposure which produces lesions. Increased pigmentation of the hair and skin is common, and the skin may develop vesicles and bullae which burst, become infected and cause scarring. The skin is also fragile and re-covers badly from trauma. It is thought that the porphyrins are photosensitizing agents because of their ability to absorb radiant energy.

The other symptoms are referable to the alimentary tract, car-diovascular system and nervous system. These are all supposedly due to episodes of demyelination. The process by which this occurs is unclear but, it is thought that the oxidized products of porphyrin and its precursors affect the intracellular metabolism of neurones throughout the body. These symptoms appear as acute attacks which may, or may not, have an identifiable precipitating cause. They are more frequent during pregnancy. Abdominal pain is of acute onset, colicky or continuous and very severe. Many patients appear to have an 'acute abdomen'. The commonest CVS abnormalities are an un-explained sinus tachycardia possibly with hypertension and auto-nomic instability. All parts of the nervous system can be affected but motor nerves are more affected than sensory, and long tracts rather more than short. The commonest disturbance is motor weakness of the limbs: in severe cases the patient may become quadriplegic with respiratory muscle paralysis. Epilepsy and mental disturbances of all types occur. There may be electrolyte changes, particularly hypo-natraemia. George III (famous for shaking hands with trees) is thought, in retrospect, to have possibly had porphyria. *It is in the pre-cipitation of these neurological symptoms that some anaesthetic agents are dangerous.* Treatment of an acute attack is the province of the specialist. Currently the patients are well hydrated, given glucose, analgesics and haematin infusions.

CLASSIFICATION

The various syndromes are described by the site of the lesion (hepa-tic or erythropoietic), the geographical distribution of disease, the clinical presentation, and the cause of the defect. Classification is therefore difficult and differs in detail from one authority to another. A simplified working classification is shown in Fig. 12.1 in which the

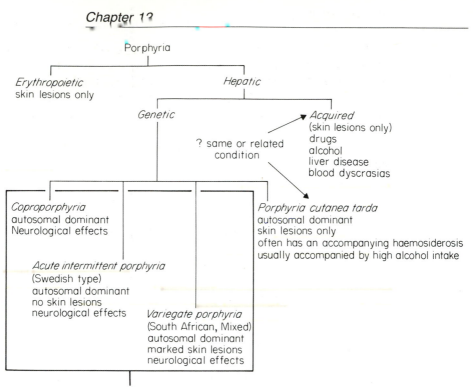

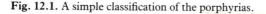

GROUPS AT RISK DURING ANAESTHESIA

Fig. 12.1. A simple classification of the porphyrias.

'at risk' groups, who exhibit neurological symptoms, are outlined. All the diseases are rare.

Acute intermittent porphyria. The history is of attacks and remissions which commence after puberty or in the early adult years (20–30 years). Many may be asymptomatic throughout their entire life. Skin lesions are absent. Psychiatric and emotional disturbances are common. Some have a history of a previous negative laparotomy. Their urine turns to a port wine colour on standing.

Variegate porphyria. This always has marked, chronic, cutaneous lesions and neurological symptoms which are similar to acute intermittent porphyria. However, the pattern of porphyrin excretion is different.

Coproporphyria. This is a very rare condition, clinically indistinguishable from acute intermittent porphyria but with dissimilar biochemistry.

ANAESTHETIC MANAGEMENT

Because of the rarity of these conditions there is a limited anaesthetic literature, and even that is at times contradictory.

376

All the 'at risk' groups with possible neurological symptoms can be screened for by a rapid urine test. This should be done on all individuals who are either themselves, or are related to, a person thought to have the condition. Once a patient is known to be positive, the anaesthetic becomes an exercise in avoiding risk factors and managing residual complications from previous attacks. Preoperative assessment needs to concentrate on the mental state, neurological deficits and the cardiovascular system. In those with cutaneous lesions, skin care, asepsis and the siting of intravenous lines is obviously important. So also is the frequency of inflation of BP cuffs and avoiding trauma induced by a face mask.

Since dehydration has itself been invoked as a trigger a preoperative dextrose (10%) infusion is sensible. Dextrose is chosen because it reputedly suppresses porphyrin enzyme activity. Drugs reported to have precipitated a crisis are *barbiturates*, sex hormones, *sulphonamides*, griseofulvin, *diazepam*, phenytoin, pentazocine, ergot preparations and possibly *pancuronium*. Drugs which are said to be safe are chlorpromazine, promethazine, droperidol, pethidine, fentanyl, morphine, nitrous oxide, the volatile agents, suxamethonium, curare, atropine and neostigmine. Abnormal neurological and cardiovascular findings should be dealt with as described elsewhere.

Unfortunately, it is possible to anaesthetize an unknown porphyric and unwittingly precipitate an acute attack, although progression to the well-developed symptomatology does not always occur. It should be thought of as a possible diagnosis in a patient who remains paralysed or comatose postoperatively, develops peripheral nerve lesions or who awakes with severe abdominal pain.

Any patient found to have porphyria needs his parents, siblings and children referring for screening.

Pregnancy

This section does not attempt to describe methods of analgesia for childbirth or anaesthesia for caesarean section, which have full coverage in many other books.

Anaesthesia during pregnancy, other than for the delivery of the baby, is required in about 2% of pregnancies. This may be for improving the survival of the foetus, e.g. insertion of Shirodkhar suture, for conditions which are aggravated by pregnancy, e.g. ovarian cysts (1 to 2300 pregnancies) or for coincidental life-threatening situations, e.g. acute appendicitis (1 in 1429 pregnancies) or more rarely intracranial tumours, beri-aneurysms, hyperthryoidism, valvular heart disease or phaeochromocytoma. The anaesthetic problems differ depending upon the gestation of the foetus.

377

First trimester

In humans, the critical period for foetal organogenesis is from 12 to 60 days. *In vitro*, and in some animal models, it has been found that anaesthetics can depress cell growth, slow cell division, cause abnormal cell division and interfere with DNA synthesis. However, in humans, in normal doses, there is no evidence that any anaesthetic agent is teratogenic, carcinogenic or adversely affects the subsequent mental and neurological development of the child. There are therefore, a wide range of premedications and general and regional anaesthetic techniques which can be used.

The maternal physiological changes of pregnancy although starting effectively with conception are not well advanced during the first trimester. The plasma and erythrocyte volumes increase progressively from the sixth week producing a small reduction in hematocrit. Of more importance is the early occurrence of a hypercoagulable state: platelets are increased by 23 000 mm^3, and the fibrinogen levels and clotting factor activities rise. Thus there is a predisposition to thromboembolic complications. Prophylaxis by the intraoperative use of stockings or pneumatic leggings is recommended. The use of subcutaneous heparin is controversial and varies from hospital to hospital.

By the end of the first trimester the ventilatory rate and tidal volume are each increased by 10%. This is disproportionate to the increase in metabolic rate so there is a fall in the $PaCO_2$. Gastric acid secretion is reduced and the risk of regurgitation is not increased until the late second or third trimester. Crash induction as a routine is unnecessary and the use of a facemask is permissible.

The main dangers to the foetus throughout pregnancy are hypoxia and acidosis. These are preventable during anaesthesia by avoiding maternal hypoxia, maternal hypotension (low placental blood flow) and excessive rises in maternal $PaCO_2$. There are therefore, obvious problems with prolonged spontaneous ventilation using volatile anaesthetics. These both drop the maternal blood pressure and cause a rise in the $PaCO_2$. If hypotension occurring during regional anaesthesia requires a vasoconstrictor, methoxamine is contraindicated because it also constricts placental blood vessels. Ephedrine is the drug of choice.

The other problem of all operative procedures carried out during pregnancy is the prevention of premature labour. Advice on the possibility of a miscarriage and the advisability of beta$_2$ adrenoceptor stimulants (salbutamol, ritodrine, terbutaline) should be sought from the obstetrician. These drugs can cause peripheral tremor, cardiac dysrhythmias, pulmonary oedema and hypokalaemia in the mother.

Their presence aggravates the incidence of <u>ventricular ectopics</u> with <u>halothane.</u> A corollary of the use of these drugs is that non-specific beta-adrenoceptor blockers should not be used to control hypertension in pregnant patients. Sedation with phenobarbitone and then hydralazine would be the treatment of choice.

Never do X-rays unless absolutely necessary.

Second trimester

These three months are the <u>best time to perform an operation if it has to be done at some time during pregnancy</u>. Always check by dates and scan reports that the pregnancy actually is in the second trimester, particularly for non-urgent surgery. When the patient is threatening to miscarry, it is often wise to delay the operation if possible, until the outcome is known.

The physiological changes in the third trimester are given below. During the second trimester they are approached gradually from the effective normality of the first trimester. The main effect these changes have on the conduct of anaesthesia which differs from the first trimester is the question of whether or not to intubate for all general anaesthetics. It is the authors' practice to manage patients early in the second trimester who have no symptoms of oesophageal reflux and who are undergoing short procedures (e.g. for insertion of Shirodkhar suture) on a face mask. All other cases are intubated.

Third trimester

The physiological changes in the mother are now well advanced and itemized below.

RS. • The minute volume increases by 40%
 • The $PaCO_2$ falls to approximately 30 mmHg (4.0 kPa)
 • The expiratory reserve volume falls by 20%
 • Breathlessness is common and reduces after the 36th week as the foetal head descends into the pelvis

CVS. • 40% increase in cardiac output
 • The resting heart rate is increased to 85–90 beats/minute
 • The total circulating haemoglobin rises by 20% but the Hb concentration falls to 11 g% at term because of the disproportionate rise in plasma volume (45%)
 • The gravid uterus can compress both the inferior vena cava and the aorta
 • Innocent systolic flow murmurs can occur

379

- There may be mild peripheral oedema from salt and water retention

GIT. • Many mothers at term experience heartburn
  - There is relaxation of the oesophageal sphincter and reduced gastric motility. The stomach can never be assumed to be empty
  - There is normally an overall weight gain of 10–12 kg.

Investigations

FBC. The Hb is usually low (see above). The white cell count is normal. The platelet count is increased by over 100 000 which, in combination with the uterus pressing on the iliac veins, predisposes to DVT and pulmonary embolism.

Plasma protein. The actual concentration declines, (albumin slightly more than globulin), but the total amount in the circulation is increased.

U & E's There should be no abnormality.

CXR. This should not be required routinely. The diaphragm is raised causing decreased vertical and increased transverse diameters of the thorax. Lung markings are more prominent due to increased blood in the pulmonary vessels. The heart is displaced laterally.

ECG. This almost invariably shows a sinus tachycardia. The change in the position of the heart may cause a large Q-wave and inverted T waves in Lead III.

ANAESTHETIC MANAGEMENT

This is identical to that for a caesarean section, and can be either regional or general. Remember the risk of regurgitation and aspiration. Give antacids to raise the pH of gastric contents. Always use a rapid induction sequence with a general anaesthetic. If there is little chance that the baby will be delivered there is no contraindication to the use of sedative premedication or opioids. If being brought from a general surgical ward, ensure that she is transported preoperatively and nursed postoperatively in the lateral position to avoid caval compression. The foetal heart rate can be monitored intraoperatively. Remind the surgeon that it is necessary to operate with a tilted or wedged table.

The puerperium

Although the peurperium strictly extends for the 6–8 weeks it takes for the pelvic organs to return to their pre-pregnancy state, the physiological changes of pregnancy (haemodynamic, ventilatory etc) return to normal within a few days. The anaesthetic considerations are mainly related to breast feeding.

Try to ensure that the mother has a private room so that she can continue to feed the baby without disturbing other patients. Organize the timing of the operation to fit in with feeding the baby shortly beforehand. During the preoperative starve avoid dehydration (which may cause the milk to dry up), by giving IV fluids if necessary.

Give an anaesthetic unlikely to cause postoperative nausea and vomiting. No anaesthetic drugs are absolutely contraindicated in patients who are breast feeding but it should be remembered that benzodiazepines and opioids are excreted in breast milk and may cause somnolence in the baby. It is unlikely with the quantities excreted that narcotics would cause ventilatory depression in the baby. Encourage early mobilization to prevent DVT.

Acquired immune deficiency syndrome (AIDS)

This is a disease of the present decade having first presented in 1981. Its incidence is increasing exponentially. There have now been 3000 cases reported in the USA and 300 in Western Europe. The largest 'at risk' groups are homosexual and bisexual men and intravenous drug addicts. Two smaller groups are Haitians and haemophiliacs.

The disease is characterized by opportunist bacterial, fungal, protozoal and viral infections in all organs of the body. Those in the chest are particularly dangerous. In addition, there is a high incidence of Kaposi's sarcoma (25% of cases). There are abnormalities of both T and B cell lymphocyte systems. Recently a Pre-AIDS syndrome has been described with fever, generalized lymphadenopathy and weight loss.

The causative virus has now been identified and it is known to be transmitted in blood and blood products. A working party has recommended that in general it is appropriate when dealing with these patients to take the same precautions as for cases of hepatitis B (see Chapter 4).

Radiotherapy

The patients considered in this group fall into two categories: those having incidental surgery during or after a course of radiotherapy, and those having anaesthesia for the radiotherapeutic procedures themselves. Their problems can be considered together.

The effect of radiation *per se* is to damage tissue. Depending on the organ affected and the dose of radiation, repair is by the inflammatory response and fibrosis or by repopulation with cells derived from the surviving pool. Modern treatments try to maximize therapeutic damage whilst minimizing the dose to normal tissues, by keeping the treatment volume to a minimum.

The procedure most likely to cause bone marrow failure and radiation sickness is whole body irradiation. This is used either to treat disseminated disease or to deliberately cause an aplastic anaemia by bone marrow depression, in which case, bone marrow transplantation follows treatment.

Any radiotherapy may precipitate radiation sickness but patients are very variable in their tolerance. The first phase of radiation sickness is at the time of the release of toxic products from necrosis of neoplasms, white blood cells and intestinal epithelium. It occurs within hours after exposure and presents with vomiting, anorexia and lethargy. Despite antiemetics, there can be associated electrolyte changes and dehydration.

Other early complications are due to the inflammatory oedema which may aggravate the symptoms of the malignancy (e.g. stridor from carcinoma of the larynx) or to rapid regression of the tumour (e.g. lymphoma causing bowel perforation because the bowel has not had time to regenerate). The complications of radiation enteritis (perforation, fistula, toxic necrosis, sepsis) occur months to years later and can necessitate laparotomy.

The depression of bone marrow is dose dependent. All cell lines are affected and although lymphopenia can occur within hours, the maximum depression of the immune system and the haemoglobin concentration is not until 3–4 weeks later. Any surgery needed in these patients should therefore be done immediately, or postponed until the bone marrow has recovered. Any patient who has had whole body radiation ought to be assumed to be immunosuppressed and treated as a case of bone marrow failure (q.v.) until proved otherwise. Defects in other organ systems are less common and should be treated appropriately.

Patients with laryngeal neoplasms usually have radiotherapy prior to surgery. Its extent depends upon the involvement of lymph nodes and the degree of local spread. Initially, after exposure, the tissues become inflamed sometimes with gross oedema of the larynx, epiglottis and pharynx. The mucosa distorts the superficial anatomy and it bleeds very easily following minor trauma (e.g. intubation). The increase in tissue oedema following extubation at this stage has been reported, on occasions, to be life-threatening. It has been suggested that extubation should be preceded by dexamethasone.

Later (after 1 month) the oedema abates and the inflammation is gradually replaced by fibrous tissue. These fibrous bands can fix tissues together, distort the anatomy, prevent adequate laryngoscopy, and make the airway difficult to manage. A smaller endotracheal tube than usual may be required. Everybody who has had radiation to the larynx must be regarded as a potentially difficult intubation and the appropriate steps must be taken.

Any patient who has had radiotherapy to the structures in the neck (including those treated with radioiodine) needs their serum thyroxine to be checked.

Radiation directed at structures on, or in, the thorax produces radiation pneumonitis and subsequent fibrosis (see Chapter 2). A subacute pneumonitis may arise at any time between 2 and 9 months after treatment. It presents with cough and dyspnoea and is often relieved by steroids. Vascular damage from radiotherapy alters the ventilation/perfusion relationship in the lungs. Arterial blood gas measurement gives a better guide to the physiological defect than does CXR. Investigations are most likely to reveal mild hypoxia and normocapnia and a restrictive pattern of breathing.

Radiation directed at structures in the mediastinum can affect the conducting system of the heart and cause fibrosis which may distort the carina and major bronchi. This has obvious implications for the use of double lumen tubes and endobronchial intubation. After irradiation several years previously (e.g. following mastectomy) there is, not infrequently, a diffuse fibrosis of the upper lobe which can mimic tuberculosis radiologically.

Irradiation of the head to prevent the growth of cerebral deposits may result in lethargy, sleepiness, anorexia and irritability. Baldness is common. To save embarrassment, allow patients to wear their wigs to the anaesthetic room.

There is very little literature on the advantages and disadvantages of any particular anaesthetic technique for these patients as regards the effectiveness of radiotherapy. It is known that for radiotherapy to be as effective as possible the target area requires a good supply of oxygenated blood. This increases the concentration of super oxides and free radicals formed. Theoretically, there is a greater chance of toxic liver damage from any compound which is metabolized in the liver which is capable of producing free radicals (e.g. halothane).

The major anaesthetic considerations (apart from the specific problems of a given condition) therefore fall into two broad categories. One is the familiar problems which are associated with repeated anaesthesia (but superimposed on potential bone marrow suppression) and the need to avoid certain agents, notably halothane. The other is the problem of administering anaesthesia at a distance, which is usually only necessary in children. The child often presents twice weekly, or even daily, for a course of treatment as a day case. The patient is usually unhappy and the parent is understandably anxious. Both need sympathy and reassurance appropriate to their positions, insight and intelligence. The choice or necessity of premedication depends upon the combination of anaesthetist, patient and parent.

It is obvious that the anaesthetist must avoid receiving radiation himself. This may imply that the patient cannot be viewed directly, but only on a television screen or through a lead-glassed window. Monitoring aids (e.g. ECG, pulse monitor, BP monitor, oxygen meter, CO_2 meter) are therefore desirable. The anaesthetist must be prepared to interrupt treatment if the adequacy of breathing is in doubt. Opinion is divided over the best anaesthetic technique. Some prefer an unintubated patient spontaneously breathing O_2, N_2O and a volatile agent whilst others prefer to maintain narcosis with IM ketamine and allow the patient to breathe air. Many anaesthetists do, however, feel that the airway is only secure enough if the patient is intubated.

Chemotherapy

Chemotherapy is used to treat a wide range of malignancies. Such patients frequently know or suspect their likely outcome. They therefore respond well to all medical personnel who take the time to explain what is going to happen in as sympathetic a manner as is appropriate for the individual. Many of them have episodes of depression or are on antidepressants (q.v.).

The main adverse effect of all these drugs is on the bone marrow, GIT, and hair follicles. Dangers are, therefore, compromised immunity, coagulation defects and anaemia (from both depressed bone marrow and GIT blood loss (see Chapter 9). Nitrous oxide appears to increase the marrow toxicity. This has come to light with attempts at perioperative chemotherapy as an adjuvant in carcinoma of the breast. It may, therefore, be advisable to avoid nitrous oxide in patients who are currently having chemotherapy.

More specific problems are that the alkylating agents can both produce pulmonary fibrosis and inhibit plasma cholinesterase and that the anti-metabolites depress both renal and hepatic function. Daunorubicin (an antibiotic which complexes with DNA) has been found to cause a dose-related cardiomyopathy which has a mortality of over 50% and has been shown, when not fatal, to last for over a year or two.

Of particular interest to the anaesthetist is bleomycin, a cytotoxic antibiotic used in the treatment of teratoma. After treatment with this drug, patients develop a peculiar sensitivity to the inspired F_IO_2, the concentrations frequently used during routine anaesthesia producing a picture indistinguishable from pulmonary oxygen toxicity. However, several reports have now demonstrated that an F_IO_2 of up to 25% is safe and that colloids rather than crystalloids as IV replacement fluids are associated with a reduced incidence of lung damage. The time when it is safe to increase the F_IO_2 after the cessation of bleomycin has not been established, a fatality having been recorded up to 1 year after stopping it.

Many patients having chemotherapy will also at some time have radiotherapy (q.v.).

FURTHER READING

Allen, S.C., Riddel, G.S. & Butchart, E.G. (1981) Bleomycin therapy and anaesthesia. *Anaesthesia*, **36**, 60–3.

Cohen, J. (1984) AIDS—a review. *Br. J. Hosp. Med.*, **31**, 250–9.

Dean, G. (1971) *The Porphyrias*. 2nd edn. Pitman Medical.

Eiseman, B. & Bond, V. (1978) Surgical care of nuclear casualties. *Surg. Gynecol. Obstet.*, **146**, 877–84.

Fell, R.H. (1980) Migraine and surgery: Avoidance of trigger mechanisms. *Anaesthesia*, **35**, 1006–7.

Kim, Y.H. & Fayos, J.V. (1981) Radiation tolerance of the cervical spinal cord. *Radiology*, **139**, 473–8.

Magnus, I.A. (1984) Drugs and porphyria. *Br. Med. J.*, **228**, 1474–5.

Pederson, H. & Finster, M. (1979) Anesthetic risk in the pregnant surgical patient. *Anesthesiology*, **51**, 439–51.

Selvin, B.L. (1981) Cancer chemotherapy: Implications for the anesthesiologist. *Anesth. Analg.*, **60**, 425–34.

Smith, G.B. & Shribman, A.J. (1984) Anaesthesia and severe skin disease. *Anaesthesia*, **39**, 443–55.

Tomlinson, A.A. (1983) Recessive dystrophic epidermolysis bullosa. *Anaesthesia*, **38**, 485–91.

Appendix: General further reading

Atkinson, R.S., Rushman G.B. & Lee J.A. (1982) *A Synopsis of Anaesthesia*, 9th edn. Wright.

Gray, T.C., Nunn, J.F. & Utting, J.E. (1980) *General Anaesthesia*, 4th edn, Vols. 1 & 2. Butterworths.

Katz, J., Benumof, J. & Kadis, L.B. (1981) *Anesthesia and Uncommon Diseases*, 2nd edn. W.B. Saunders Co.

Medicine (1978 *et seq.*) The Monthly Add-on Journal, 3rd Series. Medical Education (International) Ltd.

Miller, R.D. (1981) *Anesthesia*, Vols. 1 & 2. Churchill Livingstone.

Petersdorf, R.G., Adams, R.D., Braunwald, E. *et al.* (1983) *Harrison's Principles of Internal Medicine*, 10th edn. McGraw-Hill Book Co.

Prys-Roberts, C. (1980) *The Circulation in Anaesthesia: applied physiology and pharmacology*. Blackwell Scientific Publications.

Stoelting, R.K. & Dierdorf, S.F. (1983) *Anesthesia and Co-Existing Disease*. Churchill Livingstone.

Abbreviations

ACD	acid citrate dextose
Acetyl Co A	acetyl coenzyme A
ACTH	adrenocorticotrophic hormone
ADH	antidiuretic hormone
AF	atrial fibrillation
AHG	antihaemophilic globulin
AIDS	acquired immune deficiency syndrome
AMP	adenosine monophosphate
ALT	alanine transaminase
AP	antero-posterior
ARDS	adult respiratory distress syndrome
ASD	atrial septal defect
AST	aspartate transaminase
ATP	adenosine triphosphate
ATPS	ambient temperature and pressure saturated
A-V	atrioventricular
A-V	arterio-venous
BMR	basal metabolic rate
BP	blood pressure
BTPS	body temperature and pressure saturated
°C	degrees Centigrade
Ca^{++}	calcium
CAT	computerized axial tomography
CCF	congestive cardiac failure
CM5	chest-manubrium-V_5
CNS	central nervous system
COAD	chronic obstructive airways disease
CO_2	carbon dioxide
COMT	catechol-o-methyl transferase
CPAP	continuous positive airways pressure
CPD	citrate phosphate dextrose
CPK	creatine phosphokinase
CRF	chronic renal failure
CSF	cerebrospinal fluid
CVA	cerebrovascular accident
CVP	central venous pressure

387

CVS	cardiovascular system
CXR	chest X-ray
dB	decibel
DC	direct current
1,25-DHCC	1,25-dihydroxycholecalciferol
DIC	disseminated intravascular coagulation
DNA	deoxyribonucleic acid
dP/dt	rate of change of pressure
2,3 DPG	2,3 diphosphoglycerate
DVT	deep vein thrombosis
ECG	electrocardiogram
EDV	end diastolic volume
EEG	electroencephalogram
ERV	expiratory reserve volume
ESR	erythrocyte sedimentation rate
FBC	full blood count
FEV_1	forced expiratory volume in the first second of expiration
FFP	fresh frozen plasma
F_1O_2	fractional inspired oxygen
FRC	functional residual capacity
FSH	follicle stimulating hormone
FVC	forced vital capacity
g	gram
GFR	glomerular filtration rate
GGT	gamma glutamyl transferase
GI	gastrointestinal
GIT	gastrointestinal tract
G-6-PD	glucose-6-phosphate deficiency
GU	genito-urinary
Hb	haemoglobin
HB_sAg	hepatitis B surface antigen
HLA	human leucocyte antigen
H_2O	water
HOCM	hypertrophic obstructive cardiomyopathy
HPPF	human plasma protein fraction
ICP	intracranial pressure
ICU	intensive care unit
IM	intramuscular
IMV	intermittent mandatory ventilation
IPPV	intermittent positive pressure ventilation
IV	intravenous
IVC	inferior vena cava
JVP	jugular venous pressure
K^+	potassium

388

kg	kilogram
kPa	kilopascal
LAP	left atrial pressure
LATS	long acting thyroid stimulator
LBBB	left bundle branch block
LDH	lactic dehydrogenase
LFTs	liver function tests
LH	luteinizing hormone
LS	locomotor system
LSD	lysergic acid diethylamide
LVEDP	left ventricular end diastolic pressure
LVF	left ventricular failure
MAOI	monoamine oxidase inhibitors
MCV	mean corpuscular volume
MH	malignant hyperpyrexia
mmHg	millimetres of mercury
MSH	melanocyte stimulating hormone
MW	molecular weight
Na^+	sodium
NAD	nicotinamide-adenine-dinucleotide
NADP	nicotinamide-adenine-dinucleotide-phosphate
NB	note bene
N_2O	nitrous oxide
NS	nervous system
O_2	oxygen
ODA	operating department assistant
P_{50}	partial pressure at 50% saturation (of haemoglobin)
PA	pulmonary artery
P-A	posterior-anterior
$PaCO_2$	arterial partial pressure of carbon dioxide
PaO_2	arterial partial pressure of oxygen
PAS	para-aminosalicyclic acid
PAT	paroxysmal atrial tachycardia
PAWP	pulmonary artery wedge pressure
PDA	patent ductus arteriosus
PEEP	positive end expiratory pressure
PEFR	peak expiratory flow rate
PND	paroxysmal nocturnal dyspnoea
PRV	polycythaemia rubra vera
PTH	parathormone
$P_{\bar{v}}O_2$	mixed venous partial pressure of oxygen
RBBB	right bundle branch block
RF	regurgitant fraction
RS	respiratory system

389

RV	right ventricle
RVEDP	right ventricular end diastolic pressure
RVF	right ventricular failure
S-A	sino-atrial
SBE	subacute bacterial endocarditis
SLE	systemic lupus erythematosus
SNP	sodium nitroprusside
SVC	superior vena cava
SVT	supraventricular tachycardia
TLC	total lung capacity
TRH	thyrotrophin releasing hormone
TSH	thyroid stimulating hormone
U & Es	urea and electrolytes
UK	United Kingdom
VC	vital capacity
V_D	physiological dead space
VEs	ventricular extrasystoles
VF	ventricular fibrillation
VMA	vanillyl mandelic acid
VSD	ventricular septal defect
V_T	tidal volume
VT	ventricular tachycardia
WCC	white cell count

Index

Abbreviations 387–90
Abdominal X-rays in jaundice 171
Acid-citrate-dextrose 314
Acquired immune deficiency syndrome,
  management 381
Acromegaly 223–5
  airway management 225
  anaesthetic management 225
  examination 224
  features 223
  investigations 224–5
  preoperative considerations 224–5
Addison's disease 232–3
Adrenal glands 225–35
  adrenocortical insufficiency 232–3
  Conn's syndrome 234–5
  Cushing's syndrome 229–32
  iatrogenic adrenocortical suppression 233–4
  phaeochromocytoma 226–8
Adrenocortical insufficiency 232–3
  anaesthetic management 233
  preoperative considerations 232–3
Adrenocortical suppression, iatrogenic 233–4
Affective disorders and anaesthesia 341–2
Ageing, pattern 355–62
  see also Old age and anaesthesia
AIDS, management 381
Alanine transaminase, serum concentrations, liver
  disease 169
Alcohol abuse and anaesthesia 352–3
Aldosterone
  production, adrenal cortex 229
  secretion see Conn's syndrome
Alkaline phosphatase levels in liver disease 169
Allergic reactions to blood transfusion 316
Aminophylline, asthma, and anaesthesia 129
Amphetamines and anaesthesia 348
Amyotrophic lateral sclerosis 151
Anaemia, management 301–14
  anaesthetic considerations 311–14
    cyanosis 313
    induction 313
    maintenance 313
    peroperative phase 312–13
    postoperative phase 313
    preoperative considerations 311
    vitamin B_{12} deficiency 312
  aplastic 325–7
  blood loss, causes 301–2
  in chronic renal failure 264
  clinical setting 305–7
  corpuscular defects 310

cross-matching blood 310
examination 306
glucose-6-phosphate dehydrogenase
  deficiency 310
haemolytic 309–11
hypochromic 307
investigations 307
leukaemias 324–5
macrocytic 308
normal values 307
normochromic-normocytic 309
oxygen characteristics of blood 302–4
physiology 302–5
sickle cell
  see sickle cell syndrome
spur cell 310
Analgesics after extubation 121
Androgenic hormone production, adrenal
  cortex 229
Angina, in ischaemic heart disease 12, 39, 41
Angioneurotic oedema, and blood transfusion 316
Ankylosing spondylitis, management 281–4
  peroperative phase 283–4
  postoperative phase 284
  preoperative considerations 282–3
Anorexia nervosa 345
Antibiotics against endocarditis 74–5, 82, 89
Anticoagulants, anaesthetic considerations 77–8,
  82
Anti-depressant drugs and anaesthesia 341, 343
Anxiolytic drugs and anaesthesia 343
Aortic
  regurgitation 87–90
    aetiology 87
    anaesthetic considerations 89–90
    physiology 87–8
    preoperative considerations 88–90
  stenosis 83–7
    aetiology 83
    anaesthetic considerations 86–7
    hypotension 86
    oxygen delivery to sub-endocardium 84
    physiology 83–4
    preoperative considerations 84–6
  valve disease, mixed 90
Aplastic anaemia 325–7
  causes 325
Apnoea, obstructive, postoperative 121–2
Arterial pressure waves, monitoring and
  interpretation 25–6
Arthropathies 298–9
  bacterial 299

endocrine 299
and malignancy 299
metabolic 299
viral 298
Ascites, management 177
in portal hypertension 180, 181
Aspartate transaminase, serum concentrations,
liver disease 168–9
Asthma 125–30
anaesthetic considerations 126–8
therapeutic approaches 127
and chronic lung disease 123
dysrhythmias 128
extrinsic 125
frequency/severity 126
hypotension 128, 130
intrinsic 125–6
pneumothorax 126
salbutamol 127
severe, treatment 128–30
steroid medication 125, 126, 127
theophylline 127
ventilation 128
Ataxias, hereditary, management 151–2
Atrial
ectopics 57
fibrillation, anaesthetic management 61–2
flutter, anaesthetic management 61–2
septal defect 93–4
examination 93–4
investigations 94
tachydysrhythmias 57
Atrio-ventricular block, management 64–7
first degree 64
second degree 64
advanced (high-grade) 65–6
Mobitz type I (Wenckebach) 65
Mobitz type II 65
precautions 66
third degree 66–7
congenital 67
pacemaker implantation 67
Atropine in second degree heart block 66
Auscultation, preoperative, cardiovascular disease
7–8

Barbiturates addiction and anaesthesia 350–1
Barium meal in jaundice 171
Basal metabolic rate in old age 359
Benzodiazepines and anaesthesia 343
Beta-adrenoceptor blockade
in bronchitis and emphysema 123–4
in cardiovascular disease, preoperative
assessment 17–18
in hypertrophic cardiomyopathy 50
mode of action 17
Bethanidine, preoperative assessment 18, 19
Bifascicular blocks, description and management
69–70

Bilirubin
metabolism, drugs affecting 188
serum concentrations
in liver disease 168
in jaundice 171
Biopsy, liver, in jaundice 172
Bleeding disorders 327–30
general management 327
see also specific disorders
Bleomycin and anaesthesia 384–5
Blindness and anaesthesia 372
Blood
counts in
acute renal failure 258
anaemia 307
cardiovascular disease 8
chest diseases 107
chronic renal failure 268
epilepsy 138–9
Fallot's tetralogy 97
hypercatabolism 205
jaundice 171
malnutrition 202
portal hypertension 178
rheumatoid arthritis 276
systemic lupus erythematosus 280
cross-matching 310
effects of temperature 304
gases in
acute renal failure 258
chest diseases 107–9
hypercatabolism 206
obesity 196
polycythaemia 332
portal hypertension 179
oxygen carriage 302–4
pressure, measurement, peroperative 23–7
arterial 25–7
automated detection 24
cannulae 25–6
changes 37
direct 25–7
indirect 23–5
Korotkoff sounds 23, 24
stored, characteristics 314–15
transfusion, problems and hazards 314–18
characteristics of stored blood 314–15
complications 315–18
infected blood, transfusion 317
reactions under anaesthesia 318
re-crossmatching 316
transmission of donor infections 317
Bone marrow
depression and anaesthesia 382
failure 324–7
anaesthetic considerations 326–7
aplastic anaemia 325–7
leukaemias 324–5
Bradycardia, management 38
Breathing, spontaneous, during anaesthesia 36
Bronchial carcinoma, and anaesthesia 134

Bronchiectasis and anaesthesia 133
Bronchitis, chronic 122–4
  anaesthetic considerations 123–4
  beta-adrenoceptor drugs 123–4
  definition 122
  hypotension 124
  infections, superimposed 122–3
  pink puffer/blue bloater 123–4
  pneumothorax 124
  relation with asthma 123
  reversible component 123
  sedatives 123–4
Bronchopleural fistulae and anaesthesia 132–3
Bronchospasm
  and asthma 126, 127
  and blood transfusion 316
  in lung assessment 103
Bulbar palsy, progressive 151
Bulimia nervosa 346
Bullous conditions, and anaesthesia 131–3
Butyrophenones and anaesthesia 340

Calcium channel blockers, preoperative
  assessment 19
  mode of action 19
Carbon dioxide
  and $PaCO_2$ during general anaesthesia 37
  in peroperative considerations 117–18
Carcinoid syndrome, management 245–6
  features 245
  peroperative management 246
  preoperative assessment 246
Cardiomyopathies, management 49–51
  congestive 51
  definition 49
  hypertrophic 49–50
  obstructive 49, 50
  obliterative (restrictive) 51
Cardiovascular disease 1–101
  abnormal pulses 5
  anaesthetic considerations 33–6
    general 34
    induction 34–5
    maintenance 36–7
    premedication 34
    regional 33–4
  blood pressure measurement 23–7
    changes 37
  central venous pressure 27–8
  drugs used in treatment of 15–20
  electrocardiography, peroperative 22–3
    preoperative 8–14
  examination 3–8
  history 2–3
  incidence 1
  individual conditions 38–100
  investigations 8–15
  monitoring, principles 21–33
  pain in chest, preoperative 2–3
  peroperative management 20–37

  postoperative phase 37–8
  preoperative assessment 2–15
  pulmonary artery catheter 28–33
  risks of surgery 20–1
  stethoscopy 22
  timing of surgery 20–1
Cardiovascular system, ageing pattern 355–6
Central nervous system diseases 137–53
  see also specific diseases
Central venous pressure
  peroperative 27–8
  preoperative, cardiovascular disease 4, 6–7
    abnormalities 7
  and pulmonary artery catheter, left atrial
    pressure 27, 28–33
Cerebellar ataxia 152
Cerebrovascular accident and anaesthesia *see*
  Cerebrovascular disease
Cerebrovascular disease 140–2
  IPPV 142
  $PaCO_2$ 141–2
  peroperative considerations 141–2
  postoperative considerations 142
  preoperative considerations 141
  suxamethonium 142
Chemotherapy and anaesthesia 384–5
Chest diseases, lung assessment 102–36
  asthma 125–30
  bronchiectasis 133–4
  bronchopleural fistula 131–3
  bullous conditions 131–3
  carcinoma of bronchus 134–5
  clinical findings 106, 107
  cystic fibrosis 133
  infections 133–4
  lung function tests 110–14
  peroperative phase 115–19
  pneumothorax 131–3
    see also Pneumothorax
  postoperative phase 118–22
  preoperative considerations 102–15
  pulmonary effusions 136
  restrictive pulmonary disease 130–1
  sarcoidosis 134
  specific conditions 122–36
  see also Lung function, assessment
Chest examination and lung assessment 105–7
Chest X-rays
  cardiac outline on 9
  how to read systematically 109
  in acromegaly 224
  in acute renal failure 258
  in ankylosing spondylitis 282
  in aortic regurgitation 89
  in aortic stenosis 85
  in atrial septal defect 94
  in asthma 129
  in cardiovascular disease 8
  in chronic renal failure 268
  in coarctation of aorta 99
  in cor pulmonale 47

in the elderly 364
in enlarged thyroid 241
in Fallot's tetralogy 97
in head injuries 149
in hypertrophic cardiomyopathy 50
in hypothyroidism 237
in jaundice 171
in left ventricular ischaemia 42
in lung function, chest diseases 109–14
in mitral incompetence 82
in mitral stenosis 77
in obesity 196
in patent ductus arteriosus 96
in pneumothorax 132
in portal hypertension 179
in rheumatoid arthritis 276
in systemic lupus erythematosus 280
in ventricular septal defect 95
see also Cardiovascular: Lung: Pulmonary
Chlorpromazine and anaesthesia 339
Cholangiography in jaundice 171
Christmas disease, management 328–9
Chronic bronchitis
    anaesthetic considerations 123–4
    definition 122
    hypotension 124
    infection, superimposed 122–3
    interrelationships 122–3
    pink puffer/blue bloater 123–4
    pneumothorax 124
    reversibility 123
Chronic obstructive airways disease in lung
    anaesthetic considerations 123
    assessment 105–7
    preoperative preparation 115
    see also Obstructive airways disease, Chest
        diseases, Lung
Cirrhosis 175–6
    bilirubin metabolism 188
    causes 176
    effect of drugs 181
    induction 182
    maintenance 182–3
    management 176
    peroperative phase 181–2
    in portal hypertension 177–84
    premedication 181
    preoperative preparation 180
    see also Hepatocellular failure: Portal
        hypertension
Citrate-phosphate-dextrose 314
Citrate toxicity, blood transfusions 317
Clonidine, preoperative assessment 18
Clotting factors and liver disease 169
    in jaundice 173
    in stored blood 315
Coagulation problems after blood transfusion 318
Coarctation of aorta 98–100
    anaesthesia 99–100
    post-ductal 99
    pre-ductal 98

preoperative considerations 99
Cocaine and anaesthesia 348–9
Common cold and anaesthesia 372–3
Computed tomography in jaundice 172
Conduction defects 64–71
    see also specific defects
Congenital heart disease, management 92–100
Congestive cardiomyopathy 51
Connective tissues, diseases 274–91
Conn's syndrome 234–5
    anaesthesia for 235
    clinical features 234–5
Consent
    Jehovah's Witnesses 319
    in psychiatric illness 335–7
        certified mental patients 336
        'implied' or 'express' 335
        life threatening situation 336
        minors 336
Cor pulmonale 45–9
    acute 46
    anaesthetic management 48–9
    causes 45–6
    definitions 45
    pathophysiology 46
    preoperative considerations 47
        examination 47
        history 47
        treatment 48
    right ventricular failure 46
Coronary artery disease in old age 356
Cortisol, serum, measurement in hypothyroidism
    237
Coughing in lung assessment 103
Craniofacial dysostoses, management 293
Cushing's syndrome 229–32
    examination 230
    investigation 230
    peroperative phase 231
    postoperative phase 231–2
    preoperative considerations 230
        preparation 230–1
    sex incidence 229
Cystic fibrosis and anaesthesia 133
Cysts, lung, and anaesthesia 132–3

Dantrolene in malignant hyperpyrexia 163
Deafness and anaesthesia 371–2
Debrisoquine, preoperative assessment 18, 19
Denervation hypersensitivity 156–7
Depression
    and anaesthesia 341
    in old age 361
Dermatomyositis, management 290
Diabetes insipidus, management 222–3
Diabetes mellitus 209–21
    effect of treatment 212–13
    hyperosmolar non-ketotic diabetic coma 221
    insulin deficiency, pathology 209–13
        acute 210–11

adult (maturity onset) 210
juvenile onset 210
long-term complications 211–12
physiology 209–13
primary 210
secondary 210
lactic acidosis 221
local or general anaesthesia 214–15
peroperative phase 214
postoperative phase 215
preoperative considerations 213–14
presentation modes, and anaesthetic
    management 213–15
specific conditions, anaesthetic management
    215–21
    controlled by diet 216
    controlled by insulin 217–18
        elective surgery 217–18
        emergency surgery 218–19
    controlled by oral drugs 216–17
    in ketoacidosis 219
        anaesthetic considerations 220
        management 219–20
        presentation 219
    previously undiagnosed 216
Dialysis, anaesthetic management 269–72
    haemodialysis 269–70
    peritoneal 271–2
Diazepam elimination in old age 361
Digoxin
    administration in preoperative assessment 16
    perioperative continuance 16
    mode of action 16
    in atrial fibrillation 61
Dinamap *845*, 25
2,3-Diphosphoglycerate, intracellular levels 304–5
Disseminated intravascular coagulation
    and haemolytic reactions 316
    management and treatment 330
Diuretics, for cardiovascular disease, preoperative
    assessment 15–16
    mode of action 15
Down's syndrome, management 343
Droperidol and anaesthesia 340
Drug(s)
    abusers 346–53
        alcohol 352–3
        amphetamines 348
        barbiturates 350–1
        classification 346
        cocaine 348–9
        examination 346
        investigations 346
        LSD 349
        marijuana 349
        opioids 351–2
        preoperative considerations 346–8
            preparation 347–8
        treatment 346
        withdrawal 346
    in chronic renal failure 266

handling, in old age 361–2
    pharmacodynamics 362
    pharmacokinetics 362
and the liver 188–92
    affecting bilirubin 188
    causing enzyme induction 189
    direct toxicity 190
    halothane hepatitis 191–2
    immune mediated reactions 191
    known to cause hepatotoxicity 190
    metabolism 188–9
    relevant to anaesthesia 190
    toxicity 189–91
    preoperative assessment 15–20
    psychiatric and anaesthesia 337–41, 341–2, 343
Duchenne's muscular dystrophy 159–60
Dwarfing syndromes, problems presenting 291–3
Dyspnoea
    of cardiac origin 2
    'air hunger' 2
    assessment 2
    in lung assessment 103
Dysrhythmias
    asthma and anaesthesia 128
    management 55–64
    see also specific headings
Dystrophia myotonica 160

Eating disorders, and anaesthesia 345–6
Eaton-Lambert syndrome 159
Echocardiography
    in aortic regurgitation 89
    in mitral incompetence 82
    in mitral stenosis 77
Elderly people and anaesthesia *see* Old age and
    anaesthesia
Electrocardiography in
    acromegaly 225
    acute renal failure 258
    aortic regurgitation 89
    atrial septal defect 94
    cardiovascular disease 8–14, 22–23
        peroperative 22–23
        preoperative 8–14
            cardiac axis 13
            individual leads 13
            P wave 9
            P-R interval 9–10
            QRS complex 10–12
            Q-T interval 12
            S-T segment 12
            T wave 12
    chronic renal failure 268
    coarctation of aorta 99
    cor pulmonale 47
    Fallot's tetralogy 97
    hypertrophic cardiomyopathy 50
    hypothyroidism 237
    left ventricular ischaemia 42
    mitral incompetence 81

mitral stenosis 77
obesity 196
patent ductus arteriosus 96
peroperative 22–3
portal hypertension 179
postoperative infarction 44–5
preoperative 8–14
ventricular septal defect 94
Electroencephalogram
in epilepsy 138
in portal hypertension 179
Electrolytes in stored blood 315
Elliptocytosis 310
Emphysema 122–4
anaesthetic considerations 123–4
definition 122
hypotension 124
infections, superimposed 122–3
interrelationships 122–3
pink puffer/blue bloater 123–4
pneumothorax 124
reversibility 123
Encephalopathy in liver disease 177
clinical course 177
in portal hypertension 181
End diastolic volume in hypertrophic
cardiomyopathy 50, 51
Endocarditis, prophylaxis against 74–5
Endocrine disorders 209–47
adrenal glands 225–35
diabetes mellitus 209–21
insulinoma 221
in old age 359
parathyroid glands 243–7
pituitary gland 222–5
thyroid gland 235–42
see also specific disorders
Endoscopy in jaundice 171
in portal hypertension 179
Enzyme induction by drugs 189
Enzymes, cardiac 44
Epidermolysis bullosa and anaesthesia 373–4
Epilepsy 137
anaesthetic considerations 139–40
causes 137
clinical manifestations 137–8
grand mal 138
Jacksonian (focal) 138
petit mal 137
preoperative considerations 138–9
postoperative care 139–40
status epilepticus 140
temporal lobe 138
Etomidate in induction in cardiovascular disease
35

Factor VIII deficiency, management 328
Factor IX deficiency, management 328–9
Fallot's tetralogy 96–8
anaesthetic consideration 98

physiology 96
preoperative considerations 97–8
Febrile reactions to blood transfusion 315–16
Fentanyl in induction in cardiovascular disease 35
Fibrous dysplasias, management 293
'Floppy' valve 81
Fluid retention in portal hypertension 180
Forced expiratory volume test 110–14
Forced vital capacity test 110–14
Frank-Starling effect 28
Friedreich's ataxia 152
Functional residual capacity
in lung assessment 116, 117
in old age 357

Gall bladder, palpable, in jaundice 171
Gallamine in induction in cardiovascular disease 35
Gamma-glutyl transpeptidase levels in liver
disease 169
Gastrointestinal system in old age 358–9
Geriatric aspects of anaesthesia see Old age and
anaesthesia
Giant cell arteritis, management 288–9
Glucocorticoids see Cushing's syndrome
Glucose, blood, in diabetes 213
Glucose intolerance in old age 359
Glucose-6-phosphate dehydrogenase deficiency
310
Glyceryltrinitrate, preoperative and peroperative
assessment 20
Gout, management 293–5
Guanethidine, preoperative assessment 18, 19
Guillain-Barré syndrome 153–6
anaesthetic considerations 154–5
definition 153
symptoms 153–4
tracheostomy, management and care 155–6
complications 156
ventilatory failure 154

Haematology 301–34
anaemia 301–14
see also Anaemia
bleeding disorders 327–30
blood transfusion 314–18
see also Blood transfusion
bone marrow failure 324–7
haemoglobinopathies 319–24
Jehovah's Witnesses 319
polycythaemia 330–1
Haemochromatosis, management 333
Haemodialysis, anaesthetic management 270–1
Haemoglobin 302–5
in sickle cell syndromes 320–3
Haemoglobinopathies 319–24
sickle cell syndrome 320–3
thalassaemias 324
Haemolytic anaemia 309–11
Haemolytic reactions to blood transfusion 316–17

Haemophilia, management 328
Haemophilia B (Christmas disease), management 328–9
Haloperidol and anaesthesia 340
Halothane hepatitis 191–2
  direct toxicity 191
  hypersensitivity 192
  immune based mechanism 191
  risks 191–2
Head injuries 149–51
  fluid balance 150
  peroperative phase 150
  postoperative phase 150–1
  preoperative considerations 149–50
  regional blocks 151
Heart
  ageing pattern 355–6
  block see Atrioventricular block
Hemiblock, description and management 68–9
  in bifascicular blocks 69
Hepatic failure, acute (fulminant) 192–3
  associated conditions 192
  management 192–3
  neurological signs 192
Hepatitis, management 185–7
  acute 185
  chronic 187
  halothane 191–2
  hepatitis A 185–6
  hepatitis B 186–7
    anaesthetic procedure 187
    carriers 186
    presentation 186
    spread 186, 187
Hepatocellular failure, management 177
  ascites 177
  encephalopathy 177
  jaundice 177
Hydrocortisone, production, adrenal cortex 229
Hypercalcaemia, management 244
  causes 244
  differential diagnosis 244
Hypercatabolism 204
  background 205
  CO_2 considerations 206–7
  feeding solutions 207
  intensive care 205, 206, 207
  investigations 205
  peroperative phase 206–7
  postoperative phase 207
  preoperative considerations 205
Hyperkalaemia, preoperative management 16
Hyperosmolar non-ketotic diabetic coma 221
Hyperparathyroidism 243
Hyperpyrexia, malignant see Malignant hyperpyrexia
Hypertension
  in chronic renal failure 264, 265
  in coarctation of aorta 99
  management 38, 51–5
    anaesthetic implications 53–5

antihypertensive therapy 53–4
  clinical features 52–3
  complications 52
  physiology 51–2
  recovery period 55
  specific problems 54–5
and phaeochromocytoma 227
portal, management 177–84
  ascites 180
  'Child's grouping' 179–80
  clinical features 177
  examination 178
  induction 182
  investigations 178–9
  maintenance 183
  monitoring 183
  peroperative phase 181–2
  postoperative phase 184–5
  premedication 181
  preoperative considerations 178
    preparation 180–1
  surgery risks 179–80
pulmonary, and pulmonary artery catheter 32
Hyperthyroidism 238–40
  examination 238
  investigations 238
  peroperative phase 239–40
  postoperative phase 240
  preoperative considerations 238
    preparation 239
  thyroid crisis 240
  treatment 238
Hypertrophic cardiomyopathy 49–51
  anaesthetic considerations 50
  beta-adrenoceptor blockers 50
  end diastolic volume 50, 51
  endocarditis risk 50
  examination 49
  history 49
  investigation 50
  obstructive 49, 50
  peroperative factors 51
  physiology 50
Hypertrophy in ischaemic heart disease 39
Hyperuricaemia, management 293–5
Hypocalcaemia, management 245
  causes 245
  and citrate toxicity 317
Hypochromic anaemia 307
Hypokalaemia
  in Cushing's syndrome 230
  preoperative assessment 15
  risks in ketoacidosis 220
Hypomania and anaesthesia 341
Hypoparathyroidism 243–4
Hypotension
  in aortic stenosis 86
  asthma and anaesthesia 128
  in chronic bronchitis 124
  in emphysema 124
  in hypothyroidism 238

management 38
postural in Guillain-Barré syndrome 154
and spinal cord injury 148
Hypotensive agents, preoperative assessment 18
Hypothyroidism 235–8
anaesthetic considerations 237–8
examination 236
incidence 235
investigations 236–7
preoperative considerations 236–7
preparations 237
signs and symptoms 236

Infections
chest and anaesthesia 133–4
common cold 372–3
of the nervous system and anaesthesia 163–5
transmitting, in blood transfusion 317
Insulinoma, anaesthetic management 221
Intermittent heart blocks, description 70
Intubation
in enlarged thyroid 241–2
in spinal cord injury 147
IPPV during general anaesthesia 34, 36
Ischaemic heart disease 38–45
definitions 39
incidence 38
left ventricular 39–43
peroperative infarction 43–5
right ventricular 45
Isoprenaline in second degree heart block 66

Jaundice, management 170–5
examination 171–2
gallstones 170
in hepatocellular failure 177
induction 174
investigations 171
maintenance 174–5
monitoring 173
postoperative phase 175
premedication 173
preoperative considerations 170
preparation 172–3
renal failure 172
urine production 172–3, 174
Jehovah's Witnesses, and blood transfusion 319
Jugular venous pressure
in cardiovascular disease 4–6
in right ventricular failure 47
Junctional (nodal) rhythm 62
ECG findings 62

Ketamine in induction in cardiovascular disease 35
Ketoacidosis, presentation 219
anaesthetic considerations 220
management 219

Korotkoff sounds, peroperative 23, 24
Kashiorkor 199

Lactic acidosis 221
Laryngeal neoplasms, radiotherapy and
anaesthesia 382
Left atrial pressure and central venous pressure
28–33
Left bundle branch block, management 68
Left to right shunts, management 93–6
Left ventricular
end diastolic pressure 28–33
failure, preoperative 2, 39
hypertrophy, physiology 80
ischaemia, management 39–43
anaesthetic management 42–43
causes of insufficient oxygen supply 40
history 41–2
investigations 42
physiology 39–41
preoperative considerations 41–3
Leukaemia, management 325
Levodopa 143
Lithium and anaesthesia 340–1
Liver
disorders, management 167–93
liver function tests 167–9
and drugs 188–92
halothane 191–2
metabolism 188–9
toxicity 189–91
see also Drugs: and specific names
function tests in malnutrition 202
Locomotor system in old age 359–60
LSD and anaesthesia 349
Lung
cysts and anaesthesia 132–3
function, assessment 102–36
perioperative phase 115–19
functional residual capacity 116, 117
maximal support techniques 117–18
minimal interference techniques 115–16
postoperative phase 118–22
analgesia 121
assessment 119–20
functional residual capacity 119
initial management 119–20
IPPV 120
management after extubation 120–2
normal response 118–19
obstructive apnoea 121–2
oxygen therapy 121
posture 120–1
secretions 121
preoperative considerations 102–15
blood gases 107–9
chest examinations 105–7
clinical findings, chest disease 106, 107
dyspnoea 103
examination 104–7

history 103–4
investigations 107–14
lung function tests 110–14
medication 104
preparation 114–15
specific diseases 122–36
function tests 110–14, 122–36
in ankylosing spondylitis 283
in obesity 196
in rheumatoid arthritis 277
in systemic lupus erythematosus 280
see also Pulmonary

Malignancy and arthropathy 299
Malignant hyperpyrexia 161–3
acute case, procedure 162
dantrolene 162, 163
definition 161
hypermetabolism 161
incidence 161
known case, procedure 162
pathophysiology 161
rebound hypokalaemia 162
and unexplained tachycardia 56
Malnutrition 199–204
associated conditions 201
'at risk' group 200
examination 200–202
infection risk 204
kwashiorkor 199
marasmus 199
peroperative phase 203–4
postoperative phase 204
preoperative considerations 200–2
preparation 202–3
temperature control 204
Mandibulofacial dysostoses, management 293
Mania and anaesthesia 341
Marasmus 199
Marfan's syndrome, management 284–5
Marijuana and anaesthesia 349
Mental disorders and anaesthesia
consent 335–7
drugs 335–7
in old age 360–1
specific disorders 341–6
subnormality 342
Metabolic
acidosis, after blood transfusion 317
systems in old age 359
Methohexitone in induction in cardiovascular disease 35
Methoxamine in hypertrophic cardiomyopathy 51
Metronidazole in prolonging of warfarin half-life 78
Migraine and anaesthesia 373
Mitral
incompetence 79–83
aetiology 79–80
anaesthetic considerations 82–3
Anticoagulants 82

endocarditis 82
in old age 356
physiology 80–1
preoperative considerations 81–2
stenosis 75–9
aetiology 75
anaesthetic agents 78
anaesthetic considerations 77–9
anticoagulants 77–8
fluid management 79
monitoring 79
physiology 75–6
postoperative complications 78
preoperative considerations 76–7
valve disease, mixed 83
prolapse 80–1
Mixed aortic valve disease 90
Mixed mitral valve disease 83
Monoamine oxidase inhibitors and anaesthesia 338–9
Motor neurone disease, anaesthetic management 151
Multiple
myeloma 332–3
sclerosis 143–5
general anaesthesia 144
incidence 143
pathology 143
regional anaesthesia 144
Muscular
atrophy, progressive 151
anaesthetic considerations 151
clinical varieties 151
dystrophies 159–60
Myasthenia gravis, management 157–9
anticholinesterase treatment 157–8, 159
definition 157
postoperative phase 158–9
preoperative considerations 158
ventilation 158
Myasthenic syndrome 159
Myeloma, multiple 332–3
Myocardial infarction
perioperative 43–5
established 43
risks 20–1
postoperative 43–5
diagnosis 44–5
management 43–4
Myotonia 160
anaesthetic considerations 160
descriptions 160

Neck X-rays, lateral, in enlarged thyroid 241
Nervous system in old age 357–8
Neurofibromatosis, management 152
Neuromuscular junction, management 156–9
Neuropathies, peripheral, management 153
Neurosis, management 342
Nifedipine, preoperative assessment 19

Nitrates
  mode of action 19
  peroperative continuance 20
  preoperative assessment 19
Normochromic-normocytic anaemias 309
Nutritional disorders 194–207
  hypercatabolism 204–7
  malnutrition 199–204
  obesity 194–9

Obesity 194–9
  definition 194
  examination 195
  hypoxia 199
  induction 197–8
  investigations 196
  maintenance 198
  peroperative phase 197–8
  postoperative opioids 199
  postoperative phase 198–9
  premedication 197
  preoperative considerations 195–6
  preparation 196
Obliterative cardiomyopathy 51
Obstructive airways disease, chronic, in lung
    assessment 105–7
  chronic bronchitis 122–3
  emphysema 122–3
Old age, and anaesthesia 355–70
  ageing, patterns 355–62
  anaesthetic management 363–9
    analgesia 369
    examination 363–4
    general 365
    history 363
    hypotension 367
    investigations 364
    maintenance 366–7
    peroperative phase 364–7
    postoperative phase 368
    premedication 364–5
    preoperative considerations 363–4
    regional 365–6
    regional blocks 368
  cardiovascular system 355–6
  definition of 'geriatric' 355
  endocrine systems 359
  gastrointestinal system 358–9
  handling of drugs 361–2
  locomotor system 359–60
  mental function 360–1
  metabolic systems 359
  nervous system 357–8
  pulmonary system 357
  renal function 360
Oliguria, management 252–3
Opioids, addiction and anaesthesia 351–2
Organic cerebral syndromes, management 344–5
  anaesthetic management 345
  causes 344

Oscillotonometer, double cuff 25
Osteoarthrosis, management 297–8
Osteomalacia, management 296–7
Osteoporosis, management 296
Ostium primum atrial septal defect 93
Ostium secundum atrial septal defect 93
Oxygen
  characteristics of blood 302
  supply, myocardial, insufficient, causes 40
  therapy after abdominal and thoracic operations
    121
Oxyhaemoglobin dissociation curve 302–3

Pacemakers 71–4
  anaesthetic management 73–4
  demand 72
  electrocardiograms 73
  fixed rate 72
  permanent insertion 71–2
  preoperative considerations 72–3
  sequential 77
  temporary 71
  types 72
$PaCO_2$
  in cerebrovascular accidents 141
  in chronic renal failure 265
  during general anaesthesia 36, 37
  in ketoacidosis 220
  in lung assessment, chest diseases 107–9,
    116–18, 120
  in obesity 196
Paget's disease, management 295–296
Pain, chest, causes 2–3
  of ischaemia 3
Palpitations, preoperative 3
Panhypopituitarism, management 222
Parathormone 243
Parathyroid glands, disorders 243–7
  see also specific disorders
Parkinsonism, management 142–3
  anaesthetic considerations 142–3
  drugs 143
Paroxysmal atrial tachycardia, anaesthetic
    management 59–60
Patent ductus arteriosus, management 95–6
PCO_2 in peroperative considerations 117–18
Peak expiratory flow rate tests 110–14
PEEP during general anaesthesia 37
Peripheral nervous system 153–6
  see also specific diseases
Peripheral vascular system, ageing pattern 355–6
Peritoneal dialysis, anaesthetic management 271–2
Phaeochromocytoma 226–8
  description 226
  diagnosis 227
  hypertension 226
  incidence 226
  peroperative phase 227–8
  phentolamine 227, 228
  preoperative considerations 226

treatment 227
unsuspected case 228
Phenothiazines and anaesthesia 339
Phentolamine in phaeochromocytoma 228
Pituitary gland 222–5
Pneumothorax 131–3
  asthma and anaesthesia 126
  chest X-ray 132
  dangers in asthma 126
  dangers in chest disease and anaesthesia 124
  diagnosis 131
Poliomyelitis and anaesthesia 163–4
Polyarteritis nodosa, management 285–6
Polycythaemia, management 331–2
  rubra vera 331
Polyneuritis, subacute see Guillain-Barré
  syndrome·
Porphyria 374–7
  anaesthetic management 376–7
  'at risk' groups 377
  biochemistry 374
  classification 375–6
  symptoms 374
Portal hypertension, management 177–84
  see also Hypertension, portal
Potassium-sparing diuretics, preoperative
  assessment 15
  mode of action 15
Pregnancy 377–81
  anaesthetic management 380
  first trimester 378–9
  incidence of anaesthesia 377
  investigations 380
  puerperium 380–1
  second trimester 379
  third trimester 379–80
Prosthetic valves, management 92
Proteins, serum, in liver disease 169
Proteinuria in chronic renal failure 264
Prothrombin time
  in jaundice 173
  in liver disease 169, 171
  in mitral stenosis 77
Pseudohypoparathyroidism 243
Psychiatry and anaesthesia 335–54
  consent 335–7
  drug abusers 346–53
  drugs 337–41
    see also specific agents
  mental disorders 341–6
Pulmonary
  artery, catheter, peroperative use 28–33
    left atrial pressure 28–33
    occlusion or wedge pressure 28–33
    pulmonary hypertension 32
    rupture 31
  effusions and anaesthesia 135
  system, ageing pattern 357
  tuberculosis and anaesthesia 133–4
  valve disease, management 91–2
  see also Cardiovascular: Chest: Lung

Pulses, preoperative, cardiovascular disease 4–7

Radiotherapy and anaesthesia 381–4
  bone marrow depression 382
  early complications 382
  laryngeal neoplasms 382
  specific areas 383
  technical problems 383–4
Red cells, stored, characteristics 315
Renal
  disease 248–72
    acute renal failure 248–62
    chronic renal failure 262–72
      with dialysis 269–72
      without dialysis 262–9
    with functioning renal transplant 272
  failure, acute 248–62
    aetiology 249–50
    anaesthetic management 256–62
      general anaesthesia 260–2
        maintenance 261–2
      peroperative phase 259
        effect of anaesthesia 259
        fluid balance 260
        monitoring 259
      premedication 258
      postoperative phase 262
      preoperative considerations 256–8
        examination 257
        investigation 258
        preparation 258
      regional anaesthesia 260
    avoidance 248
    causes 249
    definition 248–9
    description 248–9
    detection in perioperative period 250–1
    established 248
    factors predisposing 251–2
    management 253–6
      conservative 254
      dialysis 255
      hyperkalaemia 253–4
      stress ulcers 255–6
      ventilatory response 255
    oliguria, management 253
    post-renal causes 250
    pre-renal causes 251
    prevention in perioperative period 250–1
  failure, chronic 263–72
    features relevant to the anaesthetist 263–6
      anaemia 264
      calcium metabolism 265
      diabetes 265
      hypertension 265
      infections 266
      management 264
      PaCO$_2$ 265
      physiology 264
      presentation 263

proteinuria 264
tetany 265
long-term dialysis 269–72
non-dialysed patients 267–9
　anaesthetic considerations, preoperative
　　267–8
　　examination 267–8
　　investigations 268
　　peroperative preparation 268
　　postoperative phase 268
　prescribing drugs 266
　transplant 272–3
function in old age 360
transplant, anaesthetic management 272–3
Reserpine, preoperative assessment 18
Restrictive cardiomyopathy 51
Restrictive pulmonary disease 130–1
Rheumatoid arthritis, management 274–9
　examination 275
　investigations 276
　peroperative phase 277–8
　postoperative phase 278
　preoperative considerations 275–6
Right
　bundle branch block management 67–8
　　in bifascicular block 69
　to left shunts, management 96–8
　ventricular failure in cor pulmonale 46
　ventricular ischaemia, management 45

Salbutamol, asthma and anaesthesia 127
Sarcoidosis and anaesthesia 133
Schizophrenia, management 343–4
Scleroderma, management 286–8
Sick sinus syndrome, anaesthetic risk 59
Sickle cell syndrome 320–3
　crises 323
　peroperative phase 322–3
　postoperative phase 323
　preoperative considerations 321–2
　sickle cell trait 321
　theoretical background 320–1
Sickle cell trait 321
Sinoatrial block 58
Sinus
　arrhythmia 56
　bradycardia, and anaesthesia 56–7
　pause, and anaesthesia 58
　tachycardia, management 55–6
Sjogren's syndrome, management 291
Skeletal deformities, congenital 291–3
Skull X-ray in acromegaly 225
Smoking, anaesthetic considerations 115
Spherocytosis 310
Spinal cord injury 145–9
　acute 145–6
　airway problems 146–7
　cardiovascular problems 147–8
　description 145
　hypotension 148

intubation 147
long standing 148–9
neurogenic pulmonary oedema 147
non-traumatic 149
peroperative 146
postoperative 148
preoperative 146
tracheostomy 147
ventilatory problems 146–7
Spinal stenosis, management 292–3
Spur cell anaemia 310
Sputum, presence and lung assessment 105
Steroid
　cover in
　　Ankylosing spondylitis 282
　　Dermatomyositis 290
　　polyarteritis nodosa 286
　　rheumatoid arthritis 275, 277
　　scleroderma 288
　　Sjogren's syndrome 291
　　SLE 279
　　temporal arteritis 289
　　Wegener's granulomatosis 289
　therapy and anaesthesia 233–4
Stethoscopy during surgery 22
Still's disease, management 291
Strokes, and anaesthesia 140–2
　peroperative considerations 141–2
　postoperative considerations 142
　preoperative considerations 141
Subacute bacterial endocarditis, prophylaxis
　against 74–5, 82, 89
Suxamethonium 142, 145, 151
　in ataxias 152
　and malignant hyperpyrexia 162
　in myasthenia gravis 158
　in myoneural junction degeneration 156, 157
Swan-Ganz catheter see Pulmonary artery
　catheter
Syncope, cardiac, preoperative 3
Systemic lupus erythematosus, management
　279–81
　examinations 279–80
　investigations 280
　peroperative phase 281
　preoperative phase 279–81
　　preparation 281
Systemic sclerosis, management 286–8

Tachycardia, management 38
Temperature, and blood oxygen 304
Temporal arteritis, management 288–9
Tension time index 40
Tetanus management 164–5
　anaesthetic considerations 165
　cardiovascular problems 165
　established case 164
　fluid balance 165
　muscular problems 164–5
　prophylaxis 164

Thalassaemias, management 324
Theophylline, asthma and anaesthesia 127
Thiazides, preoperative assessment 15
Thiopentone, in induction in cardiovascular
  disease 35
Thrombocytopenia, management 329–30
  causes 330
Thyroid
  disorders in old age 359
  enlarged 240–2
    intubation 241–2
    peroperative phase 241–2
    postoperative phase 242
    preoperative considerations 240–1
    thyroid function tests 241
  gland 235–42
    disorders, in old age 359
    enlarged thyroid 240–2
    hyperthyroidism 238–40
    hypothyroidism 235–8
    see also Hypothyroidism
    physiology 235
Thyroxine, serum, measurement in
  hypothyroidism 236
Tracheostomy 155–6
  care 155–6
  complications 156
  Guillain-Barré syndrome 154–5
  management 155
  in spinal cord injury 147
Transfusion, blood *see* Blood transfusion
Transient ischaemic attacks and anaesthesia 140
  peroperative considerations 141–2
  postoperative considerations 142
  preoperative considerations 141
Transplant, renal, anaesthetic management 272–3
Tricuspid
  incompetence
    associated disorders 91
    management 91
    physiology 91
  stenosis
    associated disorders 90
    management 90–1
    physiology 90

Tricyclic antidepressants, and anaesthesia
  337–8

Ultrasound in jaundice 172

Valves, prosthetic, management 92
Valvular heart disease 74–92
  in old age 356
  see also specific valvular diseases
Vecuronium in cardiovascular disease 35
Ventilation, asthma and anaesthesia 130
Ventricular
  conducting system 10, 11
  conduction defects, description and
    management 67–70
  depolarization 10, 11, 12–13
  dilatation, in ischaemic heart disease 39
  ectopic beats, management 63
    underlying myocardial disease 63
  septal defect, management 94–5
  tachycardia, anaesthetic management 63–4
  see also Left ventricular: Right ventricular
Verapamil, preoperative assessment 19
Vital capacity test 110–14
  reduced causes 112
Vitalograph 110–13
Vitamin B_{12} deficiency 312
Vitamin D deficiency in malnutrition 202
Vitamin K in liver disease 169
  in jaundice 173
Von Recklinghausen's disease, management 152
Von Willebrand's disease, management 329

Wandering pacemaker, risks for anaesthesia 58
Warfarin, half-life prolonged by metronidazole 78
Wegener's granulomatosis, management 289–90
Wenckebach block 65
Wolff-Parkinson-White syndrome, description
  and management 70–1
Wright's respirometer 110–11